MOSBY'S
PREP GUIDE
FOR THE
Canadian
RN Exam

Practice Questions for
Exam Success

SECOND EDITION

MOSBY'S
PREP GUIDE
FOR THE
Canadian
RN Exam

Practice Questions for Exam Success

SECOND EDITION

EDITORS

Janice Marshall-Henty
RN, BScN, MEd
George Brown College, Toronto

Jonathon Bradshaw
RN, MSN (Cand.)
George Brown College, Toronto

Dolores F. Saxton
RN, BSEd, MA, MPS, EdD

Patricia M. Nugent
RN, AAS, BS, MS, EdM, EdD

Phyllis K. Pelikan
RN, AAS, BS, MA

ELSEVIER
MOSBY

MOSBY

NOTICES

Knowledge and best practice in this field are constantly changing. As new research and expertise broaden our knowledge, changes in practice, treatment, and drug therapy may become necessary or appropriate. Readers are advised to check the most current information provided (i) on procedures featured or (ii) by the manufacturer of each product to be administered, to verify the recommended dose or formula, the method and duration of administration, and contraindications. It is the responsibility of the practitioner, relying on their own experience and knowledge of the patient, to make diagnoses, to determine dosages and the best treatment for each individual patient, and to take all appropriate safety precautions. To the fullest extent of the law, neither the Publisher nor the Author assumes any liability for any injury and/or damage to persons or property arising out of or related to any use of the material contained in this book.

The Publisher

Library and Archives Canada Cataloguing in Publication

Mosby's prep guide for the Canadian RN exam : practice questions for exam success / editors Janice Marshall-Henty ... [et al.].

Includes bibliographical references.

ISBN 978-1-926648-29-3

1. Nursing–Canada–Examinations–Study guides.
I. Marshall-Henty, Janice, 1948-

RT55.M36 2011   610.7306'920971   C2010-905150-5

Credit:
Appendix: Reprinted with permission of the Canadian Nurses Association.

Vice President, Publishing: Ann Millar
Managing Editor: Roberta A. Spinosa-Millman
Publishing Services Manager: Deborah Vogel
Project Manager: Brandilyn Tidwell
Copy Editor: Cathy Witlox
Proofreader: Wendy Thomas
Cover, Interior Design: Kim Denando
Typesetting and Assembly: SPI

Elsevier Canada
905 King Street West, 4th Floor, Toronto, ON, Canada M6K 3G9
Phone: 1-866-896-3331
Fax: 1-866-359-9534

3 4 5   15 14 13 12 11

For the people who bring joy and meaning to my life:

My parents Jack and Audrey
My beloved children Jessica and Jeremy
Their spouses Christopher and Sarah
My incredible grandchildren Carys and Peter,
My love, Scott

Preface

Mosby's Prep Guide for the Canadian RN Exam has been developed to provide nursing students with practice exams that are representative of the Canadian Registered Nurse Exam (CRNE™). As nursing educators and facilitators of exam-preparation workshops, we recognize that students not only require a broad knowledge of nursing theory, but they also need to feel confident answering the particular types of questions found on the CRNE™. For many, the problem is not a lack of nursing knowledge but rather a lack of ability to apply their knowledge in the exam situation.

You have probably purchased this text for the practice exams, but don't skip over the chapters on exam description and tips for writing questions. They provide valuable guidelines for mastering the multiple-choice questions.

Most students in their respective nursing education programs have not had sufficient experience with the specific format of the questions found on the CRNE™. The CRNE™ is unique in several important ways:

- There is a high ratio of critical-thinking questions, where all the options may be correct but one of the options is the most correct. Or many different aspects of a situation must be analyzed in order to select the most appropriate answer. This problem-solving process may be difficult for students who are used to cramming the night before an exam and then regurgitating memorized facts the next day.
- Most questions incorporate scope of practice, asking what the nurse would do in a particular situation, rather than testing knowledge of medical treatments.
- Questions are written within the framework of nursing practice in Canada. This may be a significant challenge for internationally educated nurses. In addition, most available review texts are published in the United States and are based on the National Council Licensure Examination (NCLEX), which has a different exam format from the CRNE™.

Questions included in this book are based on the *Blueprint for the Canadian Registered Nurse Examination* (CRNE™), June 2010 to May 2015. They have been authored to include preventive and primary health care, teaching and learning, professional practice, therapeutic relationships, and current developments in health care. Each question has been authored by nursing experts in the field of exam preparation, reviewed by nursing experts, and referenced to established resources.

This prep guide includes three complete practice exams. Each exam consists of 200 case and independent questions, for a total of 600 questions in the three exams. For each question, there is an explanation of why the incorrect answers are incorrect and why the correct answer is correct. You may want to write the first exam as a "diagnostic," to identify areas of weakness and get a feel for the exams. We recommend that for one of the exams, you, either by yourself or with a group of fellow students, approach it as a mock exam situation. Pretend that it is the real exam, prepare as you would for the actual day, and write the practice exam in a 4-hour time frame.

Acknowledgements

We would like to acknowledge and thank the following individuals for their time, support, and expertise in the preparation of this text:

Ann Millar, Roberta Spinosa-Millman, Martina van de Velde, and Brenda Kirkconnell of Elsevier Canada

Jennifer Cooke, RN, BScN, for her nursing and editorial expertise

John Braham of Performance Assessment Group, the "guru" of item writing

Special thanks to Cathy Witlox for her editing expertise and catching our errors

Students, clients, and fellow colleagues who have provided inadvertent inspiration for the case scenarios

Reviewers

Donna Best, RN, MN, ACNP
Associate Professor
School of Nursing
Memorial University of Newfoundland
St. John's, NL

Jennifer Cooke, RN, BScN
Professor
School of Nursing
George Brown College
Toronto, ON

Jasna K. Schwind, RN, PhD
Associate Professor
Daphne Cockwell School of Nursing
Ryerson University
Toronto, ON

Elsie Tan, RN, MSN
Senior Instructor
School of Nursing
University of British Columbia
Vancouver, BC

Joyce M. Woods, RN, BN, BA (Spec), MEd, PhD
Associate Professor
Faculty of Health and Community Studies
Mount Royal University
Calgary, AB

Contents

Chapter 1   Introduction, 1

Chapter 2   Description of the Canadian Registered Nurse Exam, 5

Chapter 3   Study and Exam Tips, 11

Chapter 4   Practice Exam 1, 21
             Case-Based Questions, 22
             Independent Questions, 38

Chapter 5   Answers and Rationales for Practice Exam 1, 53
             Case-Based Questions Answers and Rationales, 54
             Independent Questions Answers and Rationales, 77

Chapter 6   Practice Exam 2, 101
             Case-Based Questions, 102
             Independent Questions, 118

Chapter 7   Answers and Rationales for Practice Exam 2, 133
             Case-Based Questions Answers and Rationales, 134
             Independent Questions Answers and Rationales, 158

Chapter 8   Practice Exam 3, 181
             Case-Based Questions, 182
             Independent Questions, 199

Chapter 9   Answers and Rationales for Practice Exam 3, 213
             Case-Based Questions Answers and Rationales, 214
             Independent Questions Answers and Rationales, 238

Scoring Sheets, 261

Bibliography, 271

Appendix   The Canadian Registered Nurse Examination Competencies, 275

Introduction

BACKGROUND TO THE CANADIAN REGISTERED NURSE EXAM

To practise as a nurse in Canada, you must be registered, or licensed. With the exception of residents of the province of Quebec, all nursing applicants across Canada write the same Canadian Registered Nurse Exam (CRNE). The exam is administered by the individual provincial or territorial regulatory authorities. To write the exam, you must have completed an accredited nursing program or have foreign qualifications that have been assessed as being equivalent to a Canadian nursing education. In each jurisdiction, the candidates write the exam on the same day in a proctored environment. Candidates who pass the exam in their home province or territory and meet all other requirements for registration qualify to apply for registration in all other jurisdictions in Canada.

Questions on the CRNE are designed to evaluate the knowledge of generalist nurses who have just finished their education. Nursing specialties are not tested. Testable material is applicable to all sites across Canada, whether large cities with teaching hospitals or small towns with community clinics, from the Atlantic provinces to British Columbia to the northern territories. When writing the exam, you need to be able to answer questions based on the knowledge, skills, and behaviours of any nurse, not just on what you or your colleagues might have experienced in a particular setting.

The development of the exam begins with a specific blueprint, or framework. Individual questions are authored by a team of nursing experts from across Canada and are all referenced to at least two reputable resources. Each test item is reviewed, validated, and then piloted on an existing exam prior to being placed in a test bank. It takes approximately 1 to 1½ years to complete this process. Thus, most questions you encounter on the CRNE were written several years ago and contain only information found in textbooks or other authorized resources.

For each exam, questions are randomly chosen from the test bank. Individual exams are not exactly the same, so the June exam is different from the October and January exams. Others you speak with may describe past exams as having been focused, for example, on pediatric, mental health, or maternal–child nursing, but you need to remember that your exam will be different.

Each exam has a different pass mark. Some versions of the exam may be considered more difficult than others. A panel of experts determines the pass mark depending on the assessed difficulty of a particular exam. Exams considered difficult will have lower pass marks than exams that are considered easier.

You receive a mark for each correct response. Marks are not deducted for incorrect answers. The results of the exam are reported as *Pass* or *Fail*. If, for example, the pass mark for a particular exam version is 125 and you scored 125 or higher, you would pass. If, however, you scored lower than 125, you would fail. There is no bell curve applied to the exam results. In general, you need approximately 65% to pass.

The CRNE differs from the nursing licensing exam in the United States in that it focuses less on pathology and physiology and more on application and critical-thinking questions. This difference makes it preferable to use a Canadian study guide, which more closely reflects what you will experience while writing the CRNE.

A frequent worry of students who are about to write the exam is, "What happens if I fail?" With proper preparation, including management of "test stress," this outcome should not occur. Approximately 90 to 95% of first-time writers educated in Canada pass the exam. For those who received their education in other countries or for whom English is a second language, the passing rates are somewhat lower. If you do not pass on the first writing, you may rewrite the exam. All provinces and territories allow a candidate to write the exam a maximum of three times. Students who fail the exam may contact their regional regulatory bodies for information about having their paper regraded or about initiating an appeal.

HOW TO USE THIS BOOK

Mosby's Prep Guide for the Canadian RN Exam is designed to provide you with practice exams that are similar in format, content, and length to the CRNE. The value of the practice exams is that they give you the opportunity to apply your knowledge to the particular types of questions you will experience in the CRNE. You can choose to write each exam as a whole to mimic true exam conditions, or you can answer the questions individually.

Once you have answered the questions, review the correct answers and rationales. Use the exam score sheet (p. 261) to analyze your mistakes. Were there knowledge gaps? Did you misread the question? Did you add information that was not in the question? Did you misunderstand the question? Identify the frequency with which you made particular errors, and use this information as a database for further study. Perhaps you need to review certain topics, practise your math skills, or increase your reading comprehension. Remember, you are not expected to get a perfect score. If you correctly answer about 70% of the questions, you demonstrate the potential for success on the actual CRNE.

Do not use this prep guide as a source for studying content, and do not attempt to memorize any of the information from the questions in this guide. All test items on the CRNE are secure and have never been published, so the questions found in this book will not appear on the CRNE.

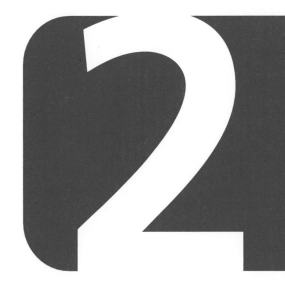

Description of the Canadian Registered Nurse Exam

The Canadian Registered Nurse Exam (CRNE) consists of 180 to 200 operational questions, plus pilot questions, in multiple-choice format. Writing time is 4 hours.

MULTIPLE–CHOICE QUESTIONS

The multiple-choice test items are written as either case-based or independent questions. Case-based questions present a health care situation along with approximately three to five questions related to the scenario. Independent, or stand-alone, items contain all the information necessary to answer the question.

Each multiple-choice question is made up of two components. The part of the item that asks the question or poses a problem is called the *stem*. The alternatives from which you are asked to select the best answer are called the *options*. There are four options; only one of the options is the correct answer. The other three options are called *distractors*. Distractors may seem to be reasonable answers but are, in fact, incorrect or incomplete.

Only one answer is correct. There are no combination options such as "1 and 2," "all of the above," or "none of the above." All questions are worth one mark. Marks are not deducted for wrong answers. Answers are coded on a scanning card, which counts the number of correct answers.

Sample Question

While receiving a blood transfusion, Mr. Ryan develops chills and a headache. What would be the nurse's initial action?

1. Notify the physician stat
2. Stop the transfusion immediately
3. Cover Mr. Ryan with a blanket and administer ordered acetaminophen (Tylenol)
4. Slow the blood flow to keep the vein open

The correct answer is 2. Mr Ryan is experiencing a transfusion reaction, thus the blood infusion must be stopped immediately.

EXAM BLUEPRINT

The CRNE is written according to a blueprint that includes competencies, levels of cognitive ability called taxonomies, age and gender, type of health care recipient, culture, health situation, and health care environment. It is not organized into sections on maternal–newborn nursing, medical-surgical nursing, pediatric nursing, mental health nursing, and so on.

COMPETENCIES

Competencies include knowledge, skills, behaviours, attitudes, and judgements that a nurse is expected to demonstrate in order to provide safe, professional care. In the exam, competencies are applied to various health situations and clients. For example, what are the safety hazards for the mental health client, the infant, or the older adult? How do you prevent the spread of infection in a hospital, a day care centre, or an immunocompromised client? Nurses learn these competencies in their education programs. There are 148 competencies in four categories. The exam asks approximately one question per competency. See the Appendix for a complete list of the CRNE competencies.

Competency Categories
Professional Practice

Professional practice means that the nurse is accountable for safe, competent, ethical nursing care. Professional practice includes legal responsibilities, scope of practice, and evidence-informed practice. Nearly one quarter of the questions on the exam (14 to 24%) will concern professional practice.

Sample Competency

Maintains clear, concise, accurate, objective, and timely documentation

Related Sample Question

Mrs. Leung was found by the nurse at 0100 hours lying on the floor beside her bed. What should the nurse document in the health record?

1. Mrs. Leung fell out of bed at 0100.
2. At 0100 hours, Mrs. Leung was found by the nurse on the floor beside her bed.

3. Mrs. Leung got out of bed at 0100 hours, slipped, and fell on the floor.
4. Mrs. Leung apparently fell out of bed at approximately 0100 hours.

The correct answer is 2.

This notation provides factual and objective documentation about the nurse's observation.

Nurse–Client Partnership

About one or two questions in ten (9 to 19% of the exam) involve the therapeutic partnership between the nurse and the client, which includes interpersonal skills, teaching–learning principles, competent cultural care, and the maintenance of professional boundaries.

Sample Competency

Uses therapeutic verbal and nonverbal communication techniques with the client

Related Sample Question

What is the most therapeutic response to Mr. Smith's question, "Am I going to die?"

1. "No, of course not."
2. "You have a very serious illness."
3. "Do you think you are going to die?"
4. "What have you been told about your illness and prognosis?"

The correct answer is 4.

This response invites Mr. Smith to discuss his understanding of his illness and provides the nurse with baseline information for further dialogue.

Health and Wellness

About one quarter or more of the exam (21 to 31%) concerns health promotion, population health, illness and injury prevention, and primary health care.

Sample Competency

Promotes healthy lifestyle practices

Related Sample Question

Which of the following lunch menus would be most appropriate and nutritious for a healthy 2-year-old child?

1. Hamburger and french fries
2. Jelly sandwich and grape soda
3. Cheese sandwich and fruit slices
4. Macaroni and cheese and cookies

The correct answer is 3.

This menu provides healthy nutrients and would appeal to a toddler.

Changes in Health

A maximum of half of the exam (40 to 50%) includes questions about clients who have health problems. Remember this when you are studying so that you do not focus all your time on care of the acutely ill client.

Competencies in this category involve care for clients who require acute, chronic, rehabilitative, or palliative care. These competencies include calculating medication doses, applying appropriate sciences to nursing practice, prioritizing interventions, selecting appropriate interventions, identifying complications, and so on.

Sample Competency

Inserts, maintains, and removes peripheral intravenous therapy

Related Sample Question

The physician order reads, "IV TKVO." What does this mean?

1. Intravenous infusion rate of 10 mL per hour
2. Intravenous infusion rate of 15 mL per hour
3. Intravenous to keep volume output
4. Intravenous rate that will maintain the patency of the infusion

The correct answer is 4.

TKVO means "to keep vein open."

TAXONOMIES OF QUESTIONS

To test your thinking abilities, questions are written at different cognitive levels: knowledge/comprehension, application, and critical thinking. Knowing the percentage of questions on the exam pertaining to each cognitive level helps to guide your studying.

Knowledge and Comprehension

The knowledge–comprehension level requires recollection of facts. For these types of questions, you are required to define, identify, or select remembered information. Knowledge questions require basic memorization. A minimum of 10% of the questions on the CRNE are of the knowledge–comprehension type.

Sample Question

Which of the following is an adverse effect of digoxin?

1. Tachycardia
2. Bradycardia
3. Diarrhea
4. Urticaria

The answer is 2, bradycardia.

To answer this question correctly, you need to have memorized the adverse effects of digoxin and the terms *tachycardia* and *bradycardia*.

Application

The application level of the intellectual process requires not only knowing and understanding information but also being able to apply it to a new situation. This level includes modifying, manipulating, or adapting information when providing client care. A minimum of 40% of the questions on the CRNE are application based.

Sample Question

Before taking Mr. Singh's vital signs, the nurse asks him if he is taking any medications. He answers, "Digoxin every morning and Tylenol in the evening." Which of the following vital sign changes might the nurse anticipate?

1. Increased blood pressure to 140/85 mmHg
2. Decreased pulse to 53 beats per minute
3. Decreased respiratory rate to 10 breaths per minute
4. Increased temperature to 38.5°C

The answer is 2, decreased pulse.

This question requires knowledge about several drugs, interpretation of vital signs, and application of this information to a particular client.

Critical Thinking

Critical-thinking questions require the most complex level of cognitive function. They ask you to analyze,

evaluate, problem-solve, or interpret data from a variety of sources before you respond to them. This often involves prioritizing nursing actions. Many refer to critical-thinking questions as "tricky" or "unfair" because the options may all be correct but only one option is considered the most important or comprehensive response. A minimum of 40% of the questions on the CRNE are critical-thinking questions.

Sample Question

The nurse is about to give Mr. Singh his morning digoxin. The radial pulse in his left arm is 45 beats per minute. What should the nurse do first?

1. Check his apical rate
2. Check the pulse in his right arm
3. Notify the physician
4. Not give the digoxin until the pulse is 60 beats per minute

The answer is 1, check his apical rate.

All the options could be correct, but checking the apical rate is the first thing the nurse should do. Consider the nursing process: validate your data.

OTHER BLUEPRINT VARIABLES

Type of Health Care Recipient

A *client* may be defined as an individual, family, population, or community.

Client Age and Gender

Questions reflect the statistical representation of Canadian populations for age and gender from preconception to older adult. Questions also reflect health situations common to each of these age groups.

Males and females are represented equally in all of the age groupings except for the over-65-years group, in which females may outnumber males.

Culture

Because Canada comprises a variety of cultural backgrounds, the CRNE integrates sensitivity and respect for diverse beliefs and values. It does not specifically test knowledge of individual cultures, other than Canada's Aboriginal, Inuit, or First Nations peoples.

Health Situation

Demographic information concerning disease morbidity and mortality provides the basis for health situations in test questions. Questions are designed to address client issues holistically, not just from a disease-based or pathology-based dimension.

Environment

The practice environment of the registered nurse (RN) includes a variety of settings. Thus, the competencies addressed in each question may be applied to any environment—clinics, hospitals, and communities—where nurses practise.

3

Study and Exam Tips

Although you may be academically well prepared to write the Canadian Registered Nurse Exam (CRNE), strategies for studying, stress management, and test taking will increase your chances of success and help to alleviate anxiety.

STUDY TIPS

It is easy to become overwhelmed as you prepare to study for the CRNE. Remember, though, that you know a lot more than you think you do. While studying is crucial, much learning is not a conscious activity. The first key to developing successful study strategies is to be realistic. Identify where you have incomplete knowledge or the need to refresh your learning.

Keep in mind that most of the questions on the exam do not merely test recalled facts, so you should try to understand the material that you read, rather than memorize it. The focus of your studies should be on principles of care and nursing interventions within a particular health situation, that is, what should the nurse do or say?

Because the exam will likely include approximately one or two questions per competency, make sure you do not get bogged down in one particular content area. For example, there may be only one competency related to diagnostic tests, so you should not spend too much time studying a comprehensive list of diagnostics.

One of the best strategies for learning is to form a study group. Self-testing and peer testing have proven to be the most effective methods for consolidating material. Have each member of the group choose a topic to teach the other members. This way, you stimulate discussion and get different perspectives on the subjects, which will help you in understanding and remembering them. If you are unable to participate in a study group, try teaching yourself the information. Rephrase or reword the written information to aid in understanding rather than memorizing.

Repetition works well for many people. If you are having trouble remembering some knowledge material, it may help to record it so that you can play it aloud while performing other activities.

Schedule your studying. Start reviewing content several months prior to the exam so that you do not feel rushed or panicked at the volume of material you need to learn. Cramming or "all-nighters" may be useful for memorizing facts, but the CRNE is an exam that requires problem-solving based on a comprehensive knowledge base. It is better to think through and analyze the material, make judgements, and determine how the subject relates to nursing. By performing these analytical and reflective processes, you are more likely to commit the information to long-term memory, which is much more reliable than your short-term memory.

To remember the strategies for studying, you can use the initialism *PQRS*, which stands for *p*lanning, *q*uestions practice, *r*epetition, and *s*elf- and peer testing.

While you study, remember to stay hydrated, eat sensibly, build in exercise breaks, and get plenty of sleep. It is also important to pursue other activities and not be involved solely in study. Research has shown that both sleep and "time out," in the form of exercise, social activities, or nutrition breaks, help to consolidate learned information.

MANAGING STRESS

Student Quotation

"If I take one more multiple-choice test, I think I may become physically ill. I won't be able to help myself. Can't they think of any other way of assessing how much we know?"

The student quoted above is setting himself up for failure because of his negativity toward the format of the test.

It is perfectly normal to feel nervous and anxious about the CRNE. You have worked hard to be successful in your nursing program, and now all that effort comes down to passing a 4-hour exam. As you prepare for the CRNE, empower yourself by developing a positive mental attitude. Henry Ford said, "Whether you think you can or think you can't. . .you're right."

Challenge your negative thoughts! Do not let them guide you.

TIPS

Become active and positive about your learning and your preparation. The more actively you plan and prepare, the more likely you will be successful. The following tips will help you manage stress:

- Try to avoid fellow students who feel overly anxious about the exam. Anxiety is like a communicable disease. You can catch it.

- Use the power of positive thinking. Build up your self-confidence by repeating to yourself, "I am well prepared. I will pass this exam."
- Practise yoga or other forms of exercise; they are great stress relievers.
- Try aromatherapy—lavender works well to promote relaxation. Sometimes just the smell will help you remember to relax and breathe.
- Eat a well-balanced diet, and get plenty of rest.

The Evening Before the Exam

Student Quotation

"The night before a test, I can't sleep. Then I worry because I can't sleep. Then I can't sleep because I'm worrying that I'm worried that I can't sleep. By morning, I'm glad to get out of bed just to stop the terrible racket in my head."

The evening before the exam, organize your clothes and exam supplies (e.g., pens, pencils, ruler, erasers, identification, watch, and bottle of water). Make sure you know the location of the exam and have arranged your transport to the exam.

Then be nice to yourself. Do something you enjoy and get a good night's sleep. Information is processed during sleep, so sleep will help you retain what you have studied. Last-minute cramming may have aided you in past test situations but is helpful only for memorizing facts. It actually decreases your ability to problem-solve the application and critical-thinking types of questions that are on the CRNE.

The Day of the Exam

Eat a healthy breakfast of protein and carbohydrates. Engage in moderate exercise if possible. If you absolutely cannot eat, try drinking a sports electrolyte solution. Although you need to be adequately hydrated, do not drink too many fluids or cups of coffee. Dress in comfortable clothes, preferably in layers, so that you can add or take off articles depending on the temperature of the exam room.

Plan to arrive at the test location at least 30 minutes ahead of the exam start time. This cushion will allow you time to relax, visit with friends, and prepare yourself mentally. However, avoid talking about the exam with your friends as conversations about it will only make you more anxious. Arriving early also gives you time for that last-minute washroom trip—stress is a potent diuretic. When you sit down in the exam room,

make a conscious effort to relax and continue your positive thinking. You may want to consider chewing gum during the exam; recent research has shown that it improves test scores.

After the Exam

After the exam, you will likely feel a sense of relief that it is over, but you may also feel the need to review questions in your head and discuss answers with your peers. Try not to dwell on this activity for too long. These post-mortems can bring you down. Remember, you have probably done better than you think!

CONTENT TO STUDY

Mosby's Canadian Comprehensive Review of Nursing is the most valuable resource for your CRNE studying. This uniquely Canadian-based review text has content created specifically for Canadian nurses, providing all you need to know about nursing in Canada—and to pass the CRNE—in one text.

Your first step in preparing for the exam is to review the 2010 Competencies (Appendix, p. 275). Notice the wording: *advocates, collaborates, supports, takes action, consults, facilitates, promotes,* and *intervenes.*

Professional Practice

The topics of the Professional Practice competencies include ethics, respect for clients, confidentiality, documentation, allocation of resources, accountability, scope of practice, rationale-based actions, professional judgement, continuous quality improvement, evidence-informed practice, abuse, action with errors or unsafe practice, conflict resolution, reflective practice, delegation, time management, partnerships, collegiality, roles of the interprofessional team, and management of resources.

Other resources for this competency include provincial standards of practice and related Web sites; Potter and Perry, *Canadian Fundamentals of Nursing*, revised fourth edition; and Keating and Smith, *Ethical and Legal Issues in Canadian Nursing*, third edition.

Nurse–Client Partnership

The topics of the Nurse–Client Partnership competencies include verbal and nonverbal communication, nonjudgemental care, therapeutic relationships, personal values, group process, sensitivity to diversity, informed consent, advocacy, alternative therapies, and teaching and learning.

Other resources for this competency include provincial standards of practice and related Web sites; Potter and Perry, *Canadian Fundamentals of Nursing*, revised fourth edition; and Arnold and Boggs, *Interpersonal Relationships*, fifth edition.

Health and Wellness

The topics of the Health and Wellness competencies include global and local health priorities, education programs, prevention strategies, resource identification, abuse prevention, disease detection, prevention of addictions, promotion of mental health, safety, healthy lifestyles, appropriate use of medications, risk factors, pandemic planning, infection control protocols, developmental transitions, sexuality, environmental safety, immunization, evidence-informed health info, and data collection techniques.

Other resources for this competency include Potter and Perry, *Canadian Fundamentals of Nursing*, revised fourth edition; Jarvis, *Physical Examination and Health Assessment*, first Canadian edition; the Health Canada Web site, www.hc-sc.ca; and the Canadian Wellness Web site, www.canadianwellness.com.

Changes in Health

The topics of the Changes in Health competencies include holistic assessment; data collection, validation, analysis, and evaluation; knowledge application from established sciences; care plans; technology application; discharge teaching; support of clients in transition; family-centred care; evaluation of client condition; prevention of complications; intervention prioritization; appropriate interventions; communication initiation with and inclusion of health team in emergencies; preparation of client for diagnostic tests; pre- and postoperative care; promotion of oxygenation, circulation, fluid balance, nutrition, parenteral and enteral nutrition, urinary elimination, bowel elimination, body alignment, mobility, tissue integrity, comfort, and sensory stimulation; medication dose calculation and evaluation of medication effects; pain management; blood administration; management of central venous access, drainage tubes, intravenous infusions, and standard precautions; intervention in changing health situations: cardiovascular, neurological, shock, respiratory, cardiac arrest, perinatal, diabetes, mental health crisis, trauma, postoperative, and

renal failure; supportive palliative and spiritual care; community resources; support of clients with chronic illness; and role in disaster planning and global health issues.

Although the CRNE is based on competencies, most resources you will be using for study are organized by topic or clinical area. The following sections outline the most common subjects within these traditional topic areas. *Mosby's Canadian Comprehensive Review of Nursing* contains all the necessary information in each section. However, should you choose to conduct further research, alternative resources are provided. When reviewing specific conditions and diseases, focus on the related nursing implications and remember to think about community-based aspects of care.

Medical-Surgical Nursing

You cannot know all diseases. Try to think globally and consider all problems associated with a system, rather than studying specific diseases. Remember that it is unlikely that you will be asked to recall specifics of disease pathology. Rather, you will need to understand effective therapies, including associated clinical skills and interventions.

- Diabetes: Types 1 and 2
- Cardiovascular: stroke, myocardial infarction, congestive heart failure, peripheral vascular disease
- Hematology: anemia, leukemias
- Gastrointestinal: colitis, colorectal cancer, constipation, diarrhea, ulcers, appendicitis
- Renal: urinary tract infections, renal failure, dialysis, incontinence
- Liver: cirrhosis, hepatitis
- Respiratory: chronic obstructive pulmonary disease (COPD), asthma, pneumonia, lung cancer, tuberculosis, common cold, atelectasis
- Musculoskeletal: arthritis, osteoporosis, fractures, chronic fatigue syndrome, scoliosis, multiple sclerosis
- Immune: acquired immune deficiency syndrome (AIDS), allergies
- Infections: methicillin-resistant *Staphylococcus aureus* (MRSA), vancomycin-resistant enterococci (VRE), *Clostridium difficile* (*C. diff.*), influenza, common cold, sepsis, epidemics, pandemics
- Sensory: cataracts, glaucoma, hearing loss
- Integumentary: burns, infestations, allergies
- Neurological: seizures, intracranial pressure, Parkinson's, spinal cord injuries

- Women's and men's sexual health: menopause, birth control, sexually transmitted infections, breast and prostate cancers
- Emergency: shock, hemorrhage, anaphylaxis

Resources include Lewis, *Medical-Surgical Nursing in Canada*, second Canadian edition, and www. sexualityandu.ca.

Maternal–Child Nursing

- Health in child-bearing years
- Fertility
- Prenatal care
- Fetal development
- Pregnancy risks and complications
- Labour and birth
- Apgar scoring
- Newborn assessment
- Preterm and newborn health problems
- Postpartum care
- Breastfeeding
- Bonding

Resources include Perry, *Maternal Child Nursing Care*, fourth edition.

Pediatric Nursing

- Family and parenting; child development, infancy to adolescence; play; safety
- Respiratory: asthma, respiratory syncytial virus (RSV), croup, cystic fibrosis
- Gastrointestinal: gastroenteritis, reflux, cleft lip and palate, appendicitis, pyloric stenosis
- Cardiovascular: atrial septal defect (ASD), ventricular septal defect (VSD)
- Hematology: sickle cell, leukemias, anemia
- Immune: human immunodeficiency virus (HIV)
- Infections and immunization: common childhood infectious diseases, schedule of vaccines
- Genitourinary: urinary tract infections
- Neurological: head injury, seizures, meningitis, hydrocephalus
- Endocrine: diabetes
- Integumentary: infestations, allergies
- Musculoskeletal: trauma, fractures, sprains and strains, arthritis, scoliosis
- Neuromuscular: cerebral palsy

Resources include *Wong's Essentials of Pediatric Nursing*, eighth edition, and the *Hospital for Sick Children Handbook of Pediatrics*, eleventh edition.

Mental Health Nursing

- Legal, ethical, interpersonal, communication, and therapeutic approaches
- Mood disorders: depression, bipolar
- Anxiety disorders: phobias, obsessive compulsive disorder
- Schizophrenias
- Personality disorders
- Substance abuse
- Cognitive disorders: dementias, Alzheimer's
- Sexual and identity disorders
- Eating disorders, body dysmorphism
- Psychiatric emergencies

Resources include Fortinash and Holoday Worret, *Psychiatric Mental Health Nursing*, fourth edition.

Diagnostic Tests

Understand the reason for the test and the appropriate health teaching for the client.

- Biopsies
- X-Rays, computed tomography (CT) scans, magnetic resonance imaging (MRI), ultrasounds, nuclear scans
- Mammograms
- Gastrointestinal scopes, bronchoscopes
- Allergy tests
- Oxygen saturation, pulmonary function tests
- Fetal tests

Resources include *Mosby's Diagnostic and Laboratory Test Reference*, seventh edition.

Laboratory Tests

Note the normal ranges and test implications.

- Complete blood count (CBC)
- International normalized ratio (INR)
- Blood sugar
- Glycosylated hemoglobin (HbA_{1c})
- Electrolytes
- Cholesterol
- Urinalysis
- Culture and sensitivity (C & S)
- Stool
- Low-density lipoprotein (LDL), high-density lipoprotein (HDL)

Resources include *Mosby's Manual of Diagnostic and Laboratory Tests*, fourth edition.

Pharmacology

Note classifications, common drugs within each classification, therapeutic effects, and precautions. You will need to know about frequently prescribed and over-the-counter drugs. In the CRNE, both the generic and brand names will be given, so you do not have to memorize both names. Knowledge regarding common herbal preparations may also be tested. Keep in mind lifespan considerations. The exam may require you to perform math calculations, so memorize your formulas and write them down when you get your exam paper. Remember, too, that calculators are not permitted.

- Analgesics and anti-inflammatories: narcotic and non-narcotic (e.g., Tylenol, nonsteroidal anti-inflammatory drugs [NSAIDs], morphine, and Demerol)
- Antacids
- Antidepressants (e.g., selective serotonin reuptake inhibitors [SSRIs])
- Antibiotics (e.g., penicillin, ampicillin)
- Anticoagulants (e.g., Coumadin, heparin)
- Antidiabetics (e.g., insulin, oral hypoglycemics)
- Antivirals
- Cardiac drugs (e.g., nitroglycerin, digoxin, antihypertensives)
- Corticosteroids (e.g., prednisone)
- Diuretics (e.g., furosemide [Lasix])
- Hormones
- Respiratory drugs (e.g., bronchodilators, inhaled steroids)
- Stool softeners and laxatives (e.g., psyllium [Metamucil], docusate sodium [Colace])
- Statins (e.g., atorvastatin [Lipitor])
- Vitamins and minerals
- Alternative, complementary, or herbal preparations

Resources include Lilley, *Pharmacology for Canadian Health Care Practice*, second Canadian edition; *Mosby's Nursing Drug Guide for Nurses*, eighth edition; and *Mosby's Handbook of Herbs and Natural Supplements*, fourth edition.

Clinical Skills

To test your clinical skills, the exam may include questions about any or all of the following: vital signs, infection control, medication administration, body mechanics, hygiene, positioning, suctioning, chest tubes, oxygen therapy, tracheostomy, intravenous initiating and maintaining, urine specimens, urinary catheters, enemas, wound care, ostomies, and first aid.

Resources include Potter and Perry, *Canadian Fundamentals of Nursing*, revised fourth edition, and Potter and Perry, *Clinical Nursing Skills and Techniques*, seventh edition.

TIPS FOR WRITING MULTIPLE-CHOICE EXAMS

Listed below are some tips for completing the multiple-choice questions particular to the CRNE:

A. Read and listen to the instructions carefully.

B. Plan your time and pace yourself. Place your watch on your desk so that you can keep track of time. You should answer approximately 25 to 30 questions in each half-hour.

C. Do not spend a lot of time on one question if you do not know the answer. Put a note in the margin and return to it later. Go on to a question that you find easy. The feeling of success will give you confidence.

D. Code responses on the scanning card as soon as you have selected your answer. Place a ruler under the corresponding question on the scanning card. Do not leave the transfer of answers to the card until the end of the exam—you may run out of time, and there is a greater chance of making a transcribing error. Only answers coded on the scanning card are counted.

E. Reading comprehension is crucial to success. Read the stem of each question carefully and make sure that you understand exactly what it asks. One of the most common test-taking errors is misreading the question. In the CRNE, important words are not highlighted, so you should identify and underline words such as *initial* or *most important* or *priority*. Take special note of any negatives such as *never* or *except*.

Sample Question

Ms. Chang is in the emergency room after being involved in a traffic accident. What would be an early sign of hemorrhagic shock?

1. Increased blood pressure
2. Pallor
3. Increased pulse
4. Shallow breathing

The key word is *early*; thus the correct answer is 3.

F. Because the majority of the questions are either at the application or critical-thinking cognitive levels, you must be prepared to problem-solve *every* question.

G. Try to answer the question before looking at the multiple-choice options.

H. Read all the options before choosing one. Do not immediately assume a response is correct without looking at all the other options; another answer may be *more correct* than the one you choose first.

I. Read each option carefully, mentally crossing out the options you know are incorrect. Choose the best option out of the ones remaining.

J. Some questions that appear to be trick questions may, in reality, measure your ability to think critically. If you believe all the options are correct, choose the one that is most comprehensive, makes the most common sense, or is the most professional answer.

Sample Question

Which of the following is most important when performing a preoperative assessment?

1. Physical assessment
2. Cardiac assessment
3. Assessment of vital signs
4. Auscultation of breath sounds

All options are valid, but answer 1 is the most inclusive.

K. To choose the most important nursing action when all of the answers appear to be correct, take the following steps:

- Read the situation and question very carefully.
- In almost all cases, consider the mnemonic *ABC* (*a*irway, *b*reathing, *c*irculation), with *airway* being the most important.
- Remember the "nursing process": collecting and validating information before acting.
- Consider safety—for the client and for yourself.
- Choose an action that can be completed quickly and safely, almost at the same time as other actions.
- Do not necessarily look for fancy answers.
- Choose simple, common-sense, safe actions.
- Choose the sickest, most unstable client as the priority.

L. A common error students make is choosing a response that might have been applicable in a specific client situation that they have experienced. Always answer according to "textbook," or standard, nursing principles.

M. Answer as you believe the perfect "textbook nurse" would answer.

N. Do not assume any information that is not given. Choose your answer based only on information in the question asked.

O. Do not panic if you have never heard of a particular disease or client situation. Apply general nursing principles to each question—the particular client health state may not matter. Candidates for the exam come from various academic backgrounds, and curricula are not identical in all universities. You are not expected to know all the answers, nor are you expected to write a perfect exam!

Sample Question

Ms. Townsend is suffering from Hick's asymmetrical dementia. Which of the following activities would be appropriate for her condition?

1. Vigorous exercise
2. Competitive games
3. Social stimulation in group activities
4. Solitary reading

Hick's asymmetrical dementia is a fictitious disorder. The care needs for a client with dementia are fundamental, so the correct response is answer 3. This is a "trick question" for the purpose of illustration. The CRNE, however, contains no trick questions.

P. Your first answer choice is usually correct. You may have learned some information subconsciously, and your first impression is often an automatic response to what you have learned. Do not second-guess yourself unless you are absolutely sure that you have misunderstood the question or provided a wrong answer. If you do decide to change an answer, ensure you completely erase the first answer from the scanning card.

Q. Select answers that are therapeutic, show respect, involve the client in care, and focus on nursing judgement rather than hospital rules or orders from other health team members.

Sample Question

Jessica tells the nurse, "I am tired of waiting for you to brush my hair. You're never here when I want you." Which of the following responses is the most appropriate for the nurse to give?

1. "I'm sorry you've had to wait. I'll get your hairbrush out for you and be back in 15 minutes to do your hair."
2. "That's not fair. I spent my lunch break with you yesterday."
3. "Jeremy down the hall is really sick, and he needs me more than you do right now."
4. "I'm doing my best, but I have a really busy assignment today."

Option 1 acknowledges the client's feelings, shows respect, and provides a clear, factual response.

Sample Question

Ms. Steele asks the nurse when she can start eating after surgery. What is the most appropriate response for the nurse to give?

1. "You'll have to ask the doctor."
2. "Tell me about your appetite."
3. "You'll likely start on clear fluids once bowel sounds can be heard."
4. "I'll have the dietitian consult with you about the most nutritious postsurgery menus."

Option 3 involves nursing judgement and directly answers the client's question.

R. Most questions will ask about actions that are based on nursing judgement rather than physician orders. However, some questions may test your knowledge of the scope of nursing practice and have as a correct response "contact the doctor." Examples of such situations include unclear or illegible orders, a specific request from a client, deteriorating client condition, and a client emergency.

S. In the case of communication questions, answers that demonstrate the nurse asking the client open-ended questions are most often correct.

Sample Question

Which of the following would elicit the best information from Mr. Loates about his pain?

1. "Do you have severe pain?"
2. "Do you have any pain?"
3. "Is your pain throbbing or stabbing?"
4. "Describe your pain to me."

Option 4 is open-ended—that is, it requires the client to give more than a one- or two-word answer. Phrasing questions in an open-ended fashion is a key component of therapeutic nursing communication.

T. Do not choose an answer because you have seen that question before and think you recall the answer. Questions on the exam may look similar to ones you have encountered during practice but will not be exactly the same. Therefore, the answer may also not be the same.

U. There is no pattern to the assigned answers. Do not change an answer because you have had too many answers in the same position.

V. If all else fails, guess. Never leave a question unanswered. You have at least a 25% chance of getting it correct.

Tips for Guessing:

1. If two of the options are similar except for one or two words, choose one of those.
Example
   Take the apical pulse
   Take the radial pulse

2. If two options have opposite meanings, choose one of those.
Example
   Vasodilation
   Vasoconstriction

3. If two quantities or mathematical calculations are similar, choose one of those.
Example
   0.14 mL
   0.014 mL

4. Choose the longest answer.

5. While there is no pattern to the answers, some studies say that in multiple-choice exams, option b or 2 is correct most of the time.

W. When you have finished the exam, be sure to check your scanning card against each of the questions to make sure that you have coded your answers correctly. Make sure the scanning card contains no marks other than those designating the options you have selected.

X. Answering 200 questions can be boring and tiring. You may find yourself becoming confused about what information relates to the question. Throughout the exam, take a mini-exercise break every 20 minutes; sip water, do neck rolls, and flex your arms and legs.

Y. Do not panic if someone leaves when you have completed only 20 questions. Most "early leavers" do not do better than exam writers who use the entire allotted time.

SUMMARY

Preparing for the exam well in advance, ensuring comprehensive content review, following the exam-taking tips, developing your reading comprehension, and maintaining a positive outlook will equip you with the necessary abilities to be successful in the CRNE.

4

Practice Exam 1

INTRODUCTION TO PRACTICE EXAMS

The practice exam questions are designed to be similar to those you will encounter in the Canadian Registered Nurse Exam (CRNE).

INSTRUCTIONS FOR PRACTICE EXAM 1

You will have 4 hours to complete the exam. The questions are presented as nursing cases or as independent questions. Read each question carefully, and then choose the answer that you think is the best of the four options presented. If you cannot decide on an answer to a question, proceed to the next question and return to this question later if you have time. Try to answer all the questions. Marks are not subtracted for wrong answers. If you are unsure of an answer, it will be to your advantage to guess.

Circle each answer in the exam book, and then transfer your answer to the scoring sheet found on p. 264. Be sure that the pencil mark completely fills the oval, but do not press so heavily that you cannot erase it if you decide to change the answer. Ensure that you are marking the question number that corresponds to the question you are answering. Make sure you do not fill in more than one oval for a question. Erase completely any answer you wish to change, and mark your new choice in the corresponding oval.

Answers to Practice Exam 1 appear on p. 54.

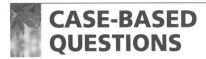

CASE-BASED QUESTIONS

CASE 1

A nurse works in a medical-surgical unit of a hospital. All client medications are dispensed by the pharmacy department in individualized single-dose packaging.

QUESTIONS 1 to 6 refer to this case.

1. What is the most accurate method for the nurse to determine she is administering the correct medication to Mr. Rickhelm?

    1. Compare the name of the drug on the pharmacy package with the prescriber's original order
    2. Ask Mr. Rickhelm to confirm he is receiving the correct medication
    3. Contact the agency pharmacy to confirm Mr. Rickhelm's medication profile
    4. Check the medication identified on the pharmacy package against information from a drug reference text or agency intranet site

2. Mr. Ogalino has been taking a brand name oral anti-infective medication at home for 6 months prior to being admitted to hospital. When the nurse brings his medications to him for the first time, he states, "What is this pink pill? I have never taken that one before." Which of the following responses by the nurse indicates safe medication administration?

    1. "This is a generic form of your regular anti-infective."
    2. "I don't know, but I'll check your medication record."
    3. "This is what your doctor has prescribed for you."
    4. "If you wish, you may refuse the medication."

3. Ms. Jasmin is a newly admitted client to the unit. The nurse prepares to administer long-acting insulin to her at 1800 hours. Ms. Jasmin tells the nurse that at home she takes this insulin at bedtime, around 2300 hours. How should the nurse respond?

    1. "I will test your blood sugar to make sure this is the best time to inject your insulin."
    2. "What is the reason you take your insulin at bedtime?"

3. "Generally the schedule for administering insulin is different when you are in hospital than when you are at home."
4. "Bedtime is not the best time for administration of long-acting insulin."

4. Ms. Corel is admitted to the unit with a diagnosis of deep-vein thrombosis. Which of the following categories of drugs is likely to be ordered?

   1. A statin
   2. An antibiotic
   3. An analgesic
   4. An anticoagulant

5. Who may legally sign the narcotics administration count sheet?

   1. A registered nurse (RN)
   2. A registered nurse or registered/licensed practical nurse (RPN/LPN)
   3. A registered nurse or a physician
   4. Any registered or regulated health care provider

6. Mrs. Aina is ordered digoxin (Lanoxin) 0.075 mg. The pharmacy dispenses digoxin 3 tablets of 0.25 mg to equal 0.075 mg. The nurse administers the provided 3 tablets of digoxin. Evaluate this action.

   1. Correct, as the digoxin has been calculated by the pharmacy
   2. Correct, as the digoxin is the same dose that the physician has ordered
   3. Incorrect, as the ordered dose of digoxin is below the therapeutic level
   4. Incorrect, as the dose administered is too high

END OF CASE 1

CASE 2

Mr. Smadu, age 19 years, was diagnosed with schizophrenia 8 months ago. His symptoms include hallucinations, delusions, flat affect, and grossly disorganized behaviour. He lives at home with his mother and his sister Shannon, both of whom work full time. His father and extended family live in another country and are not involved in his care. His

mother has asked for a visit from the community nurse to discuss concerns she has concerning her son's management at home. The nurse visits with Mr. Smadu, his mother, and his sister.

QUESTIONS 7 to 13 refer to this case.

7. Mr. Smadu's mother and sister ask the nurse what the best way is to respond when he is hearing voices. What should the nurse advise them to say?

   1. "I do not hear the voices that you hear."
   2. "Who is talking to you?"
   3. "There are no voices talking to you."
   4. "Why do you say you are hearing voices?"

8. Mr. Smadu asks for suggestions to help him cope with the voices he hears. What might the nurse suggest?

   1. To tell the voices to go away
   2. To listen to music on his headphones
   3. To distract himself by going for a walk
   4. To increase his dose of antipsychotic medication

9. Mr. Smadu's mother tells the nurse some of the neighbours are concerned that her son will be violent. They are afraid of him when he yells at the voices. What should the nurse advise Mr. Smadu's mother to tell the neighbours?

   1. "My son has a disease that causes him to hear voices, but he will never be violent."
   2. "Call the police if my son is acting in a strange manner."
   3. "Engage my son in conversation to distract him."
   4. "Do not crowd my son or get too close to him if he appears agitated."

10. Mr. Smadu is being treated with risperidone (Risperdal) 40 mg IM every 2 weeks to help manage his psychotic behaviours. What is the primary reason this drug is given to him by the intramuscular rather than oral route?

    1. It is not absorbed from the gastrointestinal tract.
    2. There is better compliance when given every 2 weeks by injection.

3. There is greater therapeutic response with the IM route.
4. The IM route decreases the incidence of tardive dyskinesia.

11. Mr. Smadu's mother asks if her son will ever get better. What is the nurse's best response to this question?

1. "About one quarter of all people with schizophrenia improve and are able to live independently."
2. "One half of people diagnosed with schizophrenia recover completely ten years from their first episode."
3. "Schizophrenia is a lifelong illness that can be managed, but he will never get better."
4. "If he doesn't get better, there are community supports to help you with his care."

12. Mr. Smadu's mother and sister tell the nurse that Mr. Smadu seems to have no interest in the world, has not followed through on his plan to return to school, and is generally not motivated to do anything. The nurse recognizes these behaviours as typical of people with schizophrenia. What is the term for these behaviours?

1. Alogia
2. Anhedonia
3. Avolition
4. Attention impairment

13. Several days after the nurse's home visit, Mr. Smadu's sister calls her because Mr. Smadu is saying that the voices are telling him to buy a gun and kill himself. How should the nurse advise Mr. Smadu's sister?

1. "Find out why he wants to commit suicide."
2. "Call 9-1-1."
3. "Take him to the mental health clinic or the hospital."
4. "I understand your concern, but although many people with schizophrenia say they are going to commit suicide, they almost never follow through."

CASE 3

A nurse specializes in infection control at a large teaching hospital. The hospital has recently had an outbreak of methicillin-resistant Staphylococcus aureus *(MRSA).*

QUESTIONS 14 to 16 refer to this case.

14. The infection control nurse must teach the staff about the spread of MRSA. Which of the following examples would be a likely mode of transmission?

1. Direct contact of an open wound with contaminated hands
2. Inhalation of aerosol particles from a person with MRSA pneumonia
3. Ingestion of contaminated food
4. Contact with blood or body fluids from a person with poor hygiene

15. Which of the following hospitalized clients has the greatest risk for acquiring MRSA?

1. Mrs. Andrews, age 65 years: pacemaker insertion
2. Andria, age 4 months: investigation of vomiting and failure to thrive
3. Mr. Anneke, age 87 years: diagnosis and assessment of possible dementia
4. Ms. Gary, age 35 years: chronic urinary tract infections secondary to spinal cord injury

16. The nurse has an open cut on his finger and is concerned about becoming infected with MRSA from his clients. What should the nurse do?

1. Keep the cut clean and cover with an occlusive adhesive bandage or tape
2. Refrain from caring for any clients with MRSA
3. Cover the cut with occlusive tape and wear gloves when performing care
4. Wash his hands before and after client contact

END OF CASE 2

END OF CASE 3

CASE 4

Denika, age 2 years, is admitted to a hospital pediatric unit. She has a severe case of eczema, which has resulted in many infected lesions. She will be receiving intravenous (IV) antibiotics.

QUESTIONS 17 to 21 refer to this case.

17. Denika has scratched her eczema to the point that she is bleeding. The nurse has repeatedly told her to stop, but she continues to scratch. The nurse decides to restrain her arms to the sides of the crib. Which explanation best describes the nurse's action?

    1. She has acted with professional accountability.
    2. She has used actions that can be interpreted as assault and battery.
    3. Denika's skin had to be protected, so the nurse acted in a prudent manner.
    4. The nurse should have asked Denika's parents for permission to restrain her.

18. Denika visits the hospital playroom. At her age, which of the following behaviours will she likely display?

    1. Building houses with blocks
    2. Being possessive of toys
    3. Attempting to stay within the lines when colouring
    4. Amusing herself with a picture book for 15 minutes

19. Denika is to receive 1 L of IV fluid per 24 hours. Using a minidrip IV set, with a drop rate of 60 drops/mL, at what rate should the IV infuse?

    1. 16 drops per minute
    2. 26 drops per minute
    3. 42 drops per minute
    4. 48 drops per minute

20. Denika is about to be discharged. The nurse advises Denika's mother to increase her fluids for several days. Her mother says Denika consistently says "no" every time she is offered fluids. What might the nurse advise Denika's mother to do?

1. "Distract her with some food."
2. "Be firm and hand her the glass."
3. "Offer her a choice of two things to drink."
4. "Explain to Denika why she needs to drink a lot of fluids."

21. Denika's mother asks the nurse when it would be appropriate to take her to the dentist for dental prophylaxis. What is the nurse's most appropriate response?

    1. Before starting primary school
    2. Between 2 and 3 years of age
    3. When Denika begins to lose deciduous teeth
    4. The next time another family member goes to the dentist

END OF CASE 4

CASE 5

A nurse works with a community midwife. One of their clients, Ms. Oliver, who is at 39 weeks gestation, plans to deliver her child at home. They receive a call from Ms. Oliver, who says that she is experiencing contractions. They make a home visit.

QUESTIONS 22 to 27 refer to this case.

22. Ms. Oliver tells the nurse, "This is the fourth time I have been pregnant. I had an abortion when I was a teenager and then delivered a baby girl when I was 20. Last year, I had a miscarriage when I was 10 weeks pregnant." How would the nurse record Ms. Oliver's pregnancy status?

    1. G.3, P.1, A.1
    2. G.3, P.0, A.2
    3. G.4, P.1, A.2
    4. G.4, P.1, A.1

23. The nurse and midwife assess that Ms. Oliver is in early labour. Which of the following components of assessment is most important for the nurse and midwife to perform?

    1. Intensity of contractions
    2. Frequency of contractions

3. Cervical dilation
4. Baseline fetal heart rate

24. Several hours later, Ms. Oliver's contractions are occurring every 50 to 70 seconds. On palpation, the fundus cannot be indented during a contraction. How would the nurse document these findings?

1. Contractions hard, approximately 1 minute apart
2. Contractions strong, 50 to 70 seconds apart
3. Ms. Oliver states that her "abdomen feels hard"; pains come every 60 seconds
4. Contractions firm, lasting 50 to 70 seconds

25. Ms. Oliver feels a gush of fluid between her legs. What should be the first action by the nurse or midwife?

1. Note the time and chart immediately
2. Assess the perineum and the fetal heart rate
3. Perform a vaginal exam
4. Check that the fluid is amniotic, not urine

26. Ms. Oliver delivers a full-term 3360-gram infant with an Apgar score of 8. What would the nurse and midwife initially do to prevent neonatal hypothermia?

1. Place the baby to the mother's breast
2. Dry the infant
3. Wrap the baby in several warmed blankets
4. Place the infant in a warmed bassinette

27. Both the midwife and the nurse are providing care to Ms. Oliver. Who is responsible for documenting care?

1. The midwife because she has contracted with Ms. Oliver to provide care for her and her infant
2. The nurse because she has a professional responsibility as an RN
3. The nurse and the midwife must each document the specific care they provide
4. The midwife can delegate the documentation regarding the delivery to the nurse

END OF CASE 5

CASE 6

Mr. Richard, age 21 years, is brought to the emergency department by the police. He has been involved in a house fire caused by his mixing volatile chemicals to make illegal street drugs. Mr. Richard has a history of intravenous drug abuse. He has sustained burns to his face and body. He is uncoordinated in his movements and verbally combative.

QUESTIONS 28 to 31 refer to this case.

28. Mr. Richard is shouting and agitated and demands to see the doctor immediately. What is the most appropriate nursing intervention?

1. Talk with him to de-escalate the behaviour
2. Monitor his behaviour to see if he becomes more agitated
3. Inform him that he will be asked to leave if he does not behave
4. Offer to take him to a quiet examination room

29. Mr. Richard is admitted to a burn unit. Which of the following observations by the nurse is a priority during the first 24 hours?

1. Wound sepsis
2. Pulmonary distress
3. Pain
4. Fluid and electrolyte imbalances

30. Mr. Richard requires an analgesic for the pain from his burns. What is the most important reason for the nurse to administer the drugs via the IV route rather than via IM injection?

1. IM injections increase the risk for tissue irritation.
2. IM injections are more painful than IV administration.
3. IV administration will ensure more effective absorption.
4. IV administration provides more prolonged relief of pain.

31. Mr. Richard has been charged by the police for his illegal drug possession and manufacturing.

A lawyer comes to visit Mr. Richard and tells the nurse that he would like to read Mr. Richard's health record. What is the most appropriate response by the nurse?

1. "You may read the chart if you get permission from Mr. Richard."
2. "You will have to get permission from the doctor."
3. "You are allowed to read the health record because Mr. Richard has been charged with a criminal offence."
4. "I am not allowed to let you read Mr. Richard's health record."

END OF CASE 6

CASE 7

Mr. Wilmot, age 23 years, has been diagnosed with cancer in his left testicle. He is admitted to hospital for the surgical removal of the testicle. Mr. Wilmot is engaged to be married in 6 months.

QUESTIONS 32 to 35 refer to this case.

32. Mr. Wilmot asks the nurse if he will still be able to father children after having his testicle removed. Which of the following responses by the nurse would be most therapeutic?

1. "The important thing is that you become healthy again. You can always adopt if children are important to you."
2. "I understand your fears. Any intervention for cancer is likely to cause infertility."
3. "I can see you are very concerned about this. Although you will still have one functioning testicle, perhaps you would like to discuss sperm banking before the surgery."
4. "There is a possibility that the surgery will make you unable to maintain an erection, which would lead to an inability to father children."

33. Mr. Wilmot tells the nurse that he feels he will not be a "real man" after the surgery, and he worries about losing his ability to perform sexually. How should the nurse respond to these concerns?

1. Ask Mr. Wilmot if he would like to meet with another man who has had the surgery.
2. Reassure Mr. Wilmot there is very little chance that he will have any problems.
3. Arrange for a psychiatrist to discuss Mr. Wilmot's sexual concerns.
4. Tell Mr. Wilmot the prognosis for this type of cancer is excellent and he need not worry.

34. Which of the following topics would the nurse include in his client teaching?

1. Once surgery and chemotherapy are completed, Mr. Wilmot can expect to lead a normal life, free of cancer.
2. Mr. Wilmot will have to take low-dose testosterone for the rest of his life.
3. Mr. Wilmot must have regular physical exams with his oncologist.
4. The likelihood of a relapse is quite high, so Mr. Wilmot must be tested every 3 months.

35. Mr. Wilmot is ready for discharge. The nurse teaches self-examination of the remaining testicle. Which of the following statements is correct?

1. Once a month in the shower, roll the testis between the thumb and first three fingers to cover the entire surface.
2. Lie flat on a bed and use circular motions with the fingers to detect any unusual lumps.
3. Shine a flashlight through the testis from the side to highlight any lesions.
4. The testis will feel like a soft-boiled egg, with the epididymis feeling smoother than the testis.

END OF CASE 7

CASE 8

A nurse is in charge on the evening shift at a long-term care facility. She is the only registered nurse working with unregulated care providers (UCPs) who have been trained to perform basic hygiene care and check vital signs. The nurse is responsible for administering medications to the 20 clients on her unit.

QUESTIONS 36 to 39 refer to this case.

36. Mr. Lok has a history of hypertension, treated with a variety of antihypertensive medications. The physician's order directs the nurse not to administer the regularly scheduled nifedipine (Adalat) if Mr. Lok's blood pressure is below 100 systolic. The UCP records a blood pressure of 120/80 for Mr. Lok. What should the nurse do?

1. Give the nifedipine
2. Check with the doctor before giving the nifedipine
3. Ask the UCP if the blood pressure reading was accurate
4. Check Mr. Lok's blood pressure before administering the nifedipine

37. Enteric-coated aspirin (ECASA) q6hr prn is ordered for Ms. Bystriska. Which of the following is a correct nursing action related to the administration of the ECASA?

1. Obtain verbal consent from Ms. Bystriska at the time of administration of the ECASA
2. Crush the tablet if she is unable to swallow it
3. Leave the ECASA at her bedside for her to take as necessary
4. Obtain a written consent that covers all medication administration

38. Mr. Gileppo is to receive insulin subcutaneously. Which would be an incorrect action by the nurse when administering the insulin?

1. Injecting it into subcutaneous abdominal tissue
2. Using a 25-gauge needle
3. Massaging the area to increase absorption
4. Pinching the tissue of the lateral aspect of the thigh

39. Ms. Banwait, a client with dementia related to Alzheimer's disease, is ordered donepezil (Aricept) to slow the progress of her disease. When the nurse offers her the donepezil, Ms. Banwait refuses to take it, stating that it upsets her stomach too much. Her husband, Mr. Banwait, insists that she take the medication. What should the nurse do?

1. Give the medication, as Ms. Banwait has dementia
2. Give the medication, as Mr. Banwait is the next of kin and is authorized to make treatment decisions
3. Do not give the medication, as it is producing adverse effects
4. Do not give the medication, as Ms. Banwait has withdrawn her consent

END OF CASE 8

CASE 9

An RN works in a family planning clinic. She provides teaching about reproductive and sexual health and birth control to a variety of clients.

QUESTIONS 40 to 44 refer to this case.

40. Ms. Eigo, age 27 years, consults the nurse regarding family planning. Ms. Eigo asks the nurse about the basal body method of calculating fertile periods in her menstrual cycle. What should the nurse tell Ms. Eigo about the basal body temperature method?

1. A woman's core temperature spikes at ovulation.
2. At about the time of ovulation, a slight decrease in temperature may occur in some women.
3. The basal body temperature of most women is elevated just prior to ovulation.
4. After ovulation, a woman's basal body temperature decreases and remains low until menstruation starts.

41. Sarah, a 16-year-old single adolescent, finds out that she is 4 weeks pregnant. She asks the nurse, "Do you think I should have an abortion?" Which of the following statements by the nurse is the most appropriate?

1. "It would probably be best for the baby and you."
2. "Do you think you would feel guilty if you had an abortion?"
3. "What do you think would be the best thing for you to do?"
4. "What do your parents want you to do?"

42. Ms. Lee is a sex-trade worker. She asks the nurse what she should use for contraception and prevention of sexually transmitted infections (STIs). Which of the following methods of prevention would be recommended by the nurse?

    1. A diaphragm
    2. A spermicide
    3. A cervical cap
    4. A female condom

43. Ms. McLeod has a positive test result for human papilloma virus (HPV). What should the nurse discuss with Ms. McLeod regarding future health care?

    1. The need to have routine Papanicolaou (Pap) tests
    2. The importance of finishing her prescribed antibiotics
    3. That she should abstain from sexual intercourse to prevent transmission
    4. If her treatment involves cryotherapy, that she will no longer be infectious to her sexual partners

44. A cardiologist has recommended to Ms. Ahmadi, age 42 years, that she should never become pregnant due to her severe congestive heart failure. Ms. Ahmadi has complied with this recommendation and asks the nurse what form of birth control would be the best option for her. What information should the nurse provide?

    1. "Your best option is the oral birth control pill."
    2. "A tubal ligation is almost 100% effective."
    3. "I'd suggest your partner have a vasectomy."
    4. "An intrauterine device is easily inserted and is an effective birth control method."

                    END OF CASE 9

CASE 10

The World Health Organization has predicted that a pandemic form of influenza will spread to Canada. A vaccine has been rapidly manufactured, and health care providers are preparing for mass immunizations and caring for acutely ill infected people.

QUESTIONS 45 to 50 refer to this case.

45. Health care workers are a priority group to receive the vaccine. A nurse is concerned about receiving this new vaccine, as the media have reported that it is not safe. What should the nurse do?

    1. Not have the vaccine because safety is in question
    2. Research reputable resources for information on the safety of the vaccine
    3. Have the vaccine in order to protect the nurse and her clients from the flu
    4. Discuss with nursing colleagues their opinions about the vaccine

46. A nurse cares for her older adult mother and has two young children. She feels that if a pandemic occurs, she will have to make a choice between caring for her clients and protecting the health of her family. What term relates to this situation?

    1. Ethical dilemma
    2. Ethical theory
    3. Moral distress
    4. Nonmaleficence

47. A nurse is aware that this pandemic situation will result in limited resource allocation. She wonders who will receive priority treatment if many acutely ill people require intensive hospital care. Which of the following guidelines would most likely be recommended?

    1. Older, frail adults receive priority care, as they are more at risk.
    2. Healthy adults receive the resources, as they are most likely to survive.
    3. The federal government legislates who the at-risk groups are for treatment.
    4. Local, provincial, federal, and international pandemic planning committees identify priorities.

48. A nurse is participating in a large community vaccine clinic. How would the nurse landmark to inject in the most appropriate muscle for older children and adults?

1. Midpoint of the lateral aspect of the upper arm, about 3 to 5 cm below the acromion process
2. The centre of the triangle of the index finger pointing to the anterior superior iliac spine and middle finger along the iliac crest toward the buttock
3. Divide the buttocks into quadrants; the site is in the middle of the upper outer quadrant
4. Middle third of the anterior lateral aspect of the thigh

49. Which of the following questions would the nurse ask prior to administering the influenza vaccine to a 20-year-old man?

1. "Are you allergic to eggs?"
2. "Are you sexually active?"
3. "Have you ever had influenza?"
4. "Are your childhood immunizations up to date?"

50. A mother brings her priority-listed asthmatic daughter to be immunized at the vaccine clinic. She also brings in her teenage son and requests that he receive the vaccine. At this time, well adolescents are not on the priority list for the vaccine. What should the nurse do?

1. Give the vaccine to the adolescent son
2. Tell the mother her teenage son is not allowed to have the vaccine
3. Inform the mother her teenage son is not at risk for getting the pandemic influenza, so he does not need to have the vaccine
4. Explain to the mother why her adolescent son is not in a priority group at present and tell her that he will likely be able to be vaccinated at a later date

END OF CASE 10

CASE 11

Ms. Smith, age 87, is admitted to a long-term care facility.

QUESTIONS 51 to 53 refer to this case.

51. Ms. Smith tells the nurse that she might as well die now, as she has no family left to care for her.

Which of the following responses by the nurse would be most therapeutic?

1. "Don't worry; you will soon make new friends here."
2. "I know it must be hard for you, but you will soon settle in."
3. "Let me get us some tea, and we can talk about how you are feeling."
4. "Why don't we go down to the lounge, and I will introduce you to some other residents."

52. Ms. Smith is mobile but spends most of her day sitting in a chair. Staff members have told her on many occasions that she needs to exercise and have explained the benefits of regular exercise for her mobility and cognitive function. Ms. Smith has said, "I am aware of the benefits of exercising, but I have never been one to enjoy exercise, and I am not going to start now." What should the nurse do?

1. Move the chair from her room so she is not able to sit in it
2. Take her to the agency exercise classes
3. Assess Ms. Smith's cognitive abilities and need for a substitute decision maker (SDM)
4. Respect her decision and continue to encourage exercise

53. Ms. Smith tells the nurse she appreciates her care and concern so much that she would like to give her a gift as a thank-you. She hands the nurse a diamond and emerald brooch. What should the nurse do?

1. Accept the gift if Ms. Smith is cognitively appropriate and aware of the value of the brooch
2. Tell Ms. Smith that since the gift is quite valuable, it is best to leave it to the nurse in her will
3. Thank Ms. Smith but explain it is against professional ethics to accept expensive gifts from clients
4. Tell Ms. Smith agency policies do not permit nurses to accept any type of gift from clients

END OF CASE 11

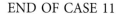

CASE 12

Mr. Hudson is a 53-year-old man who has been diagnosed with type 2 diabetes. He is referred to the nurse for education about his disease. He is somewhat overweight and requires teaching about nutrition for weight loss and diabetes management.

QUESTIONS 54 to 60 refer to this case.

54. What would be the most appropriate initial strategy for the nurse to use with Mr. Hudson at his first learning session?

    1. Provide him with a list of "dos and don'ts" about his diet
    2. Explain the need for a balanced diet to regulate his blood sugar and lose weight
    3. Ask him what behaviours he would like to change
    4. Ask him what he would like to learn from nutrition counselling

55. Which of the following would be a key concept in meal planning for Mr. Hudson?

    1. Smaller meals at frequent intervals
    2. Decreased carbohydrate intake
    3. Vitamin and mineral supplements to replace deficiencies in food intake
    4. Reduced total fat

56. Baked beans, whole grain cereals, flax seed, brown rice, and soybeans are recommended for a healthy diet. They are examples of which of the following types of carbohydrates?

    1. Simple carbohydrates
    2. Complex carbohydrates
    3. Monounsaturated carbohydrates
    4. High-glycemic-index carbohydrates

57. Mr. Hudson asks the nurse how he can lower his intake of trans fats. What should the nurse recommend?

    1. Avoiding commercially baked products, such as muffins, crackers, and cookies

    2. Choosing only lean meats, in limited amounts
    3. Using corn oil rather than canola oil for cooking
    4. Limiting egg yolks to two per week

58. Mr. Hudson asks the nurse what would be a good breakfast for him, considering his diabetes and that he would like to lose weight. Which of the following menus would be the most appropriate?

    1. One bran muffin with margarine, half a grapefruit, and a glass of orange juice
    2. A poached egg, one slice of whole-wheat toast, a glass of skim milk, and an apple
    3. Two slices of crisp bacon, scrambled eggs, and green tea
    4. One cup of raisin bran cereal with lactose-free milk and a glass of grapefruit juice

59. One month after Mr. Hudson's visit to the diabetes clinic, he calls the nurse to say that he is sick with gastroenteritis and has been vomiting. He wants to know what to do about his medications and food. How should the nurse advise Mr. Hudson?

    1. Not to take his oral hypoglycemic pills and to drink as much sweetened juice as he is able
    2. Maintain his normal diabetes medications, monitor his blood sugar every 3 to 4 hours, and drink carbohydrate fluids
    3. Contact his doctor for instructions
    4. Take half the usual dose of his oral hypoglycemic pills and sip fluids every hour

60. Mr. Hudson comes back to the clinic 3 months after his first visit. Which of the following would be the best criterion for evaluating the status of his type 2 diabetes?

    1. A weight loss of 5 kg
    2. A fasting blood-sugar reading of 6.5 mmol/L
    3. A glycosylated hemoglobin (HbA$_{1c}$) test reading of 5.9%
    4. A statement by Mr. Hudson that he feels well and is managing the disease

END OF CASE 12

CASE 13

Tiffany, age 15 years, is admitted to an eating disorders unit at a general hospital because of severe malnutrition. She has a history of self-restricted food intake and excessive exercising over the past 2 years. She is assessed to be below 60% of the expected normal body weight for her height. Her nurse performs an admission health history.

QUESTIONS 61 to 67 refer to this case.

61. The nurse asks Tiffany about her health history. What might the nurse expect Tiffany to tell her?

    1. "I feel really hot sometimes."
    2. "I stopped menstruating when I was 14."
    3. "My skin is really oily."
    4. "I get diarrhea quite often."

62. Which of the following blood tests would be most important for Tiffany?

    1. Sodium
    2. Potassium
    3. Electrolytes
    4. Chloride

63. The nurse interviews Tiffany's parents. Which of the following descriptions might her parents use for Tiffany?

    1. "We suspect she is promiscuous."
    2. "Tiffany openly discusses her anorexia with us."
    3. "She often acts out and is difficult to manage."
    4. "Tiffany is a high achiever at school."

64. The nurse takes Tiffany's vital signs later that night while Tiffany is sleeping. She discovers that Tiffany's apical rate is 41 beats per minute. What is the appropriate initial nursing intervention?

    1. Immediately notify the on-call physician
    2. Monitor the apical rate every hour until it increases and stabilizes
    3. Wake Tiffany and have her drink a glass of juice or water
    4. Bring Tiffany a snack of her preferred food

65. When Tiffany's vital signs stabilize, she is permitted to walk around the unit. The nurse plans to monitor Tiffany's physical activity. What is the primary rationale for this intervention?

    1. Adolescents with anorexia may secretly exercise as a weight-loss activity.
    2. Tiffany is so malnourished that physical activity will be harmful.
    3. Regular physical activity is an important component of the therapeutic plan.
    4. Exercise will improve Tiffany's ability to tolerate the increased nutritional intake.

66. Tiffany is scheduled to attend group sessions with the other adolescent girls on the unit who have anorexia. Tiffany says, "I don't want to sit around with a bunch of silly girls. Do I have to go?" What would be the best response from the nurse?

    1. "I think you need their support."
    2. "Let's talk about your feelings about not going to these meetings."
    3. "No, it is best to wait until you feel you really need to talk with other girls."
    4. "Yes, because the group sessions will help you cope with your anorexia."

67. Which of the following dietary goals would be appropriate for Tiffany?

    1. Tiffany will consume a high-calorie diet to promote rapid weight gain.
    2. Tiffany will eat a prescribed diet to ensure gradual weight gain.
    3. Tiffany will drink 3 L of water a day to ensure adequate hydration.
    4. Tiffany will gain 1 kg per week.

END OF CASE 13

CASE 14

A nurse works at a health information hotline. She receives a call from Ms. McColm, the mother of a 3-week-old infant.

QUESTIONS 68 to 71 refer to this case.

68. Ms. McColm is worried that her 3-week-old infant might be sick. What would be a significant manifestation of illness in an infant of this age?

   1. A red, papule-type rash on the face
   2. Long periods of sleep
   3. Grunting and rapid respirations
   4. Desire for increased fluids during the feedings

69. Ms. McColm tells the nurse her infant "feels warm." By which of the following methods would the nurse recommend that Ms. McColm take the infant's temperature?

   1. Oral
   2. Rectal
   3. Axillary
   4. Tympanic

70. Ms. McColm determines that the infant's temperature is 38.9°C. What should the nurse recommend?

   1. "Give the infant extra fluids."
   2. "Take the child to a physician."
   3. "Monitor the temperature every 4 hours for the next several days."
   4. "Administer infant acetaminophen (Tempra)."

71. The nurse documents this telephone consultation using computer charting. Which of the following is an accurate statement regarding computerized documentation?

   1. Each nurse must have an individual and secret password.
   2. Clients are not allowed to view their computerized health records.
   3. Client permission is required prior to accessing any health record.
   4. Research has shown that more documentation errors occur with computer charting.

END OF CASE 14

CASE 15

A rural community has a program to provide support to older adults to enable them to live independently for as long as possible in their own homes. A nurse leads this community initiative.

QUESTIONS 72 to 75 refer to this case.

72. Many of the nurse's clients do not have a great deal of money. What is the most important factor to consider when caring for clients who have limited financial resources?

   1. They will have decreased access to the health care system.
   2. They may have low self-esteem related to the stigma of poverty.
   3. Their basic physical needs may not be met.
   4. There is often a lack of client compliance with recommended treatment.

73. The nurse visits the home of Ms. Gash, an active 84-year-old client. Which of the following would most concern the nurse about Ms. Gash's home environment?

   1. It is a wood-frame house.
   2. There is a small throw rug on the hardwood floor.
   3. It has a microwave oven.
   4. There is electric heating from baseboard heaters.

74. Many of the nurse's clients are concerned about "moving their bowels." Which of the following recommendations would the nurse suggest to help prevent constipation in an older client?

   1. Fibre in the form of bran and fresh fruits
   2. Cellulose in the form of corn on the cob and rice
   3. Natural laxatives in the form of bananas and milk
   4. Peristalsis stimulators in the form of echinacea and feverfew

75. The local health department has issued a pollution alert on a hot, humid day. Mr. Scanlon, who has chronic obstructive pulmonary disease

(COPD), phones the nurse to ask what he should do. What should the nurse advise?

1. To stay inside his air-conditioned house
2. To carry on with his ordinary activities
3. To contact his respiratory therapist for advice
4. To increase his inhaled medications

END OF CASE 15

CASE 16

Ms. Merkel, a woman who lives in a self-sufficient religious community, has been admitted to hospital with severe pulmonary fibrosis.

QUESTIONS 76 to 78 refer to this case.

76. When providing care for Ms. Merkel, how should the nurse assess and treat her?

1. In accordance with known religious beliefs
2. According to her individually expressed needs
3. In compliance with guidelines that her family has provided
4. No differently from the other clients on the unit

77. Ms. Merkel refuses to allow Alex, a male nurse, to care for her as she says it would be considered inappropriate in her community. She insists that she have a female nurse. What should Alex do?

1. Arrange for a change-of-client assignment to a female nurse
2. Discuss with Ms. Merkel why she wishes not to have a male nurse
3. Tell Ms. Merkel that in Canadian society the rights of male nurses are respected
4. Tell Ms. Merkel she must accept him as her nurse because the charge nurse assigned him

78. Due to the severity of her illness, Ms. Merkel dies. Before performing end-of-life care for the body, what should the nurse do?

1. Arrange for Ms. Merkel's relatives to see her
2. Ensure Ms. Merkel's wishes regarding organ donation have been discussed with the family

3. Identify any cultural death rites that must be respected
4. Avoid touching the body until the religious leader has provided permission

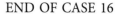

END OF CASE 16

CASE 17

Ms. Lesley, a primigravida at 40 weeks' gestation, is admitted to the birthing suite in active labour.

QUESTIONS 79 to 82 refer to this case.

79. A few hours after being admitted, Ms. Lesley becomes very restless, flushed, and irritable and perspires profusely. She states that she is going to vomit. Which stage of labour is this?

1. Late stage
2. Third stage
3. Second stage
4. Transition stage

80. Ms. Lesley delivers a healthy infant. Four hours after a vaginal delivery, she still has not voided. What should be the nurse's initial action?

1. Palpate her suprapubic area to check for distension
2. Encourage voiding by placing her on a bedpan frequently
3. Place her hands in warm water to encourage micturition
4. Inform the physician of her inability to void

81. Why will the nurse encourage Ms. Lesley to ambulate shortly after delivery?

1. It promotes respiration.
2. It increases the tone of the bladder.
3. It maintains abdominal muscle tone.
4. It increases peripheral vasomotor activity.

82. While checking Ms. Lesley on the second postpartum day, the nurse observes that Ms. Lesley's fundus is at the umbilicus and displaced to the right. What is the likely cause of this finding?

1. A slow rate of uterine involution
2. A full, over-distended bladder
3. Retained placental fragments in the uterus
4. Overstretched uterine ligaments

1. Fish
2. Canola oil
3. Whole milk
4. Omega 3 trans-fat-free soft margarine

END OF CASE 17

END OF CASE 18

CASE 18

Ms. Canseco, age 64, is admitted to hospital with a diagnosis of anginal pain.

QUESTIONS 83 to 85 refer to this case.

83. A nitroglycerin transdermal patch is prescribed for Ms. Canseco's anginal pain. Which of the following statements should be included in health teaching for Ms. Canseco?

   1. "Remove the patch at bedtime to prevent tolerance to the drug."
   2. "There are no adverse effects since the drug is delivered so slowly."
   3. "Before strenuous exercise, another patch may be cut in half and applied to prevent pain."
   4. "Used patches should be disposed of in the toilet or with biodegradable recyclable waste."

84. The nurse counsels Ms. Canseco about cholesterol in relation to atherosclerosis. What information should be included in the counselling?

   1. "Cholesterol is provided to the body entirely by dietary intake."
   2. "Cholesterol is found in many foods, from both plant and animal sources."
   3. "Cholesterol has no function in the body so must be controlled to prevent athero-sclerosis."
   4. "Cholesterol is naturally produced by the body but can increase with a high dietary intake."

85. For optimum cardiovascular health, clients should reduce the saturated fats in their diets. As part of diet counselling concerning saturated fats, which of the following foods would the nurse recommend that Ms. Canseco avoid?

CASE 19

Mr. Bangay, age 88 years, is a resident of an older-adult retirement home. Mr. Bangay's wife has advanced Alzheimer's disease and is a client in a long-term care facility in another part of the city. Mr. Bangay misses his wife and lately has shown manifestations of depression.

QUESTIONS 86 to 89 refer to this case.

86. One morning Mr. Bangay says to the nurse, "I feel terrible today." What would be the nurse's most appropriate response?

   1. "You look fine."
   2. "Do you feel ill?"
   3. "You'll feel better tomorrow."
   4. "Tell me about how you feel."

87. Mr. Bangay says to the nurse, "I wish you could have known my wife." Which response would be the most therapeutic at this time?

   1. "There are many lady residents here who would appreciate your company."
   2. "We have counsellors available to speak with you."
   3. "Her move to the long-term care facility must have made you feel very sad."
   4. "My mother had Alzheimer's, so I understand your sadness."

88. Several days later, the nurse notes Mr. Bangay's oral temperature at 0800 hours is 37.8°C. Protocol at the retirement centre is that vital signs are to be monitored every 8 hours. Which nursing action is most appropriate?

   1. Take his temperature at 1600 hours as per agency policy
   2. Take his temperature again in 2 to 4 hours

3. Call his physician for a more frequent vital signs order
4. Retake his temperature using the axillary route

89. Retirement home night-shift nurses are permitted flexible breaks. There is a lot of conflict among the team concerning how long some nurses take for their breaks. How should the nurses best resolve their conflict?

    1. Encourage each other not to take excessive time for breaks
    2. Mandate the length of breaks
    3. Report the issue to the nurse manager
    4. Collaborate on a mutually agreeable length of time for breaks

END OF CASE 19

CASE 20

Olivia, age 11 years, is taken to her physician by her parents because she has developed severe headaches. Her physician admits her to hospital for tests to rule out a brain tumour.

QUESTIONS 90 to 95 refer to this case.

90. The nurse performs a neurological exam on Olivia, which she documents on the health record. What would be the most accurate description of Olivia's general behaviour?

    1. "Behaviour appropriate for age"
    2. "Drowsy but awake and oriented to conversation"
    3. "Behaves well"
    4. "Complaining of headaches"

91. Olivia is scheduled to have a computed tomography (CT) scan. Her parents ask, "What is a CT scan?" How should the nurse answer?

    1. "A CT scan records the electrical activity of the brain."
    2. "Pulses of ultrasonic waves are sent through the brain."

3. "A dye is injected into the brain, and images are viewed on a computer."
4. "X-ray pictures are assembled by a computer and displayed as images."

92. Olivia is diagnosed with a medulloblastoma, a type of malignant brain tumour, and is scheduled for surgery. She asks the nurse if her bad headaches will go away after the operation. What is the best response by the nurse?

    1. "The operation will cure your headaches."
    2. "How bad is your headache today?"
    3. "We hope the surgery will cure the headaches, but there is a chance you will still continue to have headaches."
    4. "Are you afraid of the surgery?"

93. Olivia has surgery and is brought to the recovery room. How should the nurse position Olivia after surgery?

    1. It depends on the location of the operative site
    2. Flat with body and head in the midline
    3. Trendelenburg's position
    4. On the operative side to prevent excess bleeding

94. The nurse in the recovery room notices the presence of colourless drainage on Olivia's scalp dressing. What should be the initial action by the nurse?

    1. Circle the drainage area with a pen every hour
    2. Report the drainage to the surgeon immediately
    3. Document normal drainage on the postsurgical record
    4. Change the dressing and note any blood on the soiled gauze

95. Olivia does not recover from surgery. She becomes comatose and is transferred to a palliative care unit in the hospital. She is expected to die, and her parents do not wish resuscitation. Two weeks later at 0200 hours, the nurse finds Olivia with absent vital signs, skin discoloration, and a fixed stare. What action should the nurse take?

1. Pronounce death
2. Certify death
3. Call the physician to pronounce death and complete the death certificate
4. Remove Olivia's body to the morgue

END OF CASE 20

CASE 21

A registered nurse arrives at the cardiology unit for her 12-hour night shift. She receives the report on her clients from the 12-hour day-shift RN.

QUESTIONS 96 to 98 refer to this case.

96. Which of the following situations should the nurse attend to first when she begins her shift?

    1. A client who rings the call bell to request a sponge bath
    2. The narcotics count with the day-shift nurse
    3. A physician who requests assistance with reinsertion of a gastrostomy tube (G-tube)
    4. A client who is returning from having a CT scan

97. Ms. David is a client who is receiving palliative therapy for her end-stage cardiac disease. During the night, the physician telephones Ms. David's family to inform them that her vital signs are deteriorating and she is having episodes of apnea. They are advised to come immediately to the unit. At Ms. David's bedside, the son asks the nurse, "Do you think she will die tonight?" What is the most appropriate response by the nurse?

    1. "Why do you think she is going to die?"
    2. "You'll have to ask the doctor if she is going to die."
    3. "Would you like me to call the chaplain?"
    4. "We cannot say for sure, but it appears that she will die soon."

98. Mr. Marshall has congestive heart failure and pulmonary edema. Which of the following nursing actions would help to alleviate his respiratory distress due to these conditions?

    1. Elevate his lower extremities
    2. Encourage frequent coughing
    3. Place him in an orthopneic position
    4. Prepare him for modified postural drainage

END OF CASE 21

CASE 22

Mr. Camponi is experiencing an acute exacerbation of right-sided heart failure and has been admitted to the cardiac care unit.

QUESTIONS 99 to 100 refer to this case.

99. Which of the following nursing actions would most accurately assess the degree of Mr. Camponi's lower extremity edema?

    1. Checking for pitting in his extremities
    2. Weighing Mr. Camponi
    3. Measuring the diameter of his ankles
    4. Monitoring intake and output

100. Which of the following independent nursing actions should the nurse implement to limit the spread of Mr. Camponi's ankle edema?

    1. Restricting his fluids
    2. Elevating his legs
    3. Applying elastic bandages
    4. Performing range-of-motion exercises

END OF CASE 22

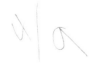

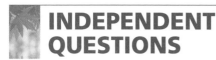

INDEPENDENT QUESTIONS

QUESTIONS 101 to 200 do not refer to a particular case.

101. Each day a nurse writes about her activities and experiences on Facebook, a social networking site. Which of the following statements best reflects professional judgement concerning her participation in Facebook?

  1. The nurse must take care never to write about clients.
  2. The nurse, according to the *Code of Ethics for Registered Nurses*, should not participate in Facebook.
  3. Participation in a social networking site is an optimum use of technology for professional development.
  4. The nurse may write about clients if she receives their verbal permission.

102. Christopher, age 13 years, has a patient-controlled analgesia (PCA) device postsurgery. Choose the statement that best indicates that his family has understood the teaching about the PCA.

  1. "We will push the button for him when he needs it."
  2. "The PCA will provide variable blood levels of the pain medication."
  3. "We should tell the nurse when we think Christopher needs to push the button."
  4. "The PCA will help Christopher have some control over his pain."

103. Ms. Levis is a newly graduated francophone nurse. Although she wrote and passed the English version of the CRNE, she does not feel comfortable speaking or understanding English. What is her professional responsibility when accepting employment as an RN in Canada?

  1. She has passed the CRNE in English; therefore, she is legally able to work in an English-speaking environment.

  2. She should obtain employment at a francophone agency until she feels confident communicating in English.
  3. She must not accept employment in a bilingual environment until she has passed a recognized English communications course.
  4. She may obtain employment at an English-speaking agency but should accept only French-speaking clients.

104. Mrs. Smirnoff, age 83 years, has advanced dementia and is not able to communicate verbally. She sustained a fractured hip, which required surgery. What is the best method of managing her postoperative level of pain?

  1. Provide her with a pediatric pain-rating scale
  2. Provide her with a PCA and show her how to use it
  3. Provide an analgesic and comfort measures as per agency protocol
  4. Provide analgesics at regular intervals and observe her behaviour

105. A young hockey player has been admitted to an observational unit after being hit hard on the head by another player's stick. How would the nurse position this client?

  1. Supine
  2. Sims
  3. Semi-Fowler
  4. With the head of the bed lowered by 15 to 30°

106. Ms. William has just had a below-the-knee amputation as a result of severe peripheral vascular disease. Nursing staff has ensured she has received the knowledge and support to make informed decisions. Although she understands the role smoking has contributed to her disease and that she will likely face further amputation if she continues to smoke, she leaves the unit regularly to go outside for a cigarette. The nurses feel helpless with her noncompliance. What nursing action is appropriate?

  1. Continue to advise and support Ms. William but do not judge her decisions

2. Suggest to Ms. William's family that they find a substitute decision maker
3. Consult with the health care team to obtain the assistance of a mediator
4. Refuse to care for Ms. William since she is being noncompliant

107. Mr. Seaberg has a tracheotomy, which requires frequent suctioning. What is the most important action by the nurse before performing suctioning?

1. Ensure he is well hydrated
2. Provide increased oxygen
3. Provide oral care
4. Ensure that clean tracheotomy ties are at the bedside

108. An RN works on a surgical unit of a hospital. On the night shift, she is "floated" to the gynecology unit, where she is assigned to women who are having therapeutic abortions. The nurse does not believe in abortions. What should she do?

1. Ask the unit manager if there are clients she could be assigned to who are not having abortions
2. Refuse to care for the women on the grounds that it is against her ethics
3. Tell the manager of her surgical unit that she is not able to float to the gynecology unit
4. Care for the women, using the time as an opportunity to provide health teaching about the dangers of abortion

109. A nurse obtains an oxygen saturation reading of 87% in a 2-hour-old full-term newborn who is not experiencing respiratory distress. What initial action should he take?

1. No action is required
2. Contact the physician
3. Administer ordered oxygen
4. Place the infant in a humidified Isolette

110. A nurse in the community visits a client who is taking a variety of complex medications, many with interactions. The client requires more education about the medications. What is the most appropriate action by the nurse?

1. Arrange a consultation with the client's pharmacist
2. Suggest that the client discuss the medications with the ordering physician
3. Research the medications and conduct a teaching session with the client
4. Obtain manufacturer's package inserts for the client to read

111. The nurse is teaching prenatal couples about therapeutic breathing techniques during labour. The nurse senses the group does not understand the information she is delivering. What would be the best action by the nurse?

1. Continue with the lesson because the group will understand as she develops the topic
2. Ask the group what they would like to learn about the effects of breathing techniques during labour
3. Change to another topic and leave breathing techniques until the following class
4. Stress to the group that this is very important information that will help them in labour

112. An older adult client in a long-term care facility often gets out of bed during the night. She has advanced osteoporosis and is unsteady on her feet. Which of the following actions by the nurse would help ensure the client's safety?

1. Ensure both side rails are up at all times
2. Ask the physician to increase her medications taken at bedtime
3. Place the bed in the lowest position and check on the client frequently
4. Place the bed against a wall, keeping the open side bed rail raised

113. An RN is caring for Mr. Green, who has recently been diagnosed with Parkinson's disease. What will the nurse teach Mr. Green's family about the manifestations of the disease?

1. He may experience mood swings.
2. His language skills will rapidly decline.

3. He may not recognize his caregivers from day to day.
4. His appetite will increase.

114. Mr. Mason, age 19 years, is a resident in a hostel for homeless people. The nurse at the hostel suspects that he is dependent on oxycodone hydrochloride (OxyContin), which he obtains illegally. During an initial interview, which of the following questions would be appropriate for the nurse to ask?

1. "How much OxyContin do you take, and what is its effect on you?"
2. "How do you get the OxyContin?"
3. "Are you aware of the legal and health implications of taking OxyContin?"
4. "Why did you start to take OxyContin?"

115. While the nurse is administering an enema, the client complains of abdominal cramping. What should be the nurse's initial action?

1. Slow the rate
2. Discontinue the procedure
3. Stop until his cramps have subsided
4. Lower the height of the container

116. A nurse in a walk-in clinic performs a health assessment on Mr. Nascad, age 81 years, and observes that he has a hand tremor. What should the nurse initially do?

1. Question Mr. Nascad about his past history and present symptoms
2. Notify the physician
3. Document this finding but recognize that most tremors are benign
4. No action is necessary as this is a common finding in older adults

117. Ms. Evans states that her last menstrual period began on June 11, but she experienced some spotting on July 8. Which date represents the nurse's calculation of Ms. Evan's expected date of delivery?

1. March 10

2. March 18
3. April 12
4. April 15

118. Mr. Gary, age 21 years, stepped on a rusty nail at a construction site where he was working for the summer. He visited the occupational health nurse, who asked him if he had been immunized against tetanus. He replied that he "had all his needles." Mr. Gary is admitted to hospital 10 days later with a diagnosis of tetanus. What is a correct statement of accountability in this situation?

1. There should have been a medical directive and protocol for the nurse to follow.
2. The nurse's judgement was adequate in view of Mr. Gary's symptoms.
3. The assessment by the nurse was incomplete; therefore, the treatment was inadequate.
4. The possibility of tetanus could not have been foreseen since Mr. Gary said he had been immunized.

119. An RN observes another nurse hitting a confused client. What should be the RN's first action?

1. Intervene in the situation
2. Report the occurrence to the nurse manager
3. Tell the nurse to leave the unit
4. Document the incident

120. Mr. Benjamin has type 1 diabetes. He asks the nurse what insulin does in the body. Which of the following statements would be the best response by the nurse?

1. "Insulin helps block extra glucose from entering the bloodstream."
2. "Insulin is necessary to help glucose get into the cells to provide energy."
3. "Insulin works with the liver to control the amount of glucose released for energy."
4. "Insulin blocks the absorption of glucose in the small intestine."

121. A community nurse who consults at a secondary school is concerned that the teenagers are drinking a lot of high-calorie, high-sugar-content

soft drinks and snacks bought from vending machines in the cafeteria. What would be the most appropriate action by the nurse?

1. Make posters to educate the teenagers about the dangers of the snacks and pop
2. Tell the school administration they must remove the vending machines
3. Host a parent–teacher meeting to promote teenagers' bringing lunches from home to eat at school
4. Consult with school administration to have the snacks and pop in the machines replaced with nutritional choices

122. An older woman is admitted to a busy medical unit. All client rooms are full, so she is placed in a bed in the hall. The woman is hard of hearing. What strategy could the nurse use to maintain confidentiality when interacting with the woman?

1. Speak in a low voice
2. Use pen and paper to communicate with the woman
3. Refrain from communicating with the woman
4. Use body language to convey information

123. An 89-year-old woman is admitted to the emergency department at 2300 hours with a diagnosis of pneumonia. She is accompanied by four adult children, all of whom say they are determined to stay at her bedside. The emergency department is very busy, and there is a rule that no more than one visitor may stay at the client's bedside. What should the nurse say to the family?

1. "You don't need to stay; your mother will be fine. I'll call if she gets worse."
2. "Only one visitor is allowed. The rest of you will have to go home."
3. "The rules of the hospital state that only one visitor is allowed."
4. "I suggest you rotate visits, ensuring one bedside visitor at a time overnight."

124. Ms. Morrissey has just been diagnosed with genital herpes. At this time, which of the following would be a priority nursing action?

1. Ensure Ms. Morrissey is tested for other sexually transmitted infections (STI)
2. Counsel Ms. Morrissey about her sexual activities
3. Discuss with Ms. Morrissey the action of ordered antiviral medication
4. Perform a mouth exam to check for oral herpes

125. Mr. Constantine is scheduled to have a sigmoido-scopy and will be performing his own preparation for the test. What will the nurse direct him to do?

1. Self-administer an enema the morning of the exam
2. Collect any stool specimens he passes prior to the procedure
3. Not have any fluids or foods for 24 hours before the exam
4. Drink the chalklike substance that will be provided to him

126. A provincial municipality has just received a report that spinach imported from another country into Canada is contaminated by *Escherichia coli* 0157, a potentially life-threatening bacterium. The spinach has already been distributed to grocery stores and has been sold to customers. What should be the priority action of the municipal officials?

1. Investigate the source of the contamination
2. Contact all groceries, advising them to remove the spinach from their stores
3. Immediately release a news bulletin for the public, warning people not to eat the spinach
4. Report the contamination to the provincial ministry of the environment

127. A student nurse asks an antenatal clinic nurse how smoking during pregnancy affects the baby. How should the nurse respond?

1. "The placenta is permeable to specific substances but not nicotine."
2. "Nicotine is addictive, and this will cause withdrawal in the fetus."

3. "Nicotine causes vasoconstriction, which will affect both fetal and maternal blood vessels."

4. "The effect is minimal as fetal circulation is separated from maternal circulation by the placental barrier."

128. The nurse is conducting a health history of a client whom she is preparing for surgery the following day. Of the following, which would be the most important question for the nurse to ask?

1. "What country are you from?"
2. "Are you taking any herbal supplements or over-the-counter medicines?"
3. "Does your diet provide adequate nutrition?"
4. "Do you have any sleep problems that might interfere with your recovery?"

129. Mr. Mehmet has metastatic lung cancer. He is refusing chemotherapy and radiation, stating his wish to use alternative therapies that do not use "poisons." What might the nurse say to Mr. Mehmet?

1. "This is not a wise decision. You are endangering your life."
2. "It is your right to decide what type of treatment you prefer."
3. "According to Canadian law, the doctor can make you take the chemotherapy."
4. "Would you like more information about scientific medical therapies and alternative treatments?"

130. Mr. Ciavello has atherosclerosis and hypertension. He has been placed on a low-salt, low-animal-fat diet. He complains that low-salt food is flavourless. What would be the nurse's best response?

1. "I'll get the dietitian to consult with you about strategies to improve the flavour of your food."
2. "You miss your favourite foods?"
3. "Salt can be very harmful to your health."
4. "Ask the doctor if you can indulge occasionally."

131. Mr. Kiros is admitted to hospital with diarrhea, anorexia, weight loss, and abdominal cramps.

A diagnosis of colitis is confirmed. Which of the following early manifestations of fluid and electrolyte imbalance should the nurse anticipate?

1. Skin rash, diarrhea, and diplopia
2. Extreme muscle weakness and tachycardia
3. Tetany with muscle spasms
4. Nausea, vomiting, and leg and stomach cramps

132. The nurse must tally a client's intake and output for 8 hours. At the time of calculation, there was 650 mL left from a 1000-mL bag of dextrose 5% in water. The client had three gastrostomy tube (G-tube) feedings of 200 mL each, plus a 50-mL flush of water at every feed. The nurse emptied the catheter bag twice, of 290 mL and 320 mL, respectively. The client had a small emesis of 25 mL. What is the intake and output?

1. Intake 930 mL, output 650 mL
2. Intake 1000 mL, output 680 mL
3. Intake 1080 mL, output 595 mL
4. Intake 1100 mL, output 635 mL

133. The nurse assesses a client's IV site and determines it is interstitial. What would be the initial action by the nurse?

1. Elevate the IV site
2. Discontinue the infusion
3. Attempt to flush the tube
4. Apply warm saline soaks to the site

134. Mr. Stephanopoulos has been admitted to the hospital with congestive heart failure. The nurse walks into his room and finds him cyanotic and unresponsive. What is the priority nursing action?

1. Call for help
2. Assess for breathing
3. Administer oxygen
4. Assess for a pulse

135. A community health nurse counsels Mr. Carter about smoking cessation. He has smoked two packages of cigarettes a day for 20 years. He says he wants to quit, but he has concerns about

withdrawal symptoms. Which of the following responses by the nurse is most therapeutic?

1. "After 24 hours, your body will be free of the physical dependency."
2. "Increasing your intake of vitamin B and vitamin C will reduce any withdrawal symptoms."
3. "You can always call the support group if your cravings get too hard to handle."
4. "I will refer you to a physician for medications to help with the symptoms of withdrawal."

136. Which of the following is a risk factor for *abruptio placentae*?

1. Cardiac disease
2. Hyperthyroidism
3. Cephalopelvic disproportion
4. Pregnancy-induced hypertension

137. Most nursing jurisdictions have a quality assurance program for their members. Which of the following statements is most important concerning nursing quality assurance (QA) programs?

1. It is a formal process that nurses engage in once each year.
2. It is an ongoing process of nurses reflecting on their practice.
3. It is a tool used by employers to evaluate their nursing employees.
4. It is a necessary component for maintaining registration.

138. Ms. Helena has been found to have an indeterminate lesion on a breast ultrasound, and her physician schedules her for a biopsy. She says to the nurse, "Why am I having a biopsy? Do I have breast cancer?" What is the best response by the nurse?

1. "Don't worry—the biopsy is being done just to make sure everything is okay."
2. "You probably do have breast cancer, and the biopsy will confirm it."
3. "Your ultrasound showed a suspicious lesion in your breast: a biopsy will determine if it is cancer."
4. "Your physician ordered the biopsy, so I don't really know why you are having it."

139. A nurse has been working alternating 12-hour day and night shifts in a busy medical surgical unit for 12 years. She is the mother of three young children. Lately, she has been experiencing nightmares about making errors in care and feels tired and overwhelmed all the time. What should be the nurse's first action?

1. Ask her manager to change her to only either day or night shifts
2. Reflect on areas of her personal and work life that can be changed
3. Make a decision to change to part-time work rather than full-time work
4. Implement healthier living habits such as sufficient sleep and improved nutrition

140. Ms. Tang, who has type 1 diabetes, is in the second half of pregnancy. Which of the following therapeutic interventions is she most likely to require?

1. Decreased caloric intake
2. Increased dosage of insulin
3. Administration of pancreatic enzymes
4. Decreased dosage of insulin

141. The nurse has been reading research articles concerning the emotional aspects of pregnancy and childbirth. Research concerning the emotional factors of pregnancy indicates which of the following reactions?

1. A rejected pregnancy will result in a rejected infant.
2. Ambivalence and anxiety about mothering are common.
3. Maternal love is fully developed within the first week after birth.
4. Most mothers experience neither ambivalence nor anxiety about mothering.

142. Mr. Patrick brings his 18-month-old son, Colm, to the clinic. He asks the nurse why his son is so difficult to please, has temper tantrums, and annoys him by throwing food from the table. What would the nurse explain to Mr. Patrick?

1. "Toddlers need to be disciplined at this stage to prevent the development of antisocial behaviours."
2. "The child is learning to assert independence, and his behaviour is considered normal for his age."
3. "This is the usual way that a toddler expresses his needs during the initiative stage of development."
4. "It is best to leave the child alone in his crib after calmly telling him why his behaviour is unacceptable."

143. Kathleen, age 2 years, is hospitalized with laryngotracheobronchitis (croup). Which would be the highest-priority nursing action when caring for Kathleen?

1. Measures to reduce fever
2. Assessment of respiratory status
3. Provision of comfort to reduce crying and bronchospasm
4. Delivery of ordered humidified oxygen

144. A 14-year-old boy is in a rehabilitation centre following a skateboard accident that caused musculoskeletal damage. He develops muscle weakness because he refuses to move. What should the nurse do to promote mobility?

1. Encourage his friends to visit every day
2. Explain that, as with sports, some pain is inevitable
3. Set strict limits to increase his compliance with the mobility plan
4. Permit him to make decisions regarding the type of activity or exercise he engages in

145. Ms. Sloane is seen by the nurse practitioner, who diagnoses that she has a bacterial infection. Which criterion should the nurse practitioner use when selecting an effective drug for the bacterial infection?

1. Ms. Sloane's toleration of the drug
2. Cost-effectiveness of the drug
3. Sensitivity of the causative organism
4. The prescriber's preference of drug

146. Baby Laszlo has had a circumcision. What is the most essential nursing observation during the immediate period after the circumcision?

1. Manifestations of infection
2. Hemorrhage
3. A shrill, piercing cry
4. Decreased urinary output

147. Ms. Price, a resident of British Columbia, develops appendicitis while on vacation in Saskatchewan. What services will the Saskatchewan health service cover for Ms. Price?

1. All hospital-provided services including medications and standard ward
2. All hospital-provided services excluding medications
3. All standard hospital services excluding specialists and intensive care
4. All health services whether or not provided by a hospital and regardless of the health care provider

148. Which of the following is an example of the implementation of primary health care by a nurse?

1. Advanced diagnostic testing
2. Correction of dietary deficiencies
3. Establishing goals for rehabilitation
4. Assisting in immunization programs

149. Mrs. Alves has experienced massive internal bleeding and is comatose. Her husband refuses to allow transfusions of whole blood because their religion prohibits blood transfusions. Which of the following interventions is the most appropriate initial action by the nurse?

1. Contact the physician so that a court order can be obtained to administer the blood
2. Have Mr. Alves sign a treatment-refusal form and notify the physician
3. Ensure that Mr. Alves understands the rationale for the transfusion and the risks of not having the transfusion
4. Institute the blood transfusion since the physician ordered it and Mrs. Alves's survival depends on volume replacement

150. Which of the following manifestations may occur in a client with atelectasis?

   1. Slow, deep respirations
   2. A dry, unproductive cough
   3. A lower than normal oral temperature
   4. Diminished breath sounds

151. Baby Sabrina is born at 32 weeks' gestation following a difficult delivery. She develops muscle twitching, convulsions, cyanosis, abnormal respirations, and a short, shrill cry. These manifestations may be due to which of the following conditions?

   1. Tetany
   2. Spina bifida
   3. Hyperkalemia
   4. Intracranial hemorrhage

152. Mr. Gautier is receiving chemotherapy for cancer of the lung. The nurse observes that he is developing ulcers in his mouth and anal region. Which of the following rationales would explain the development of the oral and rectal ulcers?

   1. Mucous membranes are generally more poorly nourished than other areas of the body.
   2. The chemotherapy causes direct irritating effects in the gastrointestinal tract.
   3. The cells in these tissues divide rapidly and are exposed to the damaging effects of the chemotherapeutic agent.
   4. Chemotherapeutic agents alter the pH of the gastric secretions, leading to ulcers.

153. Ms. Mullis sustained a fractured mandible from a motor vehicle incident. Her jaw is surgically immobilized with wires. What is a potential life-threatening problem?

   1. Infection
   2. Vomiting
   3. Osteomyelitis
   4. Bronchospasm

154. A nurse works with a medical aid agency in a developing country where dysentery is a common

problem. Which of the following is the most important method of preventing amoebic dysentery?

   1. Tick control
   2. Using mosquito nets
   3. Proper sewage disposal
   4. Proper pasteurization of milk

155. A nurse is the clinical preceptor for Wai, a foreign-educated nurse. The nurse notices that Wai does not look her clients in the eye and does not introduce herself to her clients. What should the nurse say to Wai?

   1. "In Canada, we introduce ourselves to the clients."
   2. "It is considered rude in Canada not to look people in the eye."
   3. "Why don't you look your clients in the eye or introduce yourself?"
   4. "The next time we go into a client room, let's make sure we introduce ourselves."

156. A mother decides that her son Lawrence, age 5 years, no longer requires hospitalization for his asthma because he is not experiencing respiratory distress. The attending physician has not discharged him. The mother arrives at the nursing station with Lawrence, saying she does not care if he has not been discharged; she is taking him home. What is the appropriate nursing action?

   1. Explain to the mother that if she takes Lawrence home, the appropriate child welfare authorities will be notified
   2. Tell the mother that because Lawrence is a minor, she is not allowed to discharge him against medical orders
   3. Inform the mother that agency policy does not allow them to release Lawrence into her care
   4. Ensure that the mother receives health teaching as necessary about asthma and document the situation as per agency policies

157. Mr. Hassan has just returned to the unit from the recovery room after surgery. He has an IV of dextrose 5% in water and 0.9% NaCl at

100 mL/hr, O_2 at 4 L per nasal cannula, a nasogastric tube set to low suction via a Gomco pump, and a urinary catheter to straight drainage. He was medicated with meperidine hydrochloride (Demerol) 1 hour ago and is reporting nausea. Which of the following components of assessment is the priority of the nurse when Mr. Hassan returns to the unit from the recovery room?

1. Ensure patency of the nasogastric tube and urinary catheter
2. Monitor the IV site
3. Check that the oxygen is set at the correct flow rate
4. Assess Mr. Hassan's pain and nausea

158. What is the most common cause of mortality in the adolescent years?

1. Motor vehicle accidents
2. Suicide
3. Cancers
4. Sports-related accidents

159. Mr. Edward, age 83 years, has moved into a retirement home. Mr. Martin, his life partner, visits him regularly. Which of the following statements is true regarding their sexuality?

1. They will have no sexual inhibitions because they are homosexual.
2. They will enjoy companionship more than sex.
3. They probably have become disinterested in sexual activities.
4. They will likely have an interest in sexual activity if privacy is available.

160. A third-year nursing student obtained a blood pressure of 200/120 on an 8-year-old child. She assumed that she had made a mistake in taking the blood pressure and did not report her finding to anyone. Who is responsible for this error in care?

1. The student nurse
2. The nurse working with the student
3. The teacher responsible for the student
4. Both the student and her teacher

161. What is the nurse's initial responsibility in teaching the pregnant adolescent client?

1. Informing her of the benefits of breastfeeding
2. Advising her about the proper care of an infant
3. Instructing her to watch for danger signs of pre-eclampsia
4. Discussing the importance of consistent prenatal care

162. Which of the following statements is the correct description of hemiplegia?

1. Paresis of both lower extremities
2. Paralysis of one side of the body
3. Paralysis of both lower extremities
4. Paresis of upper and lower extremities

163. Ms. Townsend has unresolved edema in her legs. Which of the following complications should the nurse assess for?

1. Proteinemia
2. Contractures
3. Tissue ischemia
4. Thrombus formation

164. Ms. Polaska has a diagnosis of systemic lupus erythematosus (SLE). Which of the following manifestations commonly occur with SLE?

1. A butterfly rash
2. Firm skin fixed to tissue
3. Muscle mass degeneration
4. An inflammation of small arteries

165. Mr. Scales expresses concern about radiation therapy for his cancer because he has heard that being exposed to radiation can cause him to develop other types of cancer. What should the nurse explain to Mr. Scales?

1. Dosage of radiation is strictly controlled.
2. Radiation doses are lowered if problems arise.
3. Good physical condition prevents problems.
4. Optimum cellular nutrition is protective.

166. Peter, age 15 years, asks his nurse why his testes are suspended in his scrotum. What would be the most appropriate response by the nurse?

1. To protect the sperm from the acidity of urine
2. To help with the passage of sperm through the urethra
3. To protect the sperm from high abdominal temperatures
4. To enable the testes to mature during embryonic development

167. An RN is counselling Mr. Olan following his vasectomy surgery. Which of the following components of health teaching is most important prior to discharge?

1. Sterilization is permanent and cannot be reversed.
2. Some impotency is to be expected for several weeks.
3. Unprotected coitus is allowed within a week to 10 days.
4. At least ten ejaculations are required to clear the tract of sperm.

168. Ms. Angelo, age 20 years, tells the nurse her menstrual periods are extremely painful, making her feel nauseated and keeping her in bed for several days. What should the nurse recommend?

1. Maintain her daily activities as much as possible
2. Make an appointment with a gynecologist
3. Take an over-the-counter drug such as ibuprofen
4. Practise relaxation of her abdominal muscles

169. Ms. McMahon is scheduled to undergo pelvic ultrasonography. What is the required preparation for this test?

1. Nothing by mouth for 8 hours prior to the test
2. A laxative the evening before and an enema the morning of the test
3. Drinking 1200 to 1500 mL of water 1 hour before the test
4. An injection of radiopaque dye immediately before the test

170. A unit nurse manager believes that consultation with her staff is unnecessary and serves only to confuse and slow down decision making on the unit. Which of the following terms would indicate her leadership style?

1. Situational
2. Laissez-faire
3. Autocratic
4. Positional

171. An RN prepares a client for coronary angiography. The client asks the reason for this test. Which of the following statements is the best response by the nurse?

1. "This test will look at the patency of the heart valves in your coronary blood flow."
2. "This exam will ensure that your heart's electrical system is operating as it should."
3. "This exam will determine the amount of blood flow through the coronary arteries to nourish your heart muscle."
4. "This exam will evaluate the strength of the left ventricle's contractions."

172. An RN performs a vaginal exam on Ms. Peteroff who is in active labour. She observes a prolapsed cord. What is the safest position for Ms. Peteroff?

1. Prone
2. Fowler position
3. Lithotomy position
4. Trendelenburg's position

173. Mr. Brendan is an intravenous heroin addict. He works in the sex trade to pay for his heroin. What would be the most important topic for health teaching?

1. Safety
2. Nutrition
3. Self-esteem
4. Legal issues

174. Ms. Hoang, who has type 2 diabetes, hypertension, and high cholesterol, tells the nurse that she takes herbal remedies. What is the most

important aspect related to herbal preparations that the nurse should discuss with Ms. Hoang?

1. Most herbal preparations are not formulated in standardized doses.
2. Herbal preparations are not regulated by Health Canada.
3. Some herbal preparations interact with prescription medications.
4. She should purchase herbal remedies from a recognized pharmacy rather than a traditional herbalist.

175. Ms. Nguyen arrives on the obstetrical unit in advanced labour. She has untreated genital herpes. What would be the danger to the infant if she were allowed to deliver vaginally?

1. Thrush
2. Systemic herpes
3. Ophthalmia neonatorum
4. Neurological complications

176. The nurse examines newborn baby Watson and notes that he has asymmetric gluteal folds. Which of the following conditions does this indicate?

1. Central nervous system damage
2. A dislocated hip
3. An inguinal hernia
4. Peripheral nervous system damage

177. Ms. Gilles, age 40 years, has just been admitted to hospital. She has bipolar disorder and is in the manic phase of her illness. Her language becomes vulgar and profane. What would be the most appropriate nursing response?

1. State, "We do not allow that kind of talk here"
2. Ignore it since the client is using it only to get attention
3. Recognize the language as part of the illness, but set limits on it
4. State, "When you can talk in an acceptable way, I will talk to you"

178. Maher is a 15-month-old infant who has a chronic renal disorder that has resulted in

numerous prolonged hospitalizations since he was born. His parents visit infrequently because they live far away; both work; and they have other children. Maher's nurse is aware that studies have shown that children who have suffered prolonged maternal deprivation early in life may demonstrate difficulty in which of the following behaviours?

1. Trusting others
2. Recalling past experiences
3. Developing age-appropriate cognitive development
4. Establishing relationships with caregivers

179. Mr. Jain, age 23 years, is a narcotics addict who is receiving methadone hydrochloride. He has undergone an emergency appendectomy. For which of the following signs of narcotic withdrawal should Mr. Jain be closely observed?

1. Piloerection
2. Agitation
3. Skin dryness
4. Lethargy

180. What is the most appropriate way to help a phobic client decrease anxiety?

1. Suggest he avoid unpleasant objects and events
2. Suggest he purposefully expose himself to fearful situations
3. Help him develop specific coping skills
4. Explore ways to introduce an element of pleasure into fearful situations

181. Ms. Alley tells the nurse that she wants to lose weight. She says she weighs 225 lb. and she wants to be 180 lb. How many kilograms does Ms. Alley want to lose?

1. 45 kg
2. 24 kg
3. 20 kg
4. 12 kg

182. Isabelle, a toddler, is brought to the emergency department by her mother, who reports that

Isabelle developed sudden hoarseness and unintelligible speech. The nurse notes that Isabelle is very distressed and anxious. What might be the first question the nurse asks Isabelle's mother?

1. "Did Isabelle have breathing problems at birth?"
2. "Has Isabelle shown previous signs of an upper respiratory tract infection (a cold)?"
3. "Is there a family history of breathing or throat problems?"
4. "Could she have aspirated something she put in her mouth?"

183. An infant has open-heart surgery for the repair of a ventricular septal defect. What would be a priority for the nurse when the child arrives in the recovery room?

1. Monitor the infant's urinary output
2. Assess the infant's pulmonary status
3. Determine the status of the operative site
4. Check the patency of the IV catheter

184. What self-care measures should the nurse advise for a 15-year-old female who experiences occasional outbreaks of acne?

1. "Scrub your face vigorously once a day."
2. "Don't eat foods such as chocolate and french fries."
3. "Always use an oil-based sunscreen when you are outside."
4. "Wash your face with mild soap and water twice a day."

185. Ms. Coutinho, a client on a long-term care unit, is immobilized. How would the nurse demonstrate the application of good body mechanics when caring for Ms. Coutinho?

1. Bending at the waist to provide power for lifting
2. Placing her feet apart to increase the stability of her body
3. Keeping her body straight when lifting to reduce pressure on her abdomen
4. Relaxing her abdominal muscles and using her extremities to prevent strain

186. What assistive device would be the most appropriate for early ambulation after hip-replacement surgery?

1. A walker
2. A cane
3. Crutches
4. A wheelchair

187. Following orthopedic surgery, Mr. Ferguson complains of pain. His nurse administers 15 mg of codeine sulphate, which has been ordered p.o., q3–4 hr prn. Two hours later, Mr. Ferguson tells the nurse he is still experiencing severe pain. What should the nurse do?

1. Report that Mr. Ferguson has an apparent idiosyncrasy to codeine
2. Tell Mr. Ferguson additional codeine cannot be given for 1 more hour
3. Request that the physician evaluate Mr. Ferguson's need for additional medication
4. Administer another dose of codeine within 15 minutes since it is a relatively safe drug

188. Moses is ordered ampicillin (Ampicin) 200 mg/kg/d. He weighs 45 kg. What dose should Moses receive every 6 hours?

1. 9.0 g
2. 4.5 g
3. 3.2 g
4. 2.3 g

189. Which of the following analgesic dosage regimens is most likely to provide optimum pain relief for a client who is 1 day postoperative from abdominal surgery?

1. "Around the clock," at intervals dependent on the length of action of the analgesic
2. "As needed" (prn), at intervals of 3 to 4 hours
3. As requested by the client and within accepted time frames
4. As assessed by the nurse

190. A nurse is teaching a group of adolescents about aspects of human sexuality. Which of the

following statements is the most correct referring to gender identity?

1. Preference for a partner of either the male or female sex
2. How one considers one's own sexual orientation
3. The internal sense of being either male or female or both male and female
4. The way one chooses to present one's gender to the world through dress and mannerisms

191. Mr. Akland, age 74, tells the nurse that because of his arthritis he is having difficulty caring for his feet. Mr. Akland has had type 2 diabetes for 7 years. Which of the following actions by the nurse would be initially most beneficial to Mr. Akland?

1. Assess Mr. Akland's movement and ability to manage his own hygiene
2. Arrange for a home care nurse to visit him
3. Ask Mr. Akland if there is a family member who could assist him
4. Suggest to Mr. Akland that he make regular appointments with his physician to monitor the condition of his feet

192. Mr. James, age 24, is HIV positive. He has been started on a new medication regimen and admits he has not been compliant with taking his drugs. Which of the following actions by the nurse would be most helpful to get Mr. James to take his medications?

1. Give him a fact sheet about human immunodeficiency virus/acquired immune deficiency syndrome (HIV/AIDS) medications so that he can understand the importance of the drugs
2. Arrange with the pharmacy to "bubble-pack" all of his medications so that he could be sure that he had taken his proper dose
3. Discuss with Mr. James how his medications might be changed to fit in with his lifestyle
4. Ask Mr. James what his reasons are for not taking his medications

193. The family of a 92-year-old man who has advanced dementia would like to care for him at

home but are overwhelmed by the care he requires. The nurse realizes they will need extensive assistance from community agencies and resources. What is the most appropriate action by the nurse?

1. Arrange a consultation with a social worker
2. Suggest that the family discuss community resources with the physician
3. Research the community agencies and conduct a teaching session with the family
4. Provide a community services pamphlet to the family

194. Which of the following procedures is correct when obtaining a throat culture from a client?

1. Have the client sit erect and swab the tonsillar area, making contact with inflamed or purulent areas but not touching the teeth, lips, or tongue
2. Have the client deep-breathe and cough, and then swab the mucus that the client has loosened
3. Have the client lie in a supine position and turn his or her head to the side; insert the swab and move it from side to side to cover as much area as possible
4. Place the client in a high Fowler position and ask him or her to lean forward with the mouth open while the swab is inserted and rotated in a clockwise movement.

195. The nurse attends a conference and hears about a new type of incontinence product. She would like to try this new product and compare it with what is currently used on the unit. What is the most appropriate initial step for the nurse?

1. Compile all available data on the new product
2. Ask the physician on the unit if she would consider ordering the new product
3. Write a research proposal and present it to the nurse manager
4. Obtain a sample of the new product and use it with clients who have provided consent

196. A client is going to the diagnostic imaging department for a magnetic resonance imaging

(MRI) scan. He has an IV running at 75 mL per hour. The nurse observes that there is 100 mL of solution remaining to be absorbed. What would be the nurse's most appropriate action to ensure that the IV is maintained while he is having the MRI?

1. Accompany the client to the MRI and change the IV solution bag when required
2. Ensure that a new IV bag of solution is sent with the client for the MRI department
3. Reduce the drip rate of the IV to 25 mL per hour before the client leaves for the MRI
4. Change the IV solution to a new bag just prior to the client leaving the unit for the MRI

197. Mr. Balasingham was identified 1 year ago to be incompetent to make decisions regarding his care. When a care decision occurs, what will happen?

1. The substitute decision maker (SDM) will make the decision.
2. His next of kin will be contacted.
3. The physician will assume responsibility for care decisions.
4. Mr. Balasingham will be provided with the opportunity to make his decision.

198. Ms. Lewis is admitted to the hospital with fever, productive cough, shortness of breath, and fatigue. A dialysis client occupies the only private room on the unit. What should the nurse do?

1. Move the dialysis client from the private room and admit Ms. Lewis to it
2. Admit Ms. Lewis to a semi-private room with a postoperative client

3. Admit Ms. Lewis to a semi-private room with a client who has cancer
4. Refuse to admit Ms. Lewis due to infection control concerns

199. A student nurse is working with an experienced registered nurse preceptor on a postpartum unit. The preceptor recommends supplementing breastfeeding with formula to a first-time mother of a full-term healthy 1-day-old infant. The student nurse is aware that supplementing breastfeeding with formula is not recommended by lactation experts. What should the student nurse do?

1. Speak with the mother in private about the benefits of breastfeeding
2. Discuss with the preceptor the best-practice research concerning not supplementing breastfeeding with bottles
3. Complain to the nursing manager about the preceptor's lack of knowledge of breastfeeding
4. Comply with the advice of the preceptor to the new mother since the preceptor is an experienced postpartum nurse

200. The nursing team leader tells another nurse to initiate an intravenous infusion with lactated Ringer's solution for a client. What would be the first action taken by the nurse?

1. Wash his hands
2. Collect the equipment for the procedure
3. Check the physician's orders
4. Inform the client of the procedure

END OF PRACTICE EXAM 1

5

Answers and Rationales for Practice Exam 1

CASE–BASED QUESTIONS ANSWERS AND RATIONALES

CASE 1

1.

1. **In order to comply with the rights of medication administration, the nurse must compare the pharmacy package with the prescriber's (usually a physician) original order to confirm that the pharmacy has prepared the correct medication for Mr. Rickhelm.**

2. Mr. Rickhelm may not know all of the medications he is receiving. The prescriber's order is the most valid resource.
3. This action is not necessary, although if a discrepancy were discovered with the prescriber's order, the pharmacy should be contacted.
4. This action will provide information about the drug but would not confirm it is the correct drug for Mr. Rickhelm.

CLASSIFICATION

Competency:
Professional Practice
Taxonomy:
Critical Thinking

2.

1. **This response answers Mr. Ogalino's question and indicates that the nurse is aware of what drug she is administering and that it is an accepted generic form of the drug.**

2. It is not responsible for the nurse to administer a drug that she neither knows the name of nor the reason it has been prescribed for Mr. Ogalino.
3. This does not answer Mr. Ogalino's question, and it is potentially dangerous for her to disregard his questioning of an unfamiliar medication.
4. This does not answer Mr. Ogalino's question, and it is potentially dangerous for him not to take a medication.

CLASSIFICATION

Competency:
Professional Practice
Taxonomy:
Application

3.

1. A blood sugar reading at 1800 hours has no value in deciding optimum time for administration of long-acting insulin.

2. **This response validates Ms. Jasmin's comment and may provide important information to the nurse for the dosing schedule.**

3. Reliance on hospital routines or policies is not an accountable response.
4. This is incorrect; if the insulin were given at 1800 hours, the peak action and potential hypoglycemia may occur in the middle of the night.

CLASSIFICATION

Competency:
Professional Practice
Taxonomy:
Application

4.

1. Statins reduce serum cholesterol levels, which are not aspects of the pathology of deep-vein thrombosis.
2. Antibiotics are used to treat bacterial infections, which are not an aspect of the pathology of deep-vein thrombosis.
3. Analgesics are used to treat pain and reduce fever. There is no indication Ms. Corel requires either.

4. **Anticoagulants, or blood thinners, are used to treat and prevent deep-vein thrombosis.**

CLASSIFICATION

Competency:
Changes in Health
Taxonomy:
Knowledge/Comprehension

5. 1. A registered nurse (RN) is not the only health care provider who can legally sign a narcotics count sheet.
   2. Registered practical nurses and licensed practical nurses are both able to sign the count sheet but are not the only health care providers who can.
   3. An RN or a physician is not the only health care provider legally able to sign a narcotics count sheet.

   4. **Regulated health care providers, such as nurses, physicians, dentists, chiropractors, and so on, are legally able to sign narcotics count sheets.**

CLASSIFICATION

Competency:
Professional Practice

Taxonomy:
Knowledge/Comprehension

6. 1. Nurses are responsible for ensuring the correct dose of medication whether or not it has been calculated by the pharmacy.
   2. The digoxin administered is not the same dose as was ordered.
   3. The administered digoxin is an overdose.

   4. **The dose of digoxin is ten times the ordered dose. It is a nursing responsibility to calculate and ensure the correct dose of every drug administered.**

CLASSIFICATION

Competency:
Professional Practice

Taxonomy:
Application

CASE 2

7. 1. **This response helps to identify it as a unique experience for Mr. Smadu, without getting into a discussion of whether it is a symptom of his schizophrenia.**

   2. It is not helpful to pretend to believe in the hallucination, even though it may be helpful for the nurse to find out more about the hallucinations.
   3. It is not helpful to Mr. Smadu to argue reality with him.
   4. Exploring with Mr. Smadu the reasons he hears voices is not helpful to him. The hallucinations are a symptom of his disease.

CLASSIFICATION

Competency:
Nurse–Client Partnership

Taxonomy:
Application

8. 1. This action will not help, as Mr. Smadu cannot control the hallucinations.

   2. **Some individuals find that listening to music on headphones helps to decrease the effect of voices.**

   3. Physical activity may help decrease some symptoms over time, but a walk is unlikely to reduce particular episodes of hearing voices.
   4. This option is unsafe.

CLASSIFICATION

Competency:
Changes in Health

Taxonomy:
Application

9. 1. Some people with schizophrenia may become violent, particularly if they are experiencing severe paranoia.
   2. There is no need to call the police unless Mr. Smadu's behaviour is threatening. The word *strange* does not adequately describe the behaviour.

CLASSIFICATION

Competency:
Changes in Health

Taxonomy:
Application

3. This action would not eliminate his hallucinations.

4. **Being too close to Mr. Smadu if he is in an agitated state may cause him to strike out to protect himself.**

10. 1. Risperidone can be given orally and is absorbed from the gastrointestinal tract.

CLASSIFICATION
Competency:
Changes in Health
Taxonomy:
Application

2. **Compliance with medication is a problem with clients who have schizophrenia. Administering the antipsychotic in a form that will provide therapeutic levels for 2 weeks aids in compliance.**

3. There is not a better response with the IM route.
4. Tardive dyskinesia is a risk regardless of the route of administration.

11. 1. **Ten years after their first episode, 25% of people are much improved and living fairly independent lives.**

CLASSIFICATION
Competency:
Changes in Health
Taxonomy:
Knowledge/Comprehension

2. One quarter, not one half, of people recover after ten years.
3. Approximately one half of people diagnosed with schizophrenia will either improve to a degree or recover.
4. This response does not address Ms. Smadu's question.

12. 1. Alogia involves decreases in thought, speech, and fluency.
2. Anhedonia is the inability to feel pleasure or happiness.

CLASSIFICATION
Competency:
Changes in Health
Taxonomy:
Knowledge/Comprehension

3. **Avolition is the inability to act on plans.**

4. Attention impairment is the inability to keep attention focused on a particular thought or activity.

13. 1. The voices have told Mr. Smadu to commit suicide. The most important action is to keep him safe.
2. This situation is not necessarily an emergency unless Mr. Smadu possesses a gun.

CLASSIFICATION
Competency:
Changes in Health
Taxonomy:
Critical Thinking

3. **Suicide precautions need to be put into effect, which means that Mr. Smadu may need to be admitted to hospital for close observation.**

4. Ten percent of all people with schizophrenia commit suicide due to feelings of torment or the voices commanding them to kill themselves.

CASE 3

14. 1. **MRSA is spread by direct contact with skin that has the bacteria or with contaminated surfaces.**

CLASSIFICATION
Competency:
Changes in Health

2. MRSA is not spread through the air by aerosol or droplet transmission.

3. MRSA is not spread via the fecal–oral route.

4. Such contact could be a possible mode of transmission; however, there is no evidence in this question that persons who did not wash their hands were colonized or infected with MRSA.

Taxonomy:

Application

---

15. 1. Open wounds are a risk factor, but hers would be a small incision. A surgical incision should not be colonized with bacteria.

2. Being an infant and the possible decreased immunity due to failure to thrive are possible risk factors but are not as great as those in answer 4.

3. Advanced age is a risk factor for MRSA, but there are no other risks.

4. **Ms. Gary has several risk factors. Those who are most at risk have chronic diseases that have been treated frequently with antibiotics. With a spinal cord injury, there is a possible increased risk for tissue breakdown and MRSA colonization on the skin.**

CLASSIFICATION
Competency:
Changes in Health
Taxonomy:
Critical Thinking

---

16. 1. These actions should be taken, but, in addition, the nurse should wear gloves.

2. If the cut is appropriately managed, the nurse has no reason to refrain from caring for clients with MRSA.

3. **Occlusive tape will cover the open cut. All nurses should wear gloves when caring for clients with MRSA.**

4. This action should be done with all clients and does not provide for additional precautions for the open cut.

CLASSIFICATION
Competency:
Health and Wellness
Taxonomy:
Critical Thinking

CASE 4

17. 1. The nurse's behaviour is unprofessional and does not account for the growth and developmental needs of children of this age.

2. **When a client is restrained inappropriately and without exploring other alternatives, the action could be considered assault and battery. If necessary, mittens are much more appropriate.**

3. Although the behaviour (scratching) needs to be decreased, the nurse can address it with the use of mittens, rather than immobilizing a child of this age.

4. Restraining Denika's hands is inappropriate whether the parents give permission or not.

CLASSIFICATION
Competency:
Professional Practice
Taxonomy:
Application

---

18. 1. This task is too advanced for toddlers and more accurate for preschoolers.

CLASSIFICATION
Competency:
Health and Wellness
Taxonomy:
Application

Answers Exam 1

2. **Common developmental norms of the toddler, who is struggling for independence, are inability to share easily, egotism, egocentrism, and possessiveness.**

3. This exercise is true of 4-year-olds.
4. One characteristic of toddlers is their short attention span; 15 minutes is too much to expect.

---

19. 1. This would be too slow to infuse the desired amount.
2. Same as answer 1.

3. $$\frac{\text{Amount of fluid} \times \text{Drop rate}}{\text{Time to infuse in hours} \times 60 \text{ min}}$$
$$\frac{1000 \times 60}{24 \times 60} = \frac{60,000}{1440} = 42 \text{ drops}$$

CLASSIFICATION
Competency:
Professional Practice
Taxonomy:
Application

4. This would be too rapid; the fluid would run out before 24 hours had elapsed.

---

20. 1. This action will not achieve the goal of giving fluids.
2. This action will not likely be successful with a toddler.

3. **Children who are expressing negativism need to have a feeling of control. One way of achieving this, within reasonable limits, is for the parent or caregiver to provide a choice of two items, rather than force one on the child.**

CLASSIFICATION
Competency:
Health and Wellness
Taxonomy:
Application

4. A toddler would not respond to intellectual reasoning, particularly regarding an activity that she does not want to do.

---

21. 1. This is too late.

2. **Denika should be taken to the dentist between 2 and 3 years of age, when most of the 20 deciduous teeth have erupted.**

CLASSIFICATION
Competency:
Health and Wellness
Taxonomy:
Knowledge/Comprehension

3. Same as answer 1.
4. This is too indefinite.

CASE 5

22. 1. This notation means three pregnancies, one living child, and one abortion.
2. This notation means three pregnancies, no living children, and two abortions.

CLASSIFICATION
Competency:
Health and Wellness
Taxonomy:
Application

3. **This notation means four pregnancies, one living child, and two abortions, and is the correct notation.**

4. This notation means four pregnancies, one living child, and one abortion.

---

23. 1. This component is important but not the priority.
     2. Same as answer 1.
     3. Same as answer 1.

     4. **Obtaining the baseline fetal heart rate is the priority in order to determine fetal health.**

CLASSIFICATION
Competency:
Health and Wellness
Taxonomy:
Critical Thinking

---

24. 1. The correct term is not *hard*. Contraction frequency should be documented in exact terms, not approximate terms.

     2. **Contractions that cause a firm fundus (i.e., one that cannot be indented) are termed *strong*. The exact frequency should be documented.**

     3. A subjective description is not necessary to assess the contraction strength. The nurse best determines this objectively. Stating that the contractions are 60 seconds apart is not accurate.
     4. The correct term is *strong*; also, contractions do not last 50 to 70 seconds.

CLASSIFICATION
Competency:
Professional Practice
Taxonomy:
Application

---

25. 1. The documentation is important but not the priority action.

     2. **The safest action is to observe the perineum to ensure that the cord has not prolapsed and to take the fetal heart rate to ensure fetal well-being.**

     3. This action may occur later but is not a priority.
     4. This action may need to be done if the nurse and midwife are not sure that the fluid is the result of the rupture of the amniotic membranes, but the most important action is to observe the perineum.

CLASSIFICATION
Competency:
Health and Wellness
Competency:
Critical Thinking

---

26. 1. This action will not prevent hypothermia although it will result in some transfer of body heat.

     2. **Evaporation of amniotic fluid on the skin causes a drop in the temperature of a newborn. Immediately drying an infant after birth is an important action to prevent hypothermia.**

     3. Blankets are useful to keep the baby warm once the baby is dry.
     4. It is not likely that there would be a warmed bassinette in a home situation; regardless, this would not be the first action.

CLASSIFICATION
Competency:
Health and Wellness
Taxonomy:
Critical Thinking

Answers Exam 1

27.   1. A contract with a midwife is not the issue. RNs must document any care they administer.
       2. The nurse must document for herself but not for another.

       3. Nurses must document any care they provide.

       4. The midwife cannot delegate her documentation to another health care provider unless it is an emergency situation.

CLASSIFICATION
Competency:
Professional Practice
Taxonomy:
Application

CASE 6

28.   1. Trying to talk Mr. Richard out of his behaviour is unlikely to be effective.
       2. Other clients need to be protected from this client. Waiting to see if the behaviour worsens is dangerous and may cause further agitation.
       3. This action may further aggravate Mr. Richard.

       4. This action separates Mr. Richard from the other clients and places him in a less stimulating environment.

CLASSIFICATION
Competency:
Nurse–Client Partnership
Taxonomy:
Application

29.   1. Wound sepsis is a possible complication but would not be evident until the third to fifth day.

       2. Inhalation burns are usually present with facial burns, regardless of their depth; the threat to life is asphyxia from irritation and edema of the respiratory passages and lungs. Breathing is the most important priority in this situation, and difficulties are most likely to occur within the first 24 hours.

       3. Pain is certainly a concern but is not the most important one within the first 24 hours.
       4. Fluid and electrolyte imbalances are a danger but do not reach their maximum until the fourth day.

CLASSIFICATION
Competency:
Changes in Health
Taxonomy:
Critical Thinking

30.   1. This statement may be true in the case of some injectable substances but is not an important consideration in this situation.
       2. While repeat intramuscular (IM) injections are more painful than intravenous (IV) administration of drugs, this is not the most important concern for Richard at this time.

       3. Damage to tissues from the burns interferes with the stability of peripheral circulation and with the effectiveness of intramuscular medications.

       4. IV administration provides more consistent blood levels of analgesic but does not necessarily provide longer pain relief than IM administration.

CLASSIFICATION
Competency:
Changes in Health
Taxonomy:
Critical Thinking

31. 1. **The client may give permission to any other person to read the health record. The only other circumstance that would allow a legal official to read the chart is the issuance of a court order.**

    2. The doctor may not give permission to read the health record.
    3. Being charged with a criminal offence does not change the legislation with regard to privacy of health information.
    4. This statement is true, but it is not the most appropriate response.

CLASSIFICATION
Competency:
Professional Practice
Taxonomy:
Application

CASE 7

32. 1. This response dismisses Mr. Wilmot's concern.
    2. This response is not necessarily true, and Mr. Wilmot will still have one testicle.

    3. **This response recognizes Mr. Wilmot's concerns and offers a positive solution while still encouraging open dialogue.**

    4. This response is not true.

CLASSIFICATION
Competency:
Nurse–Client Partnership
Taxonomy:
Application

33. 1. **This response would indicate that Mr. Wilmot's concerns are being listened to. A visit from another man who has experienced a similar treatment would allow him to get first-hand information.**

    2. This response offers false reassurance.
    3. This response would be appropriate only if Mr. Wilmot expressed a desire for psychiatric treatment.
    4. Although this response is true, it does not specifically address Mr. Wilmot's concerns.

CLASSIFICATION
Competency:
Nurse–Client Partnership
Taxonomy:
Application

34. 1. Treatment is not an absolute guarantee of a cure, and other malignancies may occur.
    2. This course of action is not required, as he will still have one functioning testicle.

    3. **Even though the cure rate is positive for testicular cancer, all clients must have routine follow-ups to monitor for relapse.**

    4. The incidence of relapse is not high.

CLASSIFICATION
Competency:
Changes in Health
Taxonomy:
Application

35. 1. **This is the correct procedure. The warmth of the water will allow the testis to be palpated more easily.**

    2. This position will not aid in feeling the testis. Circular motions are not likely to detect abnormalities.
    3. This procedure is used to examine a hydrocele.
    4. The testis should feel like a hard-boiled egg, and the epididymis is rougher.

CLASSIFICATION
Competency:
Health and Wellness
Taxonomy:
Application

CASE 8

36. 1. With the client's history of unstable and fluctuating blood pressure, the nurse needs to ensure that the blood pressure reading is accurate. Unregulated care providers (UCPs) do not have the same competencies as regulated health care workers, who have standardized education, knowledge, and skills.
     2. The doctor has written the order and has nothing to do with assessing the blood pressure at this particular time.
     3. This action will not ensure accuracy of the reading.

     4. **This action is the safest option. The nurse is accountable for her actions in administering the nifedipine and thus would be accountable for the error should the blood pressure not be what the UCP recorded. Taking and interpreting vital signs is a nursing function. Delegating such a task to a UCP, who does not have the education of a nurse, should be discussed with the hospital administration.**

CLASSIFICATION

Competency:
Professional Practice

Taxonomy:
Critical Thinking

37. 1. **Consent must be obtained for all treatments and medications. Verbal consent is appropriate prior to the administration of each dose of ECASA.**

     2. Enteric-coated tablets should not be crushed.
     3. The nurse must ensure that the client takes all ordered medication. Leaving the ECASA at Ms. Bystriska's bedside is not a responsible nursing action unless this has been predetermined as appropriate for this particular client.
     4. A written consent specifically for medication administration is not reasonable or indicated.

CLASSIFICATION

Competency:
Professional Practice

Taxomony:
Application

38. 1. This site is an appropriate subcutaneous (SC) site.
     2. This needle gauge is correct for SC injections.

     3. **Massaging the injected area is not recommended with insulin.**

     4. This technique is appropriate.

CLASSIFICATION

Competency:
Changes in Health

Taxonomy:
Application

39. 1. There is no indication that Ms. Banwait has been proven to be incapable of making decisions.
     2. There is no indication that Ms. Banwait has been judged incapable and that her husband has been designated as the substitute decision maker.
     3. The nurse would need to find out more concerning the upset stomach before withholding the medication.

CLASSIFICATION

Competency:
Professional Practice

Taxonomy:
Application

4. Ms. Banwait has withdrawn consent; therefore, the nurse is not legally permitted to force treatment on her. There is no indication that she has been deemed incapable to make decisions regarding her health care.

CASE 9

40. 1. The core temperature decreases; it does not increase.

2. In some women (but not all), there is a decrease in temperature at the time of ovulation.

3. The body temperature is elevated after ovulation, not before.
4. After ovulation, the temperature remains on an elevated plateau until 2 to 4 days before menstruation.

CLASSIFICATION
Competency:
Health and Wellness
Taxonomy:
Knowledge/Comprehension

41. 1. This response is judgemental.
2. This response is judgemental and implies that Sarah should feel guilty if she chooses to have an abortion.

3. This response is nonjudgemental and encourages Sarah to discuss her options.

4. The client is Sarah, not her parents. Sarah has the right to make her decision. However, if Sarah indicates that her parents are involved and supportive, they may be included in the discussion.

CLASSIFICATION
Competency:
Nurse–Client Partnership
Taxonomy:
Application

42. 1. A diaphragm will not prevent sexually transmitted infections (STIs).
2. Some spermicides do provide protection against some STIs, but they are generally not effective against human immunodeficiency virus (HIV), chlamydia, or cervical gonorrhea.
3. Same as answer 1.

4. A female condom is inserted by the woman prior to intercourse. If used correctly, it provides a barrier to sperm and STIs.

CLASSIFICATION
Competency:
Health and Wellness
Taxonomy:
Application

43. 1. There is a strong link between human papilloma virus (HPV) and cervical cancer, and Papanicolaou (Pap) tests are required for diagnosis. Pap tests should be performed annually.

2. Antibiotics are not effective against HPV.
3. This option is not realistic. The nurse should discuss with Ms. McLeod safe sexual practices, including the use of condoms.
4. Eradication of the virus is not considered conclusive, even after there is no visible evidence of HPV.

CLASSIFICATION
Competency:
Changes in Health
Taxonomy:
Application

44.   1. Oral birth control is very effective but not 100% effective. Ms. Ahmadi has complied with the recommendation that she use a method of birth control that is 100% effective. Also, oral contraceptives may have an effect on the cardiovascular system.

2. **All these methods are fairly effective; however, a tubal ligation (i.e., the tying of the fallopian tubes) is the most effective. A hysterectomy is the only method of birth control that is 100% effective, but surgery in someone with severe heart failure may not be recommended.**

CLASSIFICATION

Competency:
Health and Wellness

Taxonomy:
Critical Thinking

3. While a vasectomy is close to 100% effective, it is Ms. Ahmadi who should not become pregnant. There is no information that Ms. Ahmadi is in a monogamous partnership.
4. This option is not 100% effective.

CASE 10

45.   1. This outcome may occur, but the nurse should obtain factual information about the vaccine prior to making a decision.

2. **This option is the best way for the nurse to become informed of the safety and efficacy of the new vaccine. To support safe practice, it is the nurse's responsibility to seek out current information from reliable resources.**

CLASSIFICATION

Competency:
Professional Practice

Taxonomy:
Critical Thinking

3. This outcome may occur, but the nurse should research information about the vaccine prior to making a decision.
4. While it is a good idea to consult with nursing colleagues, the nurse should recognize that their opinions may not be based on fact.

46.   1. **A dilemma is defined as a situation in which one must make an uneasy and difficult choice between two alternatives. In this situation, the most ethical course of action is not clear: the nurse has a strong moral reason to support both caring for her clients and keeping her family safe.**

CLASSIFICATION

Competency:
Professional Practice

Taxonomy:
Knowledge/Comprehension

2. Ethical theory is a framework of assumptions and principles intended to guide decisions about morality.
3. Moral distress is stress caused by situations in which a person is convinced of what is morally right but is not able to act.
4. Nonmaleficence is a principle that obliges people to act so that harm to others is prevented.

CLASSIFICATION

Competency:
Professional Practice

Taxonomy:
Application

47.   1. Based on guidelines by leaders in previous pandemic planning, the priority groups were health care workers and children and adults with underlying health conditions.
2. Same as answer 1.
3. The government does not legislate who receives priority care.

4. Health care leaders and decision makers develop guidelines to help prioritize resources and identify vulnerable groups so that there is justifiable, reasonable, and fair allocation of resources and access to treatment.

48. 1. **The deltoid muscle is easily accessible and is the recommended IM site for small volume injections and routine immunizations.**

2. The ventrogluteal muscle is a safe site for IM injections for all clients; however, it is neither necessary nor practical for an immunization clinic.
3. The dorsogluteal muscle, although a traditional site for IM injections, has been associated with injury to the sciatic nerve and is not recommended.
4. The vastus lateralis is the preferred site for immunizations for infants.

CLASSIFICATION
Competency:
Professional Practice
Taxonomy:
Critical Thinking

49. 1. **Individuals who are allergic to eggs should not have the vaccine since the inactivated flu viruses are grown in chick embryos.**

2. Sexual activity has no relation to the flu vaccine.
3. Antibodies from one type of influenza do not provide immunity from another type of influenza.
4. While childhood immunizations ideally should be current, it is not necessary prior to administration of the flu vaccine.

CLASSIFICATION
Competency:
Health and Wellness
Taxonomy:
Knowledge/Comprehension

50. 1. While it is not easy to deny care to an ineligible person, the ethical use of available resources requires that the nurse refuse to give the vaccine to the adolescent at this time.
2. This statement may be true, but it does not provide a rationale for refusing the adolescent the vaccine and may cause the mother to become concerned and angry.
3. It is not necessarily true that the adolescent is not at risk for contracting this influenza; it is just that he, at present, is not in a priority group.

CLASSIFICATION
Competency:
Professional Practice
Taxonomy:
Critical Thinking

4. **The mother needs to be reassured that her adolescent son is not in a vulnerable group and that, with limited vaccine available, it must go to those people who are most at risk. The nurse also assures the mother that her son will most likely be able to receive the vaccine at a later date.**

CASE 11

51. 1. This response dismisses Ms. Smith's concerns and shows no respect for her feelings.
2. Same as answer 1.

3. **This response indicates caring and provides Ms. Smith an opportunity for her to express her feelings.**

4. Ms. Smith may not be ready to socialize with other residents.

CLASSIFICATION
Competency:
Nurse–Client Partnership
Taxonomy:
Application

52.
1. This action is neither professional nor caring and may be considered neglect.
2. Ms. Smith has stated she does not wish to participate in exercise.
3. There is no indication Ms. Smith requires a substitute decision maker (SDM). She has stated her rationale for her decision.

4. **The nurse must respect the decision of the client even if it is contrary to what the nurse believes is the "right" health care decision.**

CLASSIFICATION

Competency:
Nurse–Client Partnership

Taxonomy:
Application

53.
1. It is contrary to ethical nursing practice to accept valuable gifts from clients even if the client is cognitively appropriate.
2. Same as answer 1.

3. **This response is professional and complies with ethical guidelines for accepting gifts from clients.**

4. This is not true of all agencies as some gifts, particularly if they are for the entire nursing team, are appropriate. It also places blame on the agency rather than showing the nurse practising ethical behaviour.

CLASSIFICATION

Competency:
Professional Practice

Taxonomy:
Critical Thinking

CASE 12

54.
1. When presented early in the process, a list of "dos and don'ts" may cause resentment and impede compliance with a diet. This would be best offered later.
2. This information does need to be emphasized but may be presumptive and directive as an initial action.
3. This question presumes Mr. Hudson has behaviours that he needs to change and is not appropriate initially. In later conversations, it may be appropriate.

4. **This question is open ended, does not presume anything, involves Mr. Hudson in the nutrition plan, and puts the emphasis on his needs, not the nurse's.**

CLASSIFICATION

Competency:
Nurse–Client Partnership

Taxonomy:
Critical Thinking

55.
1. **Smaller, more frequent meals help to maintain consistent blood glucose levels.**

2. Total carbohydrate intake should be 50 to 60% of the total diet. It is the type of carbohydrate that is more important.
3. There is no evidence that a diabetic diet does not provide adequate vitamins and minerals.
4. Total fat should remain approximately the same as for the general public. It is more important to restrict the amount of saturated and trans fats, not the total fat.

CLASSIFICATION

Competency:
Health and Wellness

Taxonomy:
Application

56. 1. Simple carbohydrates include monosaccharides and disaccharides. Examples are sugars such as table sugar, honey, and fruit drinks.

2. **These foods are examples of complex carbohydrates that contain starch, glycogen, and fibre.**

3. *Monounsaturated* is a term used with fats.
4. Some of these foods have a moderate glycemic index.

CLASSIFICATION
Competency:
Health and Wellness
Taxonomy:
Knowledge/Comprehension

57. 1. **Processed foods and commercially baked products have a high trans fats content.**

2. Meat is a source of saturated fat; thus, choosing lean meat would reduce this type of fat.
3. Canola oil is an unsaturated plant fat. Trans fats are hydrogenated plant oils. Using corn oil or canola oil will not reduce trans fat intake.
4. Egg yolks are a source of cholesterol, not trans fats.

CLASSIFICATION
Competency:
Health and Wellness
Taxonomy:
Application

58. 1. The bran muffin is high in calories and may contain trans fats, as may the margarine. For diabetics, fruits are best taken whole rather than as juice since the whole fruit contains fibre. This breakfast does not contain protein or dairy products.

2. **This menu is low in calories yet contains all the food groups, providing protein, complex carbohydrates, fibre, dairy, and fruits.**

3. This menu is high in protein but contains no fibre or fruits.
4. The raisins may be high in sugar, the lactose-free milk is not necessary in a diabetic or weight-loss diet, and whole fruit would be better than juice.

CLASSIFICATION
Competency:
Health and Wellness
Taxonomy:
Critical Thinking

59. 1. Unless otherwise instructed by the physician, he should maintain his normal medication schedule.

2. **Monitoring of blood glucose will tell Mr. Hudson if he needs to adjust his diet. Unless otherwise instructed by a physician, he should maintain his normal medication schedule.**

3. It is not necessary to contact a physician for minor illnesses, unless blood sugars become unstable.
4. Same as answer 2.

CLASSIFICATION
Competency:
Changes in Health
Taxonomy:
Critical Thinking

60. 1. A weight loss of 5 kg is good and will help the diabetes but does not particularly indicate how well blood glucose has been maintained.
2. A fasting blood-sugar reading will only tell the status of the blood sugar on that particular day.

CLASSIFICATION
Competency:
Changes in Health
Taxonomy:
Critical Thinking

3. A glycosylated hemoglobin (HbA$_{1c}$) test provides an accurate long-term index of the client's average blood sugar. It is objective and reliable evidence of glucose control.

4. This method of evaluation is important but not the best. Mr. Hudson may feel well even with high blood-glucose levels. If he is not managing the diabetes, he may not want to admit this to the nurse.

CASE 13

61.   1. People with anorexia tend to have cold intolerance rather than feeling hot.

2. Women with anorexia often stop menstruating due to the loss of body fat.

3. The skin of people with anorexia tends to be dry, not oily.
4. People with anorexia have constipation rather than diarrhea.

CLASSIFICATION

Competency:

Changes in Health

Taxonomy:

Application

62.   1. This test is important but monitors only one thing.
2. This test is very important for a client with anorexia, but a test for electrolytes would include potassium.

3. An electrolytes test includes sodium, potassium, and chloride.

4. Same as answer 1.

CLASSIFICATION

Competency:

Changes in Health

Taxonomy:

Critical Thinking

63.   1. Young women with anorexia tend to avoid intimacy and are generally not sexually active.
2. Clients with anorexia more frequently deny their illness.
3. Rather than acting out, the anorexic teen often strives to be the "model child."

4. Clients with anorexia are often high achievers in school in their attempt to be perfect and have control.

CLASSIFICATION

Competency:

Changes in Health

Taxonomy:

Application

64.   1. The physician should be notified, but this is not the first action.
2. The apical rate should be monitored after fluids until it increases.

3. This is a very low apical rate and is due to low blood volume secondary to dehydration. The initial action is to increase the blood volume through the administration of fluids.

4. A snack will not increase the blood volume, and Tiffany may not want to eat.

CLASSIFICATION

Competency:

Changes in Health

Taxonomy:

Critical Thinking

65. 1. **This statement is true of teens with anorexia, and Tiffany has a history of excessive exercising. With the forced increase in food, Tiffany will fear an increase in weight, which she may attempt to counter by exercising.**

    2. Over-exercising may be harmful, but moderate exercise will be of no harm, particularly since her vital signs have stabilized.

    3. Exercise is not an important part of the therapeutic plan for a teen with anorexia.

    4. Exercise will not affect Tiffany's tolerance for food.

CLASSIFICATION
Competency:
Changes in Health
Taxonomy:
Critical Thinking

66. 1. This response may be true but is not likely to convince Tiffany to attend the sessions.

    2. **This response focuses on Tiffany's feelings rather than the group therapy itself. The group would be effective only if Tiffany is able to discuss her feelings openly.**

    3. Tiffany may never feel the need to talk with the other girls.

    4. This response offers false reassurance; group therapy with other girls who have anorexia may help Tiffany develop insight but may not help her cope with the disease.

CLASSIFICATION
Competency:
Nurse–Client Partnership
Taxonomy:
Application

67. 1. Rapid weight gain may cause cardiovascular overload and an overwhelming sense of loss of control.

    2. **Gradual weight gain is metabolically safe and will prevent the feelings of loss of control that would occur with too rapid a weight gain.**

    3. Hydration is important, but 3 L is too much. Tiffany would likely not be compliant with drinking this much fluid.

    4. This weight gain would be too fast, particularly in a person who is underweight.

CLASSIFICATION
Competency:
Changes in Health
Taxonomy:
Application

CASE 14

68. 1. This type of rash is common and usually benign in a new infant.

    2. This behaviour is not necessarily a sign of illness unless the infant cannot be roused.

    3. **Grunting and rapid respirations are abnormal behaviours in an infant. Grunting is a compensatory mechanism whereby an infant attempts to keep air in the alveoli to increase arterial oxygenation; increased respirations increase oxygen and carbon dioxide exchange.**

    4. This behaviour is a normal sign of increasing fluid requirements with growth.

CLASSIFICATION
Competency:
Changes in Health
Taxonomy:
Application

69. 1. Oral temperatures are not recommended for children under 3 years old.
2. This route is used only when no other route is possible because of the risk for rectal perforation and because it is intrusive.

> 3. **This is not invasive, and although it does not provide a core temperature, it is relatively accurate.**

4. Tympanic temperatures are not accurate with infants.

CLASSIFICATION
Competency:
Health and Wellness
Taxonomy:
Application

70. 1. Fluids will help decrease the temperature, but this is not the most important intervention.

> 2. **A temperature of 38.9°C in an infant is abnormal and indicates an infection, which could proceed rapidly to a life-threatening stage. The safest option is to seek medical attention.**

3. A temperature of 38.9°C is a concern, and the parent should not wait days for a physician's advice. The nurse has not given the parent any direction about what to do if the temperature increases.
4. Tempra will decrease the temperature, but it is more important to identify and treat the cause of the high temperature.

CLASSIFICATION
Competency:
Changes in Health
Taxonomy:
Critical Thinking

71. 1. **This statement is true. Nurses must not share or reveal their password.**

2. Clients are allowed to view their health records as per agency policy, just as would occur with paper and pencil documentation.
3. If the person accessing the health record is a member of the circle of care, permission from the client is not required.
4. There is no research to prove this statement.

CLASSIFICATION
Competency:
Professional Practice
Taxonomy:
Application

CASE 15

72. 1. Canada's health care system provides access to health care for all.
2. This statement is true but is not the most important factor.

> 3. **These clients may have to choose between food, rent, and transportation since they may not have enough money for all.**

4. There is no reason to assume these clients would not be compliant unless the treatment involved additional financial hardships.

CLASSIFICATION
Competency:
Health and Wellness
Taxonomy:
Critical Thinking

73. 1. A wood-frame house is not necessarily of concern.

> 2. **Throw rugs are hazardous, particularly on bare floors. Seniors are most at risk for falls.**

CLASSIFICATION
Competency:
Health and Wellness
Taxonomy:
Critical Thinking

3. Microwave ovens are generally safer for older adults to use than gas or electric stoves.

4. Electric baseboard heaters do not generally get hot enough to burn the skin, and this would not be the most common risk.

---

74.   **1. Fibre provides the stool with bulk and moves it through the intestine. Bran and fruits are good sources of fibre.**

2. Cellulose does help constipation, but corn on the cob may be difficult for an older adult to eat. Rice is not a good source of cellulose.

3. Bananas and milk are not natural laxatives.

4. Echinacea and feverfew are herbal remedies not indicated for constipation.

CLASSIFICATION

Competency:
Health and Wellness

Taxonomy:
Application

---

75.   **1. Staying indoors protects Mr. Scanlon from inhaling pollutants and is the safest, easiest option.**

2. If ordinary activities include outdoor activities, the client will be at risk of inhaling airborne pollutants.

3. There is no need at this time for Mr. Scanlon to consult with a respiratory therapist.

4. This suggestion is a medical decision and may not necessarily be appropriate.

CLASSIFICATION

Competency:
Health and Wellness

Taxonomy:
Application

CASE 16

76.   1. The nurse may not know what such treatment would involve. As well, the client has not stated that she wishes to be treated according to religious practices.

2. This method is client-centred care.

3. The client is the person who provides information about her own care. The family is consulted only if Ms. Merkel is not able to communicate her wishes.

4. Clients are to be cared for as individuals.

CLASSIFICATION

Competency:
Nurse–Client Partnership

Taxonomy:
Application

---

77.   **1. This action provides client-centred, culturally appropriate care.**

2. Ms. Merkel has already stated her reasons.

3. This situation is not about the nurse's rights but the client's rights.

4. This response is not culturally sensitive, client-centred care. The nurse, as a client advocate, must speak with the charge nurse about reassignment.

CLASSIFICATION

Competency:
Nurse–Client Partnership

Taxonomy:
Application

---

78.   1. The nurse must first determine with the family which cultural practices should be followed. Viewing the body may not be desired or culturally appropriate.

CLASSIFICATION

Competency:
Nurse–Client Partnership

2. Organ donation would likely have been discussed prior to Ms. Merkel's death. As she has already died, her organs will not be able to be harvested.

Taxonomy:
Critical Thinking

3. This answer is the most inclusive one.

4. There is no indication that this course of action is necessary. If it is, it would be included in information received about specific death rites in answer 3.

CASE 17

79. 1. This terminology is unclear; it does not indicate the specific stage of labour.
2. This stage lasts from the delivery of the fetus to the delivery of the placenta; the mother does not experience any physiological symptoms.
3. This stage lasts from full dilation to expulsion; a heavy bloody show and pushing are evident at this time.

CLASSIFICATION
Competency:
Health and Wellness
Taxonomy:
Knowledge/Comprehension

4. The physiological intensification of labour occurring during transition is caused by a greater energy expenditure and increased pressure on the stomach; these result in feelings of fatigue, discouragement, and nausea.

80. **1. The nurse must determine if there is a distended bladder. This physical assessment is a form of data collection and is the first step in planning care. In agencies where it is available, the nurse may also assess for urinary retention with a bladder scanner.**

CLASSIFICATION
Competency:
Changes in Health
Taxonomy:
Critical Thinking

2. This action may be a nursing intervention but is not the initial action.
3. Same as answer 2.
4. Bladder distension is fairly common after delivery. It is too soon for medical intervention; other nursing measures should be tried first.

81. 1. Vaginal deliveries should not lead to respiratory problems.
2. Bladder tone is improved by regular emptying and filling of the bladder.
3. Abdominal muscle tone is not important this soon after delivery.

CLASSIFICATION
Competency:
Changes in Health
Taxonomy:
Critical Thinking

4. There is extensive activation of the blood-clotting factor after delivery. This, together with immobility, trauma, or sepsis, encourages thromboembolization, which can be limited through activity.

82. 1. Slow uterine involution would be manifested by sub-optimum uterine descent into the pelvis.

CLASSIFICATION
Competency:
Changes in Health
Taxonomy:
Application

2. A distended bladder will easily displace the fundus upward and laterally.

3. If placental fragments were retained, in addition to being displaced, the uterus would be soft and boggy, and vaginal bleeding would be heavy.
4. From this assessment, the nurse cannot make a judgement about overstretched uterine ligaments.

CASE 18

83. **1. The patch should be removed for 10 to 12 hours each day to prevent a tolerance buildup to the medication.**

2. There are numerous adverse effects that the client may experience.
3. Patches should never be cut.
4. Neither of these options is a safe disposal method for medications. The best option is disposal in a biohazard container if available.

CLASSIFICATION
Competency:
Changes in Health
Taxonomy:
Application

84. 1. Cholesterol is produced by the body, synthesized primarily in the liver.
2. Only animal foods furnish dietary cholesterol.
3. Cholesterol is an integral part of almost every cell in the body.

4. Cholesterol is a sterol found in tissue and circulating in the blood. It can increase, in part, with diets high in saturated fats.

CLASSIFICATION
Competency:
Changes in Health
Taxonomy:
Application

85. 1. Most fish have a low fat content.
2. Canola oil contains unsaturated fat.

3. Whole milk is high in saturated fat.

4. Omega 3 is "heart healthy," and trans-fat-free margarine is low in saturated fat.

CLASSIFICATION
Competency:
Changes in Health
Taxonomy:
Knowledge/Comprehension

CASE 19

86. 1. This response dismisses Mr. Bangay's feelings.
2. This response is a closed question that may obtain either "yes" or "no" as an answer.
3. Same as answer 1.

4. This response is an open-ended question that will allow Mr. Bangay to discuss his feelings.

CLASSIFICATION
Competency:
Nurse–Client Partnership
Taxonomy:
Application

87. 1. This response is not appropriate. Mr. Bangay is grieving the absence of his wife, not looking for other female company.
2. This response presents a potential option for Mr. Bangay but does not respond to his statement.

CLASSIFICATION
Competency:
Nurse–Client Partnership
Taxonomy:
Application

Answers Exam 1

3. **This response reaffirms Mr. Bangay's grief and allows him to speak about his wife and his feelings.**

4. This response dismisses Mr. Bangay's feelings.

88.   1. This action follows the rules but does not employ nursing judgement.

2. **Mr. Bangay's temperature is above normal, especially considering he is an older adult. It is appropriate nursing judgement to monitor his temperature more frequently.**

3. The taking of vital signs does not require a physician order. It is within the scope of nursing practice.

4. This action is not necessary, and in an adult, the axillary route is not as reliable as an oral temperature.

CLASSIFICATION
Competency:
Professional Practice
Taxonomy:
Critical Thinking

89.   1. This action is not a specific resolution.
2. Collaborating rather than mandating action is likely to be more effective.
3. This action may have to occur if the issue cannot be solved.

4. **Collaboration is the most effective method of addressing conflict.**

CLASSIFICATION
Competency:
Professional Practice
Taxonomy:
Critical Thinking

CASE 20

90.   1. This documentation does not describe Olivia's behaviour.

2. **Descriptions should be simple, objective, and easily interpreted. This documentation accurately describes Olivia's behaviour.**

3. "Well" is not an accurate description of behaviour.
4. This documentation is about the headaches, not Olivia's behaviour.

CLASSIFICATION
Competency:
Professional Practice
Taxonomy:
Application

91.   1. This response describes electroencephalography.
2. This response describes echoencephalography.
3. This response is similar to a description of a positron emission tomography scan, but dye is not injected into the brain for either test.

4. **This response is the definition of a computed tomography (CT) scan.**

CLASSIFICATION
Competency:
Changes in Health
Taxonomy:
Knowledge/Comprehension

92.   1. This response may not be true.
2. This response does not answer Olivia's question.

3. **After surgery, headaches may be aggravated rather than improved. It is better to be honest and not create false hope.**

4. Same as answer 2.

CLASSIFICATION
Competency:
Nurse–Client Partnership
Taxonomy:
Application

93.   1. **The nurse should consult with the surgeon for the correct positioning since there must not be pressure on the operative site.**

2. This position is common after neurosurgery but is dependent on the operative site.
3. Trendelenburg's position may be contraindicated as with some types of surgery it may lead to increased intracranial pressure.
4. This position is incorrect as it may increase pressure on the operative site.

CLASSIFICATION
Competency:
Changes in Health
Taxonomy:
Critical Thinking

94.   1. If the drainage were sanguinous, this action would be appropriate.

2. **Colourless drainage is a sign of cerebrospinal fluid leaking from the incision site and requires physician consultation.**

3. The drainage needs to be documented, but this is not the initial action.
4. Dressings should be reinforced, not changed.

CLASSIFICATION
Competency:
Changes in Health
Taxonomy:
Critical Thinking

95.   1. **Nurses have the authority to pronounce death.**

2. There is a legal requirement for physicians to certify death. Certifying death means determining the cause of death.
3. The physician does not need to be called to pronounce death.
4. The body should not be removed to the morgue until death has been pronounced and certified.

CLASSIFICATION
Competency:
Professional Practice
Taxonomy:
Knowledge/Comprehension

CASE 21

96.   1. Assistance with bathing may be important for the client but may take time and is not the priority action.

2. **This action can be accomplished fairly quickly. To delay the count prevents the day nurse from leaving the unit.**

3. Assisting the physician to reinsert the gastrostomy tube (G-tube) may take considerable time. It is not professional to ask the day nurse to wait until this is done. Reinsertion of a G-tube is not an emergency.
4. This client must be assessed, but there is no indication that it is urgent. Assessment will require more time than the narcotics count.

CLASSIFICATION
Competency:
Professional Practice
Taxonomy:
Critical Thinking

97.   1. This response is not logical. The unit staff has called in the family because Ms. David is about to die.
2. This response deflects the question. There is no need to refer this question to a physician as the nurse has the knowledge to reply.
3. The family has not expressed a need for the chaplain. This response does not answer the question.

CLASSIFICATION
Competency:
Nurse–Client Partnership
Taxonomy:
Critical Thinking

4. **This response provides a truthful answer to the son's question.**

98. 1. Elevation of the extremities should be avoided because it increases venous return, placing an increased workload on the heart.
     2. Excessive coughing and mucus production is characteristic of pulmonary edema and does not need to be encouraged.

     3. The orthopneic position allows maximum lung expansion because gravity reduces the pressure of the abdominal viscera on the diaphragm and lungs.

     4. Positioning for postural drainage does not relieve acute dyspnea; furthermore, it increases venous return to the heart.

CLASSIFICATION

Competency:

Changes in Health

Taxonomy:

Application

CASE 22

99. 1. This action is an appropriate method of assessment but is not as accurate as measuring.
     2. Although assessing fluid balance by weighing a client is important, it does not determine the degree of edema in a specific extremity.

     3. Mr. Camponi's edema is likely to be most prevalent in his ankles. Measuring an area provides an objective assessment and is not subject to individual interpretation.

     4. Although monitoring intake and output helps in assessing fluid balance, it does not determine the degree of edema in a specific extremity.

CLASSIFICATION

Competency:

Changes in Health

Taxonomy:

Critical Thinking

100. 1. This action is taken cautiously and should be the decision of a physician.

      2. Elevation of an extremity promotes venous and lymphatic drainage by gravity.

      3. This action needs to be ordered by a physician.
      4. This action will have little effect on edema.

CLASSIFICATION

Competency:

Changes in Health

Taxonomy:

Critical Thinking

INDEPENDENT QUESTIONS ANSWERS AND RATIONALES

101. 1. **Writing about clients would be contrary to ethical and legal principles. Even if the clients were not identified by name, other identifying characteristics and knowledge of where the nurse works may breach confidentiality.**

2. There is no reason a nurse may not participate in social networking sites as long as the nurse does not breach the confidentiality of clients.
3. Social networking sites are not professionally based and therefore may not be optimum for professional development.
4. The nurse must obtain consent for each and every posting for each and every client, which may be difficult. There is a great risk for breach of confidentiality because of the casual and unstructured nature of social networking sites.

CLASSIFICATION
Competency:
Professional Practice
Taxonomy:
Application

102. 1. A family should not push the patient-controlled analgesia (PCA) device for a child unless directed to do so by the physician. Christopher is old enough to control the PCA himself.
2. The PCA provides consistent levels of medication.
3. The nurse does not need to be notified every time Christopher wants to push the button to relieve pain.

4. **Feelings of control, particularly in adolescents, are one of the documented advantages of PCAs.**

CLASSIFICATION
Competency:
Changes in Health
Taxonomy:
Application

103. 1. Legality is not the professional issue. If she is not able to communicate effectively in English, she is unable to provide safe client care.

2. **Professional responsibility includes having the ability to effectively communicate with clients. Until Ms. Levis is able to communicate effectively in English, care of English clients would be compromised.**

3. This action may be a requirement from an agency but is not a requirement for registration. The professional and ethical issue is whether she is able to communicate effectively enough to provide safe client care, not whether she has passed a course.
4. This action is not professional, safe, or practical.

CLASSIFICATION
Competency:
Professional Practice
Taxonomy:
Critical Thinking

104. 1. Clients with advanced dementia would not be capable of using this pain scale.
2. This method of delivering an analgesic is inappropriate for a client with dementia since she will likely not be able to understand how to use the PCA.
3. This action does not provide for individualized care.

CLASSIFICATION
Competency:
Changes in Health
Taxonomy:
Application

4. **Nonverbal client behaviour such as restlessness, facial grimaces, and crying may provide clues as to the effectiveness of the analgesic.**

---

105. 1. This position would not help to prevent potential cerebral edema or increased intracranial pressure.
      2. It is important to keep the head in the midline position and to prevent flexion of the neck.

      3. **This position would facilitate drainage from the head region and thus help to prevent an increase in intracranial pressure.**

      4. Lowering the head of the bed may increase intracranial pressure.

CLASSIFICATION
Competency:
Changes in Health
Taxonomy:
Knowledge/Comprehension

---

106. 1. **Ms. William has the right to make decisions regarding her disease and her life. The nurses may not agree with those decisions but must, without judgement, support the client's right to make her own informed decisions.**

      2. There is no evidence that Ms. William is not mentally competent.
      3. The choice of lifestyle is Ms. William's. A mediator is not indicated since there is no compromise to be achieved between Ms. William and the staff.
      4. This action is abandonment of the client.

CLASSIFICATION
Competency:
Professional Practice
Taxonomy:
Application

---

107. 1. This action will help to keep the secretions thin but is an ongoing action and not the most important.

      2. **Hyper-oxygenation will ensure that his oxygen level does not drop during suctioning. This action is the most important.**

      3. Oral care needs to be provided, but it is not essential before suctioning.
      4. Ties are not affected by suctioning.

CLASSIFICATION
Competency:
Changes in Health
Taxonomy:
Critical Thinking

---

108. 1. **An RN is ethically not allowed to refuse to care for certain clients; however, she can ask if she can have her assignment modified.**

      2. This action is not ethical practice and could be considered abandonment of clients.
      3. This action is not ethical and likely is not practical since she was needed on the gynecology unit.
      4. This action is not ethical or professional.

CLASSIFICATION
Competency:
Professional Practice
Taxonomy:
Application

---

109. 1. **This is a normal oxygen saturation level for a newborn infant; therefore, no action is required. If there were evidence of respiratory distress, the nurse should monitor the levels.**

      2. This action is not necessary.

CLASSIFICATION
Competency:
Changes in Health
Taxonomy:
Critical Thinking

3. This action is not necessary or desirable.

4. This action will do nothing to affect blood levels of oxygen.

---

110. 1. **The scope of practice of a pharmacist includes comprehensive knowledge of medications and health teaching about medications to clients.**

2. This action may be appropriate; however, the pharmacist likely has more in-depth knowledge of the medications and may also be more available to the client.

3. While nurses have knowledge of drugs, the pharmacist is the more appropriate resource since a pharmacist's knowledge is more comprehensive.

4. This action is not the best method to educate the client unless there are no other resources available.

CLASSIFICATION
Competency:
Professional Practice
Taxonomy:
Critical Thinking

---

111. 1. This action is based on an assumption. The nurse does not know that continuing the lesson will improve understanding.

2. **This approach follows principles of teaching and learning. The nurse will be better able to teach the group what they need to know if she determines their learning needs.**

3. The nurse does not know what it is the group does not understand about the presentation of breathing techniques. Changing the topic does not address the issue and may cause the group to perceive that breathing techniques are not important.

4. This approach will not increase the understanding of the information. The nurse must determine the perceived learning needs of the group.

CLASSIFICATION
Competency:
Professional Practice
Taxonomy:
Application

---

112. 1. This action is a form of restraint. Canadian health care follows a philosophy of "least restraint." Clients must be individually and frequently assessed for the need for side rails.

2. The client might become more confused, a state that would be considered a chemical restraint.

3. **This would be the best choice for the client's safety. With the bed in the lowest position, it is likely a fall would not cause injury to the client. If the nurse checks on the client frequently, she may be able to assess for wakefulness and confusion.**

4. This action restricts the client's movement and is a restraint.

CLASSIFICATION
Competency:
Professional Practice
Taxonomy:
Application

---

113. 1. **Fluctuations in mood are common in the early stages of Parkinson's disease as the client deals with the emotional stress of the diagnosis.**

2. This manifestation will occur later in the disease process.

CLASSIFICATION
Competency:
Changes in Health

3. This manifestation occurs much later in the disease process.

4. There is no reason for an increase in appetite.

Taxonomy:
Knowledge/Comprehension

---

114.   **1. The primary health issue for the nurse and Mr. Mason is to assess the extent of the chemical dependence.**

2. This question addresses a legal issue and may break trust between Mr. Mason and the nurse.

3. Mr. Mason is likely to be aware of the legal and health issues related to his substance abuse. This question serves no purpose.

4. This question can be explored at a further date. The initial assessment is to determine the extent of the dependency.

CLASSIFICATION
Competency:
Nurse–Client Partnership
Taxonomy:
Critical Thinking

---

115.   1. Slowing the rate decreases the pressure but does not eliminate it.

2. Cramps are not a reason to discontinue the enema entirely; temporary clamping of the tubing usually relieves the cramps, and the procedure can be continued.

3. Administration of additional fluid when a client complains of abdominal cramps adds to discomfort because of additional pressure. By clamping the tubing for a few minutes, the nurse allows the cramps generally to subside. Then the enema can be continued.

4. This action will reduce the flow of the solution, in turn decreasing pressure, but may not reduce the cramping.

CLASSIFICATION
Competency:
Changes in Health
Taxonomy:
Critical Thinking

---

116.   **1. The nurse needs to have further assessment information prior to action. More data are required. He must find out if this is a new finding or if Mr. Nascad has had any previous tremors.**

2. The physician may need to be notified, but this is not the first step.

3. This statement is true, and the finding should be documented, but the nurse needs more data before assuming the tremor is benign.

4. This statement is not necessarily true. The cause of the tremor needs to be investigated.

CLASSIFICATION
Competency:
Changes in Health
Taxonomy:
Critical Thinking

---

117.   1. This calculation is incorrect.

2. To answer this question correctly, you must know Nägele's rule, which is to subtract 3 months and add 7 days to the first day of the last menstrual period. The information about spotting is a distracter, but the stem clearly states that June 11 was the date of the last normal menstrual period. With this calculation, the correct response is March 18.

3. Same as answer 1.

4. Same as answer 1.

CLASSIFICATION
Competency:
Health and Wellness
Taxonomy:
Application

118. 1. A medical directive and protocol would not have changed the accountability of the nurse.
   2. The nurse's assessment was not thorough in regard to determining the last date of immunization.

   3. **The nurse's data collection was not adequate because no questions were specifically asked concerning when the most recent tetanus inoculation occurred. The nurse failed to support the life and well-being of a client.**

   4. It was essential to determine the date of the last tetanus immunization; for a "tetanus-prone" wound, such as a puncture from a rusty nail, some form of tetanus immunization is usually given.

CLASSIFICATION
Competency:
Professional Practice
Taxonomy:
Critical Thinking

119. 1. **The first action by the RN must be to stop the abuse. This is achieved by intervening in the situation.**

   2. This action will be done but is not the first action.
   3. This action is possible but is not the first action.
   4. Same as answer 2.

CLASSIFICATION
Competency:
Professional Practice
Taxonomy:
Critical Thinking

120. 1. This statement is not accurate.

   2. **Insulin assists the transport of glucose through the cell membrane.**

   3. Same as answer 1.
   4. Same as answer 1.

CLASSIFICATION
Competency:
Changes in Health
Taxonomy:
Knowledge/Comprehension

121. 1. This action is appropriate, but it is likely the teens already are aware of the health hazards of the snacks and make poor choices regardless.
   2. This action is possible; however, the school administration may be reluctant to take this major step, particularly as schools sometimes receive monies from the snack companies.
   3. It is a good idea to have a parent–teacher meeting, but there are many teens who may not be able to bring lunches, and bringing one may not prevent them from also purchasing snacks and drinks at school.

   4. **This action is likely to be the most successful option. If the high-sugar snacks and pop are not in the machines, the students will not be able to purchase them.**

CLASSIFICATION
Competency:
Health and Wellness
Taxonomy:
Critical Thinking

122. 1. The woman is hard of hearing so would not be able to hear what the nurse says.

   2. **Provided the information on the paper was destroyed at the end of the shift, although not ideal, this is the most logical mechanism to ensure confidentiality.**

CLASSIFICATION
Competency:
Professional Practice
Taxonomy:
Application

3. This action is not ethical practice.

4. It is not likely body language would be able to convey pertinent information about care.

---

123. 1. It is not compassionate care to state that the mother does not need to have her children stay with her. The nurse does not know that the client will be fine.

2. While the nurse has the authority to enforce the visiting hours, the family may view this action as only caring about rules, not the care of their mother.

3. Same answer as 2.

4. This solution provides the family with an option of all being with their mother at some point during the night and allows the nurse to minimize noise and disruptions for other clients.

CLASSIFICATION

Competency:

Professional Practice

Taxonomy:

Application

---

124. **1. A client who has contracted one sexually transmitted infection (STI) will frequently have other STIs. Some are asymptomatic. Depending on reported symptoms, testing would be advised for gonorrhea, chlamydia, HIV, and syphilis. If other STIs are diagnosed, they will require treatment.**

2. Counselling implies there is a problem with the client's sexual activities, and this is not known. Transmission of genital herpes and other STIs needs to be discussed, but this is not the priority.

3. This needs to be discussed, as well as the fact the herpes cannot be cured, but is not the priority.

4. Although not necessarily common, it is possible to transfer herpes from the genital area of a partner during oral sexual activity. It is unlikely an exam would be warranted: Ms. Morrissey would be well aware of having oral herpes (cold sores), which would appear on her lips, not in her mouth.

CLASSIFICATION

Competency:

Changes in Health

Taxonomy:

Critical Thinking

---

125. **1. To permit adequate visualization of the mucosa during the sigmoidoscopy, the bowel must be cleansed with a nonirritating enema before the exam.**

2. Stool will be eliminated from the colon by an enema before the exam. Collecting a stool specimen serves no purpose.

3. Because only the lower bowel is being visualized, it is unnecessary and debilitating to place these restrictions on the client; clear liquids and a laxative may be given the day before to limit fecal residue.

4. The client does not drink such a substance in preparation for a sigmoidoscopy.

CLASSIFICATION

Competency:

Changes in Health

Taxonomy:

Knowledge/Comprehension

---

126. 1. This action must be done but is not the priority action.

2. Same as answer 1.

CLASSIFICATION

Competency:

Health and Wellness

3. The priority must be to warn the public not to eat this food. A news bulletin is the quickest way to inform the public of the hazard to their health.

Taxonomy:
Critical Thinking

4. Same as answer 1.

---

127. 1. The placenta is permeable to certain substances, which may include nicotine.
2. There is no evidence that the fetus becomes addicted to nicotine.

3. Heavy cigarette smoking or continued exposure to a smoke-filled environment causes both maternal and fetal vasoconstriction, resulting in fetal growth retardation and increased fetal and infant mortality.

CLASSIFICATION
Competency:
Health and Wellness
Taxonomy:
Knowledge/Comprehension

4. The fetal circulation is separate from the maternal circulation; however, nicotine can cross the placental barrier.

---

128. 1. It is important to know a client's culture, but the country of origin does not necessarily apply to culture. It is more important to assess for any risk factors, such as the use of herbal therapies.

2. Herbal supplements and over-the-counter medicines may have adverse effects that interfere with clotting after surgery and may have interactions with other drugs.

CLASSIFICATION:
Competency:
Health and Wellness
Taxonomy:
Critical Thinking

3. It is important that a client be adequately nourished before surgery, but the client's general health status should reflect this. This question is poorly worded for obtaining complete information about nutrition.
4. Sleep is important for healing after surgery but is not the most important factor at this time.

---

129. 1. While this statement may be true, it will shut down any communication between the nurse and the client.
2. This statement is true, but the client needs information about all types of treatment. This response by the nurse neglects the client's health and chances of survival.
3. This statement is not true.

CLASSIFICATION
Competency:
Nurse–Client Partnership
Taxonomy:
Application

4. The client may be basing his decision on inadequate information. It is the nurse's responsibility to provide the client with the knowledge he needs to make an informed decision.

---

130. 1. This response provides a solution for Mr. Ciavello's complaint about flavourless food and is an appropriate referral to another health care provider.

CLASSIFICATION
Competency:
Professional Practice
Taxonomy:
Critical Thinking

Answers Exam 1

2. This response is inappropriate; Mr. Ciavello does not mention specific foods.

3. The nurse should first acknowledge Mr. Ciavello's feelings and then assess his level of knowledge before imparting such information.

4. This response suggests that adherence to the prescribed medical regimen is unnecessary.

---

131.   1. These symptoms do not indicate an electrolyte imbalance.

2. **Potassium, the major intracellular cation, functions with sodium and calcium to regulate neuromuscular activity and contraction of muscle fibres, particularly the heart muscle. In hypokalemia, these symptoms develop, and they may be life threatening.**

3. These symptoms would indicate hypocalcemia, which does not generally occur with colitis.

4. Nausea and vomiting might occur with a prolonged potassium deficit; however, this is not an early sign. Leg and abdominal cramps occur with potassium excess, not deficit.

CLASSIFICATION
Competency:
Changes in Health
Taxonomy:
Knowledge/Comprehension

---

132.   1. This result is a miscalculation.

2. Same as answer 1.

3. Same as answer 1.

4. **This calculation is correct and is outlined in the chart below.**

	Intake (mL)		Output (mL)
IV fluid	350	Urine	290
G-tube feedings	600	Urine	320
Water	150	Emesis	25
TOTAL	1100		635

CLASSIFICATION
Competency:
Professional Practice
Taxonomy:
Application

---

133.   1. Elevation does not change the position of the IV cannula; the infusion must be discontinued.

2. **When an IV infusion is infiltrated, it should be removed to prevent swelling, possible damage of the tissues, and pain.**

3. This action would add to the infiltration of fluid.

4. Soaks may be applied, if ordered, after the IV is removed.

CLASSIFICATION
Competency:
Changes in Health
Taxonomy:
Application

---

134.   1. **The sequence for cardiopulmonary resuscitation should be maintained regardless of the setting or diagnosis. The nurse will need assistance in providing emergency care to the client; therefore, calling for help is the priority action.**

2. This action should be taken after the call for help.

CLASSIFICATION
Competency:
Changes in Health
Taxonomy:
Critical Thinking

3. Oxygen should be administered if Mr. Stephanopoulos is assessed to be breathing.
4. The assessment of a pulse is determined after the assessment of the airway.

---

135. 1. The physical craving for nicotine may last for months.
2. Increased vitamin intake may be beneficial but will not reduce withdrawal symptoms.
3. This suggestion will be helpful but will not reduce his withdrawal symptoms.

4. This is practical advice that addresses Mr. Carter's concern.

CLASSIFICATION
Competency:
Health and Wellness
Taxonomy:
Application

---

136. 1. Generally, cardiac disease does not cause *abruptio placentae*.
2. Hyperthyroidism may cause endocrine disturbance in the infant but does not affect the blood supply to the uterus.
3. Cephalopelvic disproportion may affect the delivery of the fetus but does not affect the placenta.

4. Pregnancy-induced hypertension leads to vasospasms; this, in turn, causes the placenta to tear away from the uterine wall (*abruptio placentae*).

CLASSIFICATION
Competency:
Changes in Health
Taxonomy:
Knowledge/Comprehension

---

137. 1. Some jurisdictions may request annual official proof of compliance with quality assurance (QA) programs. However, ongoing and continuous quality assurance is essential to maintaining competency.

2. Most quality assurance programs are based on the principle of lifelong learning, daily reflection, and continuous improvement in competency. Self-assessment, a common component of QA programs, is never static nor formally scheduled.

CLASSIFICATION
Competency:
Professional Practice
Taxonomy:
Critical Thinking

3. While some employers do use a QA tool, its primary purpose is not employee evaluation.
4. While some jurisdictions require nurses to participate in QA programs to maintain registration, their primary purpose is not registration maintenance.

---

138. 1. This response is not necessarily true and negates Ms. Helena's feelings.
2. This response is not necessarily true and may alarm Ms. Helena unnecessarily.

3. This response is a truthful and factual answer to Ms. Helena's question.

CLASSIFICATION
Competency:
Nurse–Client Partnership
Taxonomy:
Application

4. This response implies that the nurse does not have the necessary knowledge to discuss the biopsy with Ms. Helena.

139. 1. This action may be a solution but is not the first action the nurse should take.

2. **The nurse must first reflect on what is happening in her life and how it can be changed so she does not succumb to burnout. Implementing strategies without a complete understanding of what needs to be changed is not likely to be effective.**

CLASSIFICATION

Competency:

Health and Wellness

Taxonomy:

Critical Thinking

3. The nurse must first assess the stressors in her life. She may not be able to afford to work part time.

4. This action is likely to happen, but the nurse must first assess her eating and sleeping habits to determine what changes need to be made.

140. 1. Caloric intake is increased to meet the demands of the growing fetus.

2. **As pregnancy progresses, there are usually alterations in glucose tolerance and in the metabolism and use of insulin. The result is an increased need for exogenous insulin.**

CLASSIFICATION

Competency:

Changes in Health

Taxonomy:

Knowledge/Comprehension

3. Pancreatic enzymes or hormones other than insulin are not taken by diabetics.

4. Same as answer 2.

141. 1. This statement is untrue; often the maternal instinct is nurtured by the sight of the infant.

2. **Almost all mothers, including multiparas, report some ambivalence and anxiety about their ability to be good mothers.**

CLASSIFICATION

Competency:

Health and Wellness

Taxonomy:

Knowledge/Comprehension

3. This statement is untrue; it may take a much longer time.

4. This statement is untrue; ambivalent feelings are universal in response to mothering.

142. 1. This statement is untrue; excessive discipline leads to feelings of shame and self-doubt, the major crisis at this stage of development.

2. **The psychosocial need during the early toddler age is the development of autonomy. The toddler objects strongly to discipline.**

CLASSIFICATION

Competency:

Health and Wellness

Taxonomy:

Application

3. The sense of initiative is attained during the preschool age, not the toddler age.

4. It is frightening for a child to be left alone; it leaves the child with feelings of rejection, isolation, and insecurity.

143. 1. This action is important, but maintenance of respiration has priority.

CLASSIFICATION

Competency:

Changes in Health

2. **Laryngeal spasms can occur abruptly; patency of the airway is determined by a constant assessment for symptoms of respiratory distress.**

Taxonomy:
Critical Thinking

3. Same as answer 1.
4. Same as answer 1.

---

144. 1. This action does not ensure movement but social interaction.
2. Although this statement may be true, it may not be motivating and may make the boy feel less masculine.
3. Limit setting meets the security needs of young children. Adolescents do not respond well to strict rules.

4. **Decision making fosters and supports independence, a developmental need of the adolescent. It also increases a sense of self-worth and control.**

CLASSIFICATION
Competency:
Health and Wellness
Taxonomy:
Application

---

145. 1. Although this criterion is considered, the selection of drugs is based primarily on the ability of the drug to destroy the specific organism.
2. This criterion may be a factor if Ms. Sloane does not have a medical insurance plan, but it is not the most important factor.

3. **When the causative organism is isolated, it is tested for susceptibility (sensitivity) to various antimicrobial agents. When an organism is sensitive to a medication, the medication is capable of destroying the organism.**

CLASSIFICATION
Competency:
Professional Practice
Taxonomy:
Critical Thinking

4. Although the ordering practitioner's preference is considered, the selection of drugs is based primarily on the ability of the drug to destroy the specific organism.

---

146. 1. It is too soon to observe for signs of infection.

2. **The surgical site is an extremely vascular area, and the infant must be closely observed for bleeding.**

CLASSIFICATION
Competency:
Changes in Health
Taxonomy:
Critical Thinking

3. The infant is likely to cry during the procedure, but with an analgesic and comforting, the pain should be managed. A shrill, piercing cry is indicative of central nervous system difficulty.
4. Urinary output is assessed but is not the most essential nursing action in the initial postoperative period.

---

147. 1. **These services are the ones covered under provincial health care plans and are transferable between provinces under the *Canada Health Act*.**

CLASSIFICATION
Competency:
Health and Wellness
Taxonomy:
Knowledge/Comprehension

2. Medications administered while in hospital are covered.
3. Specialists and intensive care services are covered under provincial plans.

4. Not all health services or health care providers are covered under provincial plans.

---

148. 1. This intervention is a tertiary intervention.
2. This intervention is a secondary intervention.
3. Same as answer 1.

4. **Immunization programs prevent the occurrence of disease and are considered primary interventions.**

CLASSIFICATION
Competency:
Health and Wellness
Taxonomy:
Application

---

149. 1. This alternative does not have a legal basis.
2. Some agencies may require a treatment-refusal form, but law does not require this. The physician will need to be notified but not until the nurse has discussed the risks and benefits with Mr. Alves.

3. **Since Mrs. Alves is unconscious, her husband is the substitute decision maker (SDM). The substitute decision maker must act as he assumes his wife would wish. The nurse's responsibility in this consent situation is to ensure that he is aware of the risks and benefits of the refusal of treatment.**

4. This action is not legal or professional.

CLASSIFICATION
Competency:
Professional Practice
Taxonomy:
Critical Thinking

---

150. 1. A client would have rapid, shallow respirations to compensate for poor gas exchange.
2. Atelectasis may cause a loose, productive cough.
3. Atelectasis may cause an elevated temperature.

4. **Because atelectasis involves the collapsing of the alveoli distal to the bronchioles, breath sounds would be diminished in the lower lobes.**

CLASSIFICATION
Competency:
Changes in Health
Taxonomy:
Knowledge/Comprehension

---

151. 1. This condition is caused by hypocalcemia. It is manifested by exaggerated muscular twitching.
2. This condition is an obvious defect of the spinal column; it is easily recognized.
3. Elevated potassium causes cardiac irregularities.

4. **Intracranial bleeding may occur in the subdural, subarachnoid, or intraventricular spaces of the brain, causing pressure on vital centres; clinical signs are related to the area and degree of cerebral involvement.**

CLASSIFICATION
Competency:
Changes in Health
Taxonomy:
Knowledge/Comprehension

---

152. 1. The state of nourishment would be applicable to all cells.
2. This effect is not caused by direct irritation; most agents are administered parenterally.

CLASSIFICATION
Competency:
Changes in Health
Taxonomy:
Knowledge/Comprehension

3. Many chemotherapeutic agents function by interfering with the replication of deoxyribonucleic acid (DNA) associated with normal cellular reproduction (mitosis). The normal rapid mitosis of the stratified squamous epithelium of the mouth and anus results in their being powerfully affected by the drugs.

4. Chemotherapeutic agents do not alter the pH of gastric secretions.

---

153. 1. This problem is unlikely to be life threatening.

2. Vomiting may result in aspiration of the vomitus because it cannot be expelled. This could cause pneumonia or asphyxia.

3. Same as answer 1.
4. Bronchospasm is not a common risk with wiring of the jaw.

CLASSIFICATION
Competency:
Changes in Health
Taxonomy:
Critical Thinking

---

154. 1. Dysentery is not a tick-borne disease.
2. Malaria, not dysentery, is transmitted by mosquitoes.

3. *Entamoeba histolytica*, the organism that causes amoebic dysentery, is transmitted through excreta.

4. This organism is not transmitted via milk.

CLASSIFICATION
Competency:
Health and Wellness
Taxonomy:
Application

---

155. 1. This approach may be perceived to be punitive and aggressive.
2. This approach is not supportive and implies that Wai is rude.
3. This approach may be inferred to be culturally insensitive and too forward.

4. Communicating directly may appear to be aggressive and insensitive to the foreign-trained nurse. This approach is supportive and culturally respectful.

CLASSIFICATION
Competency:
Nurse–Client Partnership
Taxonomy:
Application

---

156. 1. This action is not necessary unless there is evidence that the mother is abusive or neglectful or if Lawrence's asthma is severe enough that his life is in danger if he is discharged.
2. This statement is not true.
3. The mother is his legal guardian; thus, agency policies would not prevent her from taking him home.

4. The mother is Lawrence's legal guardian and may discharge him. The important action is to ensure that she understands how to care for his asthma so that she can manage it at home. The nurse should ensure that the event is documented according to agency policies.

CLASSIFICATION
Competency:
Professional Practice
Taxonomy:
Critical Thinking

---

157. 1. This action is important but not the priority.
2. Same as answer 1.

CLASSIFICATION
Competency:
Changes in Health

3. All options could be correct, but respiratory assessment is the most crucial at this time.

Taxonomy:

Critical Thinking

4. Same as answer 1.

---

158. 1. Motor vehicle accidents are the most common cause of death among adolescents.

CLASSIFICATION

Competency:

Health and Wellness

Taxonomy:

Knowledge/Comprehension

2. Suicide is the second most prevalent cause of death.
3. Cancers are not the most common cause of death.
4. Sports injuries do occur but are not the most common cause of death.

---

159. 1. Sexual inhibitions are individual and not related to sexual orientation.
2. While companionship is important, it should not be assumed that it is any more important than sexual activity.
3. Sexual interest and activity do not cease in the older adult.

CLASSIFICATION

Competency:

Health and Wellness

Taxonomy:

Application

4. Sexual responses do not cease in the older adult. Older adults have an interest in sexual activities when a suitable partner and privacy are available.

---

160. 1. Student nurses are responsible and accountable for their own actions. A third-year student is fully prepared to take and interpret blood pressure readings.

CLASSIFICATION

Competency:

Professional Practice

Taxonomy:

Critical Thinking

2. The nurse should reasonably expect a third-year student to take and interpret a blood pressure reading.
3. The teacher is responsible only if she has given a client assignment that is beyond the expected knowledge and skills of the student. Blood pressure reading is not beyond the skill of a third-year student.
4. Same as answer 3.

---

161. 1. This teaching should come later in pregnancy but not before ascertaining the client's feelings about breastfeeding.
2. This teaching can be done in the latter part of pregnancy and reinforced during the postpartum period.
3. This teaching will have to be done, but it is not the priority intervention.

CLASSIFICATION

Competency:

Health and Wellness

Taxonomy:

Critical Thinking

4. It is not uncommon for adolescents to avoid prenatal care; many do not recognize the deleterious effect that a lack of prenatal care can have on them and their babies.

---

162. 1. Paresis is a weakness or partial paralysis.

CLASSIFICATION

Competency:

Changes in Health

Taxonomy:

Knowledge/Comprehension

2. Hemiplegia is paralysis of one side of the body.

3. Paraplegia is the paralysis of both lower extremities and the lower trunk.
4. This statement describes quadriplegia.

163.
1. This complication would not result from long-term edema.
2. Same as answer 1.

3. **Oxygen perfusion is impaired during prolonged edema, leading to tissue ischemia.**

4. Same as answer 1.

CLASSIFICATION
Competency:
Changes in Health
Taxonomy:
Knowledge/Comprehension

164.
1. **The connective tissue degeneration of SLE leads to the involvement of the basal cell layer, producing a butterfly rash over the bridge of the nose and in the malar region.**

2. This manifestation occurs in scleroderma.
3. This manifestation occurs in muscular dystrophy, which is characterized by muscle wasting and weakness.
4. This manifestation occurs in polyarteritis nodosa, a collagen disease affecting the arteries and nervous system.

CLASSIFICATION
Competency:
Changes in Health
Taxonomy:
Knowledge/Comprehension

165.
1. **Radiation in controlled doses is therapeutic. When uncontrolled or in excessive amounts, it is carcinogenic.**

2. Therapeutic and controlled doses are used regardless.
3. Physical status does not affect the outcome of radiation therapy.
4. The nutritional status of the cells does not influence radiation's effect.

CLASSIFICATION
Competency:
Changes in Health
Taxonomy:
Knowledge/Comprehension

166.
1. Sperm do not move through the urine; they are found in semen.
2. Sperm are motile and achieve motility by motion of their flagella; they move from the epididymis to the vas deferens to the ejaculatory ducts to the urethra.

3. **Sperm cells are very fragile and can be destroyed by heat, resulting in sterility.**

4. During this period, the testes are not suspended.

CLASSIFICATION
Competency:
Health and Wellness
Taxonomy:
Application

167.
1. Although it is considered a permanent form of sterilization, there has been some success reversing the procedure.
2. The procedure does not affect sexual functioning.
3. Precautions must be taken to prevent fertilization until absence of sperm in the semen has been verified.

4. **Some spermatozoa will remain viable in the vas deferens for a variable time after vasectomy.**

CLASSIFICATION
Competency:
Health and Wellness
Taxonomy:
Application

168.   1. Although diversion is a method of altering pain perception and nausea, Ms. Angelo needs to see a physician for management of her dysmenorrhea.

   2. Ms. Angelo's symptoms may be serious and are compromising her lifestyle. She needs to consult a physician for treatment to correct the dysmenorrhea.

   3. Although ibuprofen may help with the pain, she initially needs to consult a physician.
   4. Voluntary relaxation of the abdominal muscles does not cause cessation of uterine pain.

CLASSIFICATION
Competency:
Changes in Health
Taxonomy:
Application

169.   1. This action is not required.
   2. Same as answer 1.

   3. A full bladder is necessary so that the pelvic organs can be clearly visualized.

   4. Same as answer 1.

CLASSIFICATION
Competency:
Changes in Health
Taxonomy:
Knowledge/Comprehension

170.   1. Situational indicates a flexibility depending on the situation.
   2. Laissez-faire is a relaxed and nondirective form of leadership.

   3. Autocratic indicates that the leader uses power and position to govern according to his or her own priorities.

   4. Positional is not a recognized form of leadership.

CLASSIFICATION
Competency:
Professional Practice
Taxonomy:
Knowledge/Comprehension

171.   1. The coronary blood flow is unconnected to the heart valves.
   2. This statement is a description of electrocardiography.

   3. The catheter examines the condition of the coronary arteries. This statement provides a simple explanation of what a coronary artery is.

   4. The strength of contractions is not measured in angiography.

CLASSIFICATION
Competency:
Changes in Health
Taxonomy:
Knowledge/Comprehension

172.   1. This position does not relieve the pressure of the oncoming head on the cord.
   2. This position may increase the pressure of the presenting part on the cord.
   3. The pressure of the presenting part on the cord is not relieved in this position.

   4. A position in which the mother's head is below the level of the hips helps to decrease the compression of the cord and therefore maintains the blood supply to the infant.

CLASSIFICATION
Competency:
Changes in Health
Taxonomy:
Application

173. 1. Mr. Brendan is involved in high-risk behaviour that causes danger to his health. Safety topics would include, for example, safe sex, use of clean needles, physical safety, and signs of sexually transmitted infections.

2. Mr. Brendan likely has poor nutrition, but this is not as important as safety.
3. Mr. Brendan likely has poor self-esteem, but this is not as important as safety.
4. Mr. Brendan likely is aware of the legal issues surrounding his work and heroin use.

CLASSIFICATION
Competency:
Health and Wellness
Taxonomy:
Critical Thinking

174. 1. Although some herbal preparations may not have standardized dosages, this is not the most important aspect to discuss with Ms. Hoang.
2. This statement is presently true, although the government may move to regulate herbal preparations; however, it is not the most important aspect to discuss with Ms. Hoang.

3. Some combinations of prescription drugs and herbal preparations interact. It is important that the health care provider be aware of all medications a client is taking, whether prescription or herbal. Ms. Hoang should be aware of the potential interactions.

4. This statement is not necessarily true.

CLASSIFICATION
Competency:
Health and Wellness
Taxonomy:
Critical Thinking

175. 1. Monilia, not herpes, causes thrush.

2. The infant may acquire the herpes infection from the vaginal birth, putting the infant at risk for systemic herpes, which has a very high mortality.

3. Chlamydia and gonorrhea, not herpes, are the most common causes of ophthalmia neonatorum.
4. Neurological complications may result from the infant's systemic herpes infection, but this is a late stage of the illness.

CLASSIFICATION
Competency:
Changes in Health
Taxonomy:
Knowledge/Comprehension

176. 1. Impaired reflex behaviour and a shrill cry indicate central nervous system damage.

2. Asymmetry of the gluteal dorsal surface of the thighs and inguinal folds indicates congenital dislocation of the hip; folds on the affected side appear higher than those on the unaffected side.

3. An inguinal hernia is evidenced by the protrusion of the intestine into the inguinal sac.
4. Peripheral nervous system damage would be manifested by limpness or flaccidity of the extremities.

CLASSIFICATION
Competency:
Changes in Health
Taxonomy:
Knowledge/Comprehension

177. 1. This statement shows little understanding or tolerance of the illness.
2. Ignoring the behaviour is a form of rejection; the client is not using the behaviour for attention.

CLASSIFICATION
Competency:
Changes in Health

3. Recognizing the language as part of the illness makes it easier to tolerate, but limits must be set for the benefit of the staff and other clients. Setting limits also shows the client that the nurse cares enough to stop the behaviour.

Taxonomy:
Application

4. This statement demonstrates a rejection of the client and little understanding of the illness.

---

178. 1. A child learns to trust others by having his needs met in infancy. A child who has been maternally deprived is unlikely to have developed trust.

2. Studies do not address this issue.
3. Some cognitive delay may be expected with prolonged hospitalization, but with appropriate care in hospital, cognitive milestones should ultimately be met.
4. These children frequently develop relationships with primary caregivers in place of the mother and father.

CLASSIFICATION
Competency:
Nurse–Client Partnership
Taxonomy:
Knowledge/Comprehension

---

179. 1. This symptom is not related to methadone hydrochloride reduction.

2. When methadone is reduced, a craving for narcotics may occur. Without narcotics, anxiety will increase, agitation will occur, and the client may try to leave the hospital to get drugs.

3. Same as answer 1.
4. This symptom may occur with a methadone hydrochloride overdose.

CLASSIFICATION
Competency:
Changes in Health
Taxonomy:
Application

---

180. 1. A person must learn to cope with unpleasant objects and events.
2. Exposure to fearful situations without a plan of coping mechanisms may increase anxiety.

3. Learning a variety of coping mechanisms helps reduce anxiety in stressful situations.

4. Fearful situations can never be viewed as pleasurable.

CLASSIFICATION
Competency:
Changes in Health
Taxonomy:
Application

---

181. 1. This calculation is incorrect.
2. Same as answer 1.

3. Correct calculation:
225 lb. − 180 lb. = 45 lb.
45 lb. ÷ 2.2 lb./kg = 20.45 kg, which rounds down to 20 kg

4. Same as answer 1.

CLASSIFICATION
Competency:
Professional Practice
Taxonomy:
Application

182.   1. An anomaly at birth would not likely produce the clinical signs listed and would be evident before the toddler years.
2. Acute respiratory infection usually has a gradual onset.
3. In view of the sudden onset of clinical signs and the age of the child, a hereditary condition is unlikely.

4. **All of the questions could be correct, but this question is the first the nurse should ask as it is the most likely. Respiratory tract obstructions generally occur in the larynx, trachea, or major bronchi (usually right). Hoarseness may indicate a vocal cord injury. Unintelligible speech may indicate interference in the flow of air out of the respiratory tract or obstruction or injury to the larynx. It is common for toddlers to choke on small objects.**

CLASSIFICATION
Competency:
Changes in Health
Taxonomy:
Critical Thinking

183.   1. It is too soon for output to be a priority; however, it certainly must be assessed later.

2. **A patent airway and adequate pulmonary ventilation are always priorities after surgery.**

3. This action is important, but adequate ventilation is the priority.
4. The IV lines would be checked once the airway, breathing, and circulation are determined to be functioning well.

CLASSIFICATION
Competency:
Changes in Health
Taxonomy:
Critical Thinking

184.   1. Vigorous scrubbing irritates the skin and increases the likelihood of an outbreak.
2. There may be no link between food and acne. Each individual should assess if any particular food causes an outbreak.
3. Sunscreen should be used, but oil-based sunscreens block the pores.

4. **Only mild soap and water are necessary; washing should be gentle in order not to irritate the skin tissues.**

CLASSIFICATION
Competency:
Changes in Health
Taxonomy:
Application

185.   1. Bending at the waist should be avoided because it strains the lower back muscles; the power for lifting should be supplied by the muscles of the thighs and buttocks.

2. **Placing the feet apart creates a wider base of support and brings the centre of gravity closer to the ground. This improves stability.**

3. Pressure on the abdomen is prevented by tightening the abdominal and gluteal muscles to form an internal girdle; keeping the body straight does not reduce strain on the abdominal musculature.
4. Relaxing the abdominal muscles with physical activity increases strain on the abdomen.

CLASSIFICATION
Competency:
Professional Practice
Taxonomy:
Application

186.   1. **A walker requires only partial weight bearing of the affected limb and gives the most overall support to the individual.**

    2. A cane requires full weight bearing of the affected limb.
    3. Crutches are used only when there should be no weight bearing.
    4. A wheelchair is not appropriate because it does not promote the regaining of strength in the affected limb.

CLASSIFICATION
Competency:
Changes in Health
Taxonomy:
Critical Thinking

---

187.   1. There are no data to support this. The amount of medication was probably inadequate for the client's pain tolerance level.
    2. The nurse should not ignore the client's need for pain relief.

    3. **The nurse made the assessment that the medication was ineffective in relieving Mr. Ferguson's pain for the duration ordered. This information should be communicated to the physician for evaluation.**

    4. The physician's order is for administration q3–4hr prn. It should be given only within these guidelines.

CLASSIFICATION
Competency:
Changes in Health
Taxonomy:
Application

---

188.   1. This calculation is incorrect.
    2. Same as answer 1.
    3. Same as answer 1.

    4. **Correct calculation:**
    200 mg/kg/d $\times$ 45 kg = 9000 mg/d
    9000 mg/d $\div$ 4 doses/d = 2250 mg = 2.25 g, which rounds up to 2.3 g

CLASSIFICATION
Competency:
Professional Practice
Taxonomy:
Application

---

189.   1. **In most cases, administration of pharmacological agents at regular intervals rather than as needed is preferable. Pain is easier to prevent than to treat. The round-the-clock approach alleviates pain before it becomes severe and can facilitate an earlier recovery.**

    2. Same as answer 1.
    3. Many clients are reluctant, for many reasons, to request pain medication and thus would not receive optimum pain management.
    4. While nurses should be expert at evaluating client pain, it is better to prevent pain from occurring rather than treating the pain.

CLASSIFICATION
Competency:
Changes in Health
Taxonomy:
Critical Thinking

---

190.   1. This statement refers to a personal choice and is not indicative of gender identity.
    2. How a person considers his or her own sexual orientation is not related to gender identity.

    3. **This statement offers the correct interpretation of gender identity. It is how a person identifies as being male, female, or a combination. It begins as soon as a person is aware of the difference in the sexes.**

    4. Same as answer 1.

CLASSIFICATION
Competency:
Health and Wellness
Taxonomy:
Critical Thinking

191. 1. **The nurse needs to perform an initial thorough assessment. Based on this assessment, the nurse will be able to arrange suitable physical aids or the services of a foot care specialist.**

2. An assessment needs to be performed prior to arranging nursing care.
3. The assessment is the initial action.
4. Although regular physician's appointments are important, they do not address Mr. Akland's immediate concern.

CLASSIFICATION
Competency:
Professional Practice
Taxonomy:
Critical Thinking

192. 1. A fact sheet is not the most appropriate teaching tool at this time. The nurse needs to know why he is not taking his drugs.
2. There is no reason to suppose his noncompliance is due to confusion about doses or times.
3. There is no reason to suppose lifestyle interferes with the regimen.

4. **The nurse must first find out from Mr. James if there is a specific reason for his noncompliance. Initially, with HIV medication regimens, the adverse effects are unpleasant. Supporting Mr. James until the adverse effects are reduced is very important and will help him be compliant.**

CLASSIFICATION
Competency:
Changes in Health
Taxonomy:
Critical Thinking

193. 1. **The social worker is the correct health care provider to advise and arrange for community services. It is part of social workers' scope of practice.**

2. The physician may be able to assist, but the social worker is the best choice.
3. This action takes time for the nurse if he is not well acquainted with the community services. It is more appropriately within the scope of the social worker's practice.
4. This action may help the family, but if they are feeling overwhelmed, then the best action is to provide the personal assistance of a social worker who can best facilitate support.

CLASSIFICATION
Competency:
Professional Practice
Taxonomy:
Critical Thinking

194. 1. **This procedure is correct for obtaining the culture.**

2. This method will obtain only mucus, not a culture of the pharynx.
3. The client is much more likely to gag in a supine position.
4. It would be difficult to insert the swab with the client's head forward.

CLASSIFICATION
Competency:
Health and Wellness
Taxonomy:
Application

195. 1. **The nurse must first gather all possible information (nursing process) about the new product prior to taking action.**

2. A physician does not necessarily have to be involved nor give permission for the ordering of an incontinence product.
3. This action is premature. The information must be compiled first and then discussed with the nurse manager.
4. The nurse may not independently conduct an action such as this without permission from hospital leaders.

CLASSIFICATION
Competency:
Professional Practice
Taxonomy:
Critical Thinking

196. 1. It may not be necessary for the nurse to accompany the client to the magnetic resonance imaging (MRI) scan, and doing so just to change an IV bag is not appropriate use of personnel.

2. Only if the nurse has previously consulted with the personnel in the MRI department and has been assured the bag can be changed would this action be appropriate.

3. It may not be appropriate to reduce the rate of the IV.

4. This action is the safest and most logical.

CLASSIFICATION
Competency:
Professional Practice
Taxonomy:
Critical Thinking

---

197. **1. Once a client has been identified as being incompetent to make decisions, the identified SDM becomes the decision maker based on what the client would have wished had he been capable of making an informed decision.**

2. There is no need for the next of kin to be contacted unless he or she is the SDM.

3. The physician is not responsible to make the care decisions unless it is an emergency.

4. Mr. Balasingham has been identified as incompetent, thus this action is not appropriate.

CLASSIFICATION
Competency:
Professional Practice
Taxonomy:
Application

---

198. **1. Ms. Lewis requires isolation as she likely has a communicable disease. The dialysis client must be moved to free up the room for isolation.**

2. Ms. Lewis requires isolation and should not share a room with another client.

3. This would be particularly hazardous as the cancer client may be immune suppressed, thus more likely to contract a communicable disease.

4. This action is not professional. Ms. Lewis has been admitted and requires care.

CLASSIFICATION
Competency:
Professional Practice
Taxonomy:
Application

---

199. 1. This approach is not professional. While the information may assist the mother with breastfeeding, it does not solve the problem of the preceptor advocating an outdated practice. In addition, the mother may be confused by receiving different advice from the twxo nurses.

2. This approach is the professional choice. Even though the preceptor is an experienced postpartum nurse, she may not be aware of best practice regarding breastfeeding and supplementing with bottles of formula. It is in the best interest of the preceptor and the mother for the student to question and discuss the issue.

CLASSIFICATION
Competency:
Professional Practice
Taxonomy:
Critical Thinking

3. This is adversarial and not professional.

4. The student nurse has a professional responsibility to question outdated or inaccurate practice, even if the nurse preceptor has more experience.

200. 1. This action must be done but is not the first action.
2. Same as answer 1.

3. **If the nurse is performing the action, he is responsible for ensuring that it has been ordered by the physician. In some jurisdictions, a nurse may initiate an intravenous infusion without a physician order, but only normal saline solution is permitted.**

CLASSIFICATION
Competency:
Professional Practice
Taxonomy:
Critical Thinking

4. Same as answer 1.

END OF ANSWERS AND RATIONALES TO PRACTICE EXAM 1

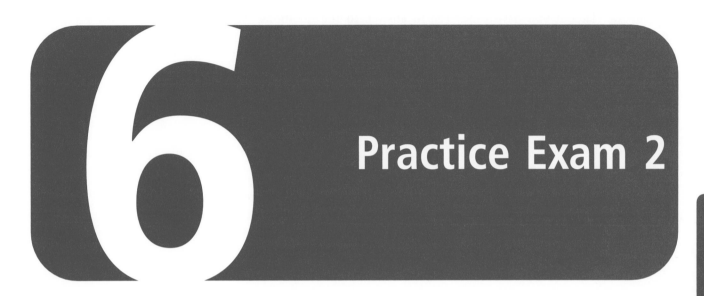

6

Practice Exam 2

INSTRUCTIONS FOR PRACTICE EXAM 2

You will have 4 hours to complete the exam. The questions are presented as nursing cases or as independent questions. Read each question carefully, and then choose the answer that you think is the best of the four options presented. If you cannot decide on an answer to a question, proceed to the next question and return to this question later if you have time. Try to answer all the questions. Marks are not subtracted for wrong answers. If you are unsure of an answer, it will be to your advantage to guess.

Circle each answer in the exam book, and then transfer your answer to the scoring sheet found on p. 266. Be sure that the pencil mark completely fills the oval, but do not press so heavily that you cannot erase it if you decide to change the answer. Ensure that you are marking the question number that corresponds to the question you are answering. Make sure you do not fill in more than one oval for a question. Erase completely any answer you wish to change, and mark your new choice in the corresponding oval.

Answers to Practice Exam 2 appear on p 134.

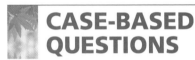

CASE-BASED QUESTIONS

CASE 1

A nurse is facilitating a cardiac rehabilitation group for ten men who have recently been discharged from the hospital post–myocardial infarction (MI). She will provide teaching and guidance about heart-healthy living.

QUESTIONS 1 to 5 refer to this case.

1. An important topic to be covered during the first class is the pathophysiology of a heart attack. What would be the most appropriate teaching technique to start the teaching session?

    1. Ask each group member what he or she knows about myocardial infarctions
    2. Conduct a brief overview, with visual aids, about what happens during a heart attack
    3. Distribute pamphlets that provide complete information about MIs
    4. Organize a role-playing activity for group members to demonstrate what happens during a heart attack

2. The nurse performs a health assessment on each of the men, many of whom are obese. Which of the following assessments is most indicative of a diagnosis of obesity?

    1. Waist-to-hip ratio
    2. Ratio of total body weight to height
    3. Weight over the 85th percentile on standard adult growth charts
    4. Hydrostatic weight

3. The nurse teaches a client about a heart-healthy diet. What recommendation should the nurse include in the teaching?

    1. "Eat at least two servings of fruit and vegetables a day."
    2. "Portion your dinner plate to ½ vegetables, ¼ starch, and ¼ protein."
    3. "Limit fat intake to 35% of your total calories."
    4. "Replace complex carbohydrates with simple carbohydrates."

4. Many of the group members have hypertension. The nurse provides nutrition counselling regarding reducing their dietary sodium. Which of the following recommendations would offer the most effective advice for controlling salt intake?

    1. "Use a salt substitute."
    2. "Read nutrition labels on all bought foods."
    3. "Avoid adding salt when cooking."
    4. "Purchase only foods advertised as having reduced sodium."

5. The nurse engages the men in active learning by having them evaluate various menus. Which of

the following should they choose as the best low-sodium, low-calorie meal?

1. Salmon steak with lemon, baked sweet potato, green salad with vinegar dressing
2. 250 g of pasta with tomato sauce, whole-wheat roll, salad with low-calorie dressing
3. Breaded fish on a multi-grain bun with tartar sauce and baked beans
4. Ham and cheese omelette, avocado salad, and chicken broth

END OF CASE 1

CASE 2

Mr. Poulos, age 80, has periorbital cellulitis of his left eye and requires intravenous (IV) antibiotics. A saline lock was inserted in the emergency department, and Discharge Services has arranged for him to have home nursing care twice a day to infuse the medication and monitor the cellulitis.

QUESTIONS 6 to 12 refer to this case.

6. The home care nurse visits Mr. Poulos. After introducing himself, which of the following actions should he next perform?

   1. Wash his hands
   2. Examine the saline lock
   3. Check the medications
   4. Assess the cellulitis

7. The pharmacy has prepared preloaded syringes of the antibiotics. Which of the following actions is the correct nursing responsibility for the administration of the preloaded syringes?

   1. The nurse must call the pharmacist to confirm the drug and dosage.
   2. The nurse is not permitted to administer syringes that another health care provider has prepared.
   3. The nurse must perform the rights of medication administration.
   4. The nurse must confirm the labelling on the syringe against the physician order.

8. Mr. Poulos's eye is swollen and irritated and has an exudate that causes crusting. He asks the nurse what he should do as a comfort measure. Which of the following measures would be the most effective?

   1. Apply a cold compress every 4 hours
   2. Apply a warm saline compress as necessary
   3. Wear sunglasses to protect his eye from light
   4. Keep the eye patched at all times

9. Mr. Poulos lives alone in his own home. The cellulitis has affected his vision, and he finds it difficult to see. What question should the nurse ask him?

   1. "Do you have family to help you?"
   2. "Would you like a visiting homemaker to help with your daily activities?"
   3. "Are you able to cook your meals and clean the house?"
   4. "How are you managing with making meals and household chores?"

10. One of the antibiotics administered to Mr. Poulos is vancomycin. The nurse is aware that vancomycin requires therapeutic serum levels, which have not been ordered by the physician. In this situation, what is the nurse's responsibility?

    1. Contact the physician to discuss an order for vancomycin levels
    2. Draw blood from Mr. Poulos for vancomycin levels
    3. Instruct Mr. Poulos to go to a community laboratory to have blood drawn for the levels
    4. Consult with the nursing team leader concerning the most appropriate action

11. On the nurse's subsequent visit, Mr. Poulos states that his arm feels itchy close to the insertion site of the saline lock. Which of the following actions would be the nurse's first priority?

    1. Stop the infusion
    2. Check a medication reference for adverse effects of the antibiotics

3. Check the labelling on the syringes to ensure the correct drug and correct dose
4. Assess the insertion site

12. Mr. Poulos has completed 7 days of antibiotics. The physician determines that he will not require a 10-day course. Six preloaded syringes remain. Which of the following statements would be the best advice from the nurse on how Mr. Poulos should dispose of them?

    1. "You should throw the syringes in the garbage."
    2. "You should empty the syringes into a sink."
    3. "You should return the syringes to the pharmacy."
    4. "I will take them and dispose of them for you."

END OF CASE 2

CASE 3

Several clients on a surgical floor begin to have frequent and uncontrollable watery stools. The hospital infection control specialist believes that this may be an outbreak of Clostridium difficile. *Ms. Patel, who is day 1 post–major surgery, is among the affected clients.*

QUESTIONS 13 to 15 refer to this case.

13. The nurse must collect a stool sample from Ms. Patel for *Clostridium* toxin assay. How should the nurse properly collect the specimen?

    1. Have Ms. Patel defecate into a specimen container
    2. Collect the stool from a clean bedpan or incontinence pad
    3. Obtain a stool sample after Ms. Patel has defecated in the toilet
    4. Apply an adult incontinence diaper to Ms. Patel

14. Ms. Patel is very weak and continues to have episodes of watery diarrhea occurring every 1 to 2 hours. Which of the following concerns is the most important for the nurse to assess for first?

    1. Fluid and electrolyte imbalance
    2. Potential for systemic infection

3. Perianal excoriation
4. Cardiovascular decompensation

15. Ms. Patel observes specific hygiene practices. In her culture, the left hand is used to perform unclean procedures. How would the nurse provide culturally competent care to Ms. Patel?

    1. Allow Ms. Patel to guide the nurse in hygiene practice
    2. Have Ms. Patel perform self-care hygiene after each bowel movement
    3. Use her right hand to hold the bedpan and the left to clean the perineal area
    4. Wash her hands before touching Ms. Patel

END OF CASE 3

CASE 4

Mr. and Mrs. Corrigan attend childbirth education classes at a birthing centre. Mrs. Corrigan is 30 weeks' gestation in her first pregnancy.

QUESTIONS 16 to 19 refer to this case.

16. Mrs. Corrigan says to the nurse, "I'm worried about gaining too much weight because I have heard that weight gained in pregnancy never comes off." Which of the following statements would be the nurse's best response?

    1. "A weight gain of approximately 7 to 8 kg is recommended."
    2. "If you have gained over 5 kg at this stage, you should probably start a low-calorie diet."
    3. "Don't worry about gaining weight. You need to be more concerned about the health of your baby."
    4. "An 11- to 15-kg weight gain is recommended to allow for proper growth of your baby. It should not cause you to be overweight afterward."

17. The nurse teaches Mrs. Corrigan and her husband about labour. At what point after Mrs. Corrigan's labour has started should the nurse tell them they should go to the birthing centre?

1. When the contractions are 10 to 15 minutes apart
2. When she has a bloody show and back pressure
3. When her membranes rupture or contractions are 5 to 8 minutes apart
4. When the contractions are 2 to 3 minutes apart and she cannot walk about

18. Mr. and Mrs. Corrigan ask the nurse what the difference is between true and false labour. Which of the following statements regarding true labour would be correct information for the nurse to give them?

   1. It accomplishes progressive cervical dilation.
   2. It occurs immediately after the membranes rupture.
   3. It will stop if she walks around.
   4. It becomes less uncomfortable if she lies on her side.

19. Mrs. Corrigan asks the nurse if her small breasts will affect her ability to breastfeed. What would be the nurse's best response?

   1. "Everybody can be successful at breastfeeding."
   2. "You seem to have some issues with breastfeeding."
   3. "The size of your breasts will not affect your milk production."
   4. "The amount of fat and glandular tissue in the breasts determines the amount of milk produced."

END OF CASE 4

CASE 5

A nurse who works at a community pediatric clinic is responsible for performing health assessments, teaching parents, and administering immunizations.

QUESTIONS 20 to 24 refer to this case.

20. A father asks why his 14-month-old daughter must receive a rubella vaccination. Which of the following responses by the nurse provides accurate information?

   1. "Because rubella is a severe disease in childhood."
   2. "To prevent pregnant women from contracting rubella."
   3. "Because it is the law in Canada."
   4. "To prevent your daughter from having serious side effects, such as encephalitis, which may occur with rubella."

21. One of the routine immunizations the nurse administers is the *Haemophilus influenzae* type B (Hib) vaccine. Why is the Hib vaccine given to infants?

   1. It reduces the incidence of meningitis.
   2. It eliminates the risk of influenza.
   3. It prevents the contraction of hepatitis.
   4. It increases the general immune system of the infant.

22. The nurse performs a health assessment on a 1-year-old boy. She takes his vital signs, including blood pressure. Which of the following readings would reflect a normal blood pressure for a 1-year-old child?

   1. 65/40 mm Hg
   2. 90/52 mm Hg
   3. 109/64 mm Hg
   4. 120/70 mm Hg

23. The parents of 19-month-old Ravi ask the nurse what they should do if he develops a fever. What would be the best advice for the nurse to give to the parents?

   1. "If his temperature is over 38°C, you should take him to the doctor."
   2. "If his temperature is over 39°C, you should administer liquid ibuprofen and sponge his skin with alcohol."
   3. "The fever does not necessarily have to be treated, but if Ravi is not feeling well, you may give him liquid acetaminophen according to the directions on the box."

4. "If the fever lasts more than 24 hours, you should consult your pediatrician."

24. The nurse counsels the parents of Yuri, age 12 months, about diet and nutrition. Which of the following foods would be the best source of iron for Yuri?

    1. Milk
    2. Lamb
    3. Orange juice
    4. Mineral-fortified cereal

END OF CASE 5

CASE 6

Ms. Blackhawk, a 27-year-old mother of two young children, requires investigation of weakness in her arms and legs, blurred vision, tinnitus, and increased emotional lability. She has been transported from her small northern community to a regional health centre.

QUESTIONS 25 to 27 refer to this case.

25. Ms. Blackhawk is scheduled for a number of tests to determine a diagnosis. She begins to cry, telling the nurse that she misses her family and is worried about how her husband and children will cope without her. Which of the following responses by the nurse would be most therapeutic?

    1. "I'm sure your husband will manage. Sometimes we don't give dads the credit we should."
    2. "I can see you are upset; perhaps you would like to speak with a chaplain about your concerns."
    3. "Perhaps we could ask your husband to give you a call every evening before the children go to bed so you can talk to them."
    4. "I understand how hard this must be for you, but right now you must concentrate on getting well yourself."

26. Ms. Blackhawk is diagnosed with primary relapsing multiple sclerosis (MS). Depressed

about her diagnosis, she asks the nurse if she thinks she will live to see her children become adults. Which of the following responses by the nurse would be both honest and therapeutic?

    1. "There is a possibility you will live to see them as teenagers."
    2. "Progression of the disease is individual, and with new medications and therapies, you may be healthy for many years."
    3. "I am not comfortable giving you any guess about how long you may live."
    4. "Don't worry about that. I am sure you will be around for a long time to come."

27. Ms. Blackhawk tells the nurse that because of her illness, she has often felt too tired to prepare dinner for her family. They have been eating fast foods, and she is concerned about the effects this is having on her and her family's health. Which of the following nursing responses would be the most therapeutic?

    1. "It is important that your diet include fibre to avoid constipation."
    2. "Perhaps your husband and your children could help prepare meals."
    3. "With children, as long as they have milk and eat some protein, they will be fine."
    4. "You must stop eating fast foods because they are low in nutritive value."

END OF CASE 6

CASE 7

Mr. Bricker has been admitted to hospital for treatment following a diagnosis of leukemia.

QUESTIONS 28 to 31 refer to this case.

28. The laboratory results indicate that Mr. Bricker is neutropenic. This state would place him at greater risk of developing which of the following conditions?

    1. Infection
    2. Internal bleeding
    3. Anemia
    4. Anorexia

29. As part of his chemotherapy regimen, Mr. Bricker is to receive prednisone (Apo-Prednisone). Which of the following adverse effects might he experience?

    1. Alopecia
    2. Anorexia
    3. Weight loss
    4. Mood changes

30. Mr. Bricker is scheduled to receive cranial radiation. His family asks the nurse why he requires radiation when he is already receiving chemotherapy. Which of the following statements would be the nurse's best response?

    1. "It will improve his quality of life."
    2. "Radiation reduces the risk of systemic infection."
    3. "It helps to avoid metastasis to his lymph system."
    4. "Radiation prevents central nervous system involvement."

31. The chemotherapy causes Mr. Bricker to develop stomatitis. Which of the following interventions would his nurse implement?

    1. Frequent rinsing of his mouth with mouthwash
    2. Using foam-tipped applicators for mouth care
    3. Having him brush three times a day with a toothbrush
    4. "Swish and spit" mouth rinsing with hydrogen peroxide

END OF CASE 7

CASE 8

A nurse working in a facility that provides electroconvulsive therapy (ECT) is preparing Mr. Ahmed for his first treatment.

QUESTIONS 32 to 34 refer to this case.

32. The nurse should ensure Mr. Ahmed is provided with what information prior to the ECT?

    1. "Sleep will be induced, so you will not feel the ECT."
    2. "There will be some permanent memory loss as a result of the treatment."
    3. "ECT can be frightening, so it is best not to ask any questions."
    4. "With new methods of administration, the treatment is totally safe."

33. Which of the following statements by the nurse about the ECT may help to decrease Mr. Ahmed's anxiety?

    1. "The treatments will make you feel better."
    2. "You will not be alone during the treatment."
    3. "A period of amnesia will follow the ECT."
    4. "There is no need to be afraid."

34. Which nursing intervention would be most appropriate after Mr. Ahmed has awakened from his first ECT?

    1. Bring him a lunch tray
    2. Orient him to time and place and tell him that he has just had an ECT treatment
    3. Get him up and out of bed as soon as possible and back into the unit's routine
    4. Take his blood pressure and pulse rate every 5 minutes until he is fully awake

END OF CASE 8

CASE 9

Ms. Da Costa, age 64 years, has been admitted to a respiratory unit with manifestations of dyspnea and chest tightness. She has a tentative diagnosis of chronic obstructive pulmonary disease (COPD).

QUESTIONS 35 to 37 refer to this case.

35. Ms. Da Costa is scheduled for a number of diagnostic tests. Which of the following tests would be most conclusive in diagnosing COPD?

    1. Pulmonary function tests
    2. Arterial blood gases
    3. Electrocardiography
    4. Chest radiography

Practice Exam 2

36. Ms. Da Costa has been a cigarette smoker for more than 30 years. Her oxygen saturation registers 89%. How should the nurse interpret this reading?

    1. This reading is slightly low, but considering the client's age, it is acceptable.
    2. This reading may be normal for a client with COPD.
    3. This reading indicates that oxygen therapy should be started immediately.
    4. This reading is normal for a client with dyspnea.

37. Ms. Da Costa is very anxious about exercising. Which of the following actions by the nurse would be the most effective in decreasing her anxiety level?

    1. Thoroughly explaining the reasons for, and the scope of, the exercise program
    2. Ensuring that Ms. Da Costa has portable oxygen and practical footwear
    3. Walking with Ms. Da Costa to help maintain an appropriate pace and increase her confidence
    4. Asking the physician to prescribe a mild anti-anxiety medication

END OF CASE 9

CASE 10

Ms. Jansen is admitted to the medical intensive care unit due to an acute, severe attack of colitis. It is determined that she is in the early stages of septic shock as a result of a perforated colon.

QUESTIONS 38 to 41 refer to this case.

38. Which of the following clinical manifestations might indicate Ms. Jansen is in the compensatory (early) stage of septic shock?

    1. Hypotension, hypothermia
    2. Restlessness, increased heart rate
    3. Bradycardia, increased respiratory rate
    4. Decreased response to stimuli, cold and clammy skin

39. Ms. Jansen's condition rapidly deteriorates. She becomes pale, with mottled skin and unstable vital signs. Which of the following actions would be most important for the nurse to implement?

    1. Administer high-flow oxygen
    2. Establish a secondary IV line
    3. Perform an arterial puncture for blood gases
    4. Insert an oral airway

40. Fluid resuscitation is commenced on Ms. Jansen. Which of the following manifestations is the most important for the nurse to observe for during fluid replacement?

    1. Chills and fever
    2. Further hypotension
    3. Signs of circulatory overload
    4. Anuria

41. The physician instructs the nurse to insert an indwelling urinary catheter in Ms. Jansen. What is the primary reason for the catheter?

    1. The bladder will need to be drained because of the rapid fluid infusion.
    2. There will be urine retention and overflow as a result of the shock and excess fluids.
    3. Ms. Jansen will be incontinent of urine, which will contaminate the treatment area.
    4. The catheter is used to accurately monitor urine output.

END OF CASE 10

CASE 11

Mr. Donny, age 21, is admitted to hospital with a gunshot wound to his right femur. Because the injury occurred during an armed robbery, he is handcuffed to the bed and is guarded by two police officers. Mr. Donny does not speak English.

QUESTIONS 42 to 44 refer to this case.

42. Mr. Donny requires cleansing of his wound. His nurse speaks the same language as Mr. Donny but has been told by the police and her nursing team leader she must not speak this language with

Mr. Donny. What is the most appropriate action by the nurse?

1. Comply with police direction and not speak with Mr. Donny
2. Inform the police she will explain the wound cleansing to Mr. Donny in his language
3. Consult agency policies for directions
4. Explain the treatment of the wound to Mr. Donny in English

43. There is a great deal of media attention about the armed robbery and the condition of Mr. Donny. Many phone calls are coming to the unit, and the nurse needs to know how to respond to these calls. What is the priority consideration for the nurse in this situation?

1. Nurses are not permitted to speak with the media about a client.
2. The client must be consulted about his wishes for release of information to the media.
3. Agency spokespeople are permitted only to confirm that the client has been admitted to their facility.
4. The police control what information may be released to the media.

44. Both of Mr. Donny's hands are handcuffed to the bed rail. The nurse notices that the skin under the handcuffs is broken and bleeding. What should the nurse do?

1. Ask the police to remove both handcuffs so that skin care may be given
2. Provide skin care while the handcuffs are in place
3. Have the police officer remove one handcuff at a time and provide care
4. Do not provide skin care unless the area becomes infected

END OF CASE 11

CASE 12

Neville, age 11 years, has type 1 diabetes. Recently his blood sugars have been unstable, so he is admitted to hospital.

QUESTIONS 45 to 48 refer to this case.

45. Neville is placed in a two-bed room. Which of the following children would be the best roommate for him?

1. A 12-year-old girl with colitis
2. An 8-year-old boy with asthma
3. An 11-year-old girl with a fractured femur
4. A 10-year-old boy with rheumatoid arthritis

46. The physician orders 20 units of Humulin R insulin for Neville. The vial reads, "1 mL = 100 U of Humulin R insulin." An insulin syringe is not available. Which of the following amounts, measured in a regular syringe, should the nurse administer?

1. 0.2 mL
2. 0.3 mL
3. 0.4 mL
4. 0.6 mL

47. As part of the teaching plan, the nurse will review with Neville his need for insulin. During which of the following times will the dose of insulin likely decrease?

1. At the onset of puberty
2. When an infection is present
3. When there is emotional stress
4. When active exercise is performed

48. Which of the following topics should be included when teaching Neville about his type 1 diabetes?

1. "Always carry a concentrated form of glucose."
2. "Weigh all food on an accurate gram scale."
3. "Candies, sweets, and fast foods are not allowed in your diet."
4. "Eat crackers, cheese, or an apple if you feel dizzy and confused."

END OF CASE 12

CASE 13

Mr. Gordon, age 36, has schizophrenia. He has been admitted to hospital because he is experiencing an acute psychotic episode.

QUESTIONS 49 to 51 refer to this case.

49. Mr. Gordon states that he knows the police are out to kill him. Which of the following medical terms would best describe what Mr. Gordon is experiencing?

    1. An illusion
    2. A delusion
    3. Autistic thinking
    4. A hallucination

50. Mr. Gordon is refusing all food because he believes that it is being poisoned. Which of the following nursing interventions would be most appropriate to implement?

    1. Taste the food in Mr. Gordon's presence
    2. Suggest that food be brought in from home
    3. Tell Mr. Gordon that the food is not poisoned
    4. Tell Mr. Gordon that tube feedings will be started if he does not begin to eat

51. The nurse explores with Mr. Gordon his fear that his food is being poisoned. Which of the following statements would be the most appropriate?

    1. "You really know the food is not poisoned, don't you?"
    2. "You feel someone wants to poison you?"
    3. "Your fear is a symptom of your illness."
    4. "You'll be safe with me. I won't let anyone poison you."

END OF CASE 13

CASE 14

A nurse works in a rehabilitation hospital. On her days off, she operates a private business providing specialized foot care for people in their homes.

QUESTIONS 52 to 56 refer to this case.

52. The nurse visits Mr. and Mrs. Marsh, a couple in their 80s who live independently in their home. At the first visit, she completes a health history. What information would be most important for

the nurse to determine prior to cutting the toenails of Mr. and Mrs. Marsh?

    1. Any history of peripheral vascular disease
    2. Any recent respiratory infections
    3. Nutritional status
    4. Signs of dementia or memory impairment

53. The nurse begins by soaking the feet of Mr. and Mrs. Marsh in basins of warm water. What is the primary reason to soak feet prior to care?

    1. It is a comfort measure for the client.
    2. The water softens nails and thickened epidermal cells.
    3. Soaking will enable the nurse to assess blood flow to the extremities.
    4. It will decrease the odour associated with the feet of older adults.

54. The nurse shortens the couple's toenails. Which of the following is the correct technique for shortening toenails?

    1. Cut the nails straight across with nail clippers
    2. File the nails with an emery board
    3. Clip the nails in an arc around the toe
    4. Cut the nails with sharpened pedicure scissors

55. Mr. Marsh asks the nurse why she changes gloves after completing his feet and before starting with his wife's. Which of the following statements would be the best response by the nurse?

    1. "It is a best practice guideline for foot care."
    2. "I need to use separate gloves for you and your wife."
    3. "I feel more comfortable using a clean pair of gloves with every client."
    4. "Gloves prevent transmission of possible fungal infections."

56. The nurse realizes that many of her clients in the rehabilitation hospital could use her foot-care services when they are discharged home. What would be an appropriate and professional way to inform them of her business?

1. Ask the director of care at her facility if she might post information on the unit bulletin board
2. Provide the clients with her business card
3. Tell the clients that they will require foot care when they get home and give them her business number
4. Provide foot care to clients who are about to be discharged and inform them that they could receive the same care from her when they are at home

END OF CASE 14

CASE 15

Sam, age 9 years, was playing at an unsupervised construction site with his friends when he fell on a 25-cm spike that punctured his chest. He is brought to the emergency department by ambulance.

QUESTIONS 57 to 60 refer to this case.

57. On admission to the emergency department, Sam is experiencing shortness of breath, dizziness, and pain in his chest. His lips and nail beds are cyanotic. The spike is protruding from the fifth intercostal space in the left axillary line. What will be the initial priority emergency treatment?

1. Remove the spike and cover the wound with an occlusive bandage
2. Establish intravenous access to prepare for fluid resuscitation
3. Administer high-flow oxygen
4. Remove Sam's shirt to assess the injury

58. The nurse performs a respiratory assessment on Sam. It is provisionally presumed that Sam has a pneumothorax. What might be an expected finding?

1. Diminished breath sounds on the left side
2. Muffled, distant heart sounds
3. Wheezing and crackling on expiration
4. Increased air entry on the nonaffected side

59. The physician in the emergency department prepares to insert a chest tube into Sam. He unwraps

a sterile tray that includes a scalpel. Sam becomes extremely upset, screaming and saying he is not going to let the doctor cut him with "that knife." Which of the following statements by the nurse would be most therapeutic and calming for Sam?

1. "The spike hurts you more than the knife will."
2. "I will stay with you."
3. "What is it you are afraid of?"
4. "We will put some special medicine on your skin so that you won't feel the knife."

60. The chest tube is inserted and attached to a disposable plastic drainage system (Pleur-evac). What is a nursing responsibility for care of Sam's chest tube system?

1. Ensure there is vigorous bubbling in the water seal chamber
2. Make sure all connections are secure and taped
3. Routinely strip and milk the chest tubes
4. Keep all tubes above the level of Sam's chest

END OF CASE 15

CASE 16

Mr. Stein, age 26 years, is in the manic phase of his bipolar disorder. He has been admitted to hospital because of increasing hyperactivity and erratic behaviour.

QUESTIONS 61 to 64 refer to this case.

61. Mr. Stein becomes loud, noisy, and disruptive in the client lounge. The nurse tells him to be quiet or he will be put in isolation. What are the legal implications of this situation?

1. The statement by the nurse constitutes a threat.
2. Isolation is justified for Mr. Stein's own protection.
3. Mr. Stein's behaviour is to be expected and should be ignored.
4. Because of his disease, Mr. Stein cannot be held responsible for not understanding instructions.

62. While the nurse is talking with Mr. Stein in the client lounge, he continues his disruptive behaviour and starts to use profane and vulgar language. How should the nurse respond?

    1. Have him leave the lounge so that he does not upset the other clients
    2. Tactfully include other clients in providing group censure for his behaviour
    3. Refuse to talk to Mr. Stein when he is speaking in this manner
    4. Ask Mr. Stein to limit the use of vulgarity but continue the conversation

63. That evening, Mr. Stein physically assaults another client on the unit. What precautions by the nursing staff would have been most appropriate to prevent this situation?

    1. Mr. Stein should have been sedated with tranquilizers because he was known to have erratic behaviour.
    2. Mr. Stein should have been placed in restraints because of his history of hyperactivity.
    3. Mr. Stein should have been put in a secure, segregated unit, rather than an open ward, because of his disruptive behaviour.
    4. The nursing staff should have provided close observation because they knew Mr. Stein's behaviour was volatile.

64. Two days later, Mr. Stein demands to be allowed to go downtown to shop. Because he is an involuntary admission who is legally not allowed to leave the facility, which of the following statements by the nurse would be the best response?

    1. "You are not stable enough to leave the unit."
    2. "You'll have to ask your doctor."
    3. "Not right now. I don't have a staff member to go with you."
    4. "You are not permitted to leave the unit. What do you need?"

END OF CASE 16

CASE 17

A nurse who is trying on clothes at a shopping mall sees a pregnant woman lying on the floor of the change room, moaning. The woman tells her that the baby is "coming now."

QUESTIONS 65 to 70 refer to this case.

65. What should be the nurse's first action?

    1. Call for help
    2. Examine the woman's perineum
    3. Ask her how often the contractions are coming
    4. Check to see if the membranes have ruptured

66. The woman's apprehension is increasing, and she asks the nurse what is happening. The nurse tells her not to worry, that she is going to be all right, and everything is under control. What is a correct evaluation of the nurse's statements?

    1. Adequate, since there does not need to be any further explanation
    2. Proper, since the client's anxieties would be increased if she knew the dangers
    3. Correct, since this is reassuring to the woman
    4. Questionable, since the woman has the right to know what is happening and why

67. Following a gush of bloody liquid, the woman precipitously delivers a full-term male infant. What should be the nurse's first action?

    1. Establish an airway for the baby
    2. Ascertain the condition of the fundus
    3. Quickly tie and cut the umbilical cord
    4. Assess for hemorrhaging in the mother

68. The nurse assesses the baby's heart rate. Which of the following ranges represents the normal range of heart rate for an infant within 3 minutes after birth?

    1. 100 to 200 beats per minute
    2. 130 to 190 beats per minute
    3. 120 to 160 beats per minute
    4. 80 to 130 beats per minute

69. As the nurse places the baby in the woman's arms immediately following delivery, the mother asks, "Is he normal?" What would be the most appropriate response by the nurse?

    1. "Most babies are normal. Of course he is."
    2. "He must be all right. He has such a good, strong cry."
    3. "I think so because there were no complications during the delivery."
    4. "Let us both look him over."

70. The ambulance and paramedics arrive on the scene. As the paramedic examines the baby, he instructs the nurse to start an IV line on the mother and infuse a bolus of dextrose 5% in water. The mother is not hemorrhaging. What would be the nurse's best response to the paramedic?

    1. "I am not allowed to initiate an IV."
    2. "I am not permitted to carry out orders from a paramedic."
    3. "I will start the IV and document this as an emergency."
    4. "I do not think an IV is necessary and will not do this."

END OF CASE 17

CASE 18

Ms. Connor returned from a holiday in Central America two weeks ago. She visits a local health clinic because she feels nauseated and very tired. She has a temperature of 37.9 °C.

QUESTIONS 71 to 75 refer to this case.

71. The assessment by the nurse indicates that Ms. Connor may have contracted hepatitis A. Which of the following manifestations are indicative of hepatitis A?

    1. Nausea and right upper quadrant pain
    2. Right flank pain and hunger
    3. Hypotension and bradycardia
    4. Confusion and hypothermia

72. It is confirmed that Ms. Connor has a hepatitis A infection. She asks the nurse if this means that she will have to be hospitalized. Which of the following responses would answer this question most completely?

    1. "Hospitalization and isolation will be required until the contagious period is over."
    2. "Hospitalization will not be required, but quarantine in your home will be necessary."
    3. "Hospitalization is not required unless you are unable to look after yourself or are incontinent of stool."
    4. "There are no special restrictions other than enteric precautions, which I will explain."

73. Ms. Connor asks the nurse if this infection will cause permanent liver damage. Which of the following responses from the nurse would be most appropriate?

    1. "With hepatitis A, normal liver function should return with no complications."
    2. "As with all forms of hepatitis, long-term liver damage will occur."
    3. "You will not have liver damage provided you comply with the special diet and drink alcohol only in moderation."
    4. "The medication you will be prescribed will prevent damage to the liver."

74. Clients with hepatitis often have anorexia. Which of the following dietary recommendations would the nurse suggest to Ms. Connor?

    1. "Eat a high-carbohydrate diet and limit protein intake."
    2. "You will require supplemental nutrition for a number of weeks."
    3. "Have several small meals a day that include foods you like."
    4. "Eat the most nutrient-rich meal in the morning, when you are not as nauseated."

75. Which of the following measures would have been most effective in preventing Ms. Connor from contracting viral hepatitis A or B?

1. Hand hygiene
2. Proper personal hygiene
3. Prophylactic immunization
4. Environmental sanitation

END OF CASE 18

CASE 19

Seven-year-old Kofi has sickle-cell anemia and has been admitted to hospital during a vaso-occlusive crisis.

QUESTIONS 76 to 79 refer to this case.

76. Kofi is to receive 3000 mL of IV fluid over a 12-hour shift. Using a minidrip IV set, with a drop rate of 60 drops/mL, at what rate should the IV infuse?

    1. 25 drops/hr
    2. 36 mL/min
    3. 250 mL/hr
    4. 360 drops/hr

77. When the nurse checks Kofi during the night, he finds that Kofi has wet the bed. What should the nurse do?

    1. Have Kofi help him remake the bed
    2. Gently tell Kofi that he is too old to be having "accidents"
    3. Put incontinence pants on Kofi
    4. Change Kofi's clothes and bedding and help him back to bed

78. Kofi's parents are upset and say to the nurse, "We should never have had Kofi. We have given him this disease." What is the most therapeutic response by the nurse?

    1. "It must be very hard to see your son in pain."
    2. "It is not your fault Kofi has sickle-cell disease."
    3. "I know how you feel."
    4. "Do your other children have sickle-cell disease?"

79. Several days later, Kofi is well enough to visit the hospital playroom. During a game of tag with another client, Kofi complains of feeling dizzy. What should the nurse's initial response be?

    1. Check his pulse and blood pressure
    2. Have him sit down
    3. Call for help
    4. Assist him to his room

END OF CASE 19

CASE 20

Mr. Wogan, age 62, has been treated for depression for the past ten years. He has recently shared with his friends and family that he has been thinking more and more about suicide. Mr. Wogan is admitted to the psychiatric unit of a hospital.

QUESTIONS 80 to 83 refer to this case.

80. Which of the following questions would the nurse find most beneficial to evaluate Mr. Wogan's potential for suicide?

    1. Ask him about his plans for the future
    2. Ask other clients if Mr. Wogan has discussed suicide
    3. Ask the family if Mr. Wogan has ever attempted suicide
    4. Ask Mr. Wogan if he has thoughts about and a plan for harming himself

81. Mr. Wogan confides to the nurse that he has a plan to kill himself. What has likely motivated him to confide in the nurse?

    1. He wishes to frighten the nurse.
    2. He wants attention from the staff.
    3. He feels safe and can share his feelings with the nurse.
    4. He is fearful of his own impulses and is seeking protection from them.

82. Mr. Wogan is placed on suicide precautions. Which of the following measures would be the most therapeutic way to provide for his safety?

1. Not allow him to leave his room
2. Remove all sharp or cutting objects
3. Give him the opportunity to vent his feelings
4. Assign a staff member to be with him at all times

83. Mr. Wogan asks the nurse, "Why am I being watched round the clock, and why am I not allowed to move around the unit as I like?" Which of the following would be the nurse's best response?

    1. "Why do you think we are observing you?"
    2. "What makes you think that we are observing you?"
    3. "We are concerned that you might try to harm yourself."
    4. "Your doctor has ordered it, and she is the one you should ask about it."

END OF CASE 20

CASE 21

Mr. Patterson, age 72 years, has his eyes examined at the eye clinic. He reports that he occasionally has a dull headache in the morning and a mild pain in his left eye and that his peripheral vision is not as good as it used to be.

QUESTIONS 84 to 86 refer to this case.

84. It is determined that Mr. Patterson has open-angle glaucoma. He says that he thinks his father also had trouble with his eyes, and he eventually went blind. He asks the nurse if this will happen to him. Which of the following responses by the nurse would be accurate regarding glaucoma?

    1. "With treatment, it is unlikely that you will lose your vision."
    2. "Your vision will decrease over time, especially at night, but you will not lose it altogether."
    3. "With this type of glaucoma, it is impossible to say what the outcome for your vision will be."
    4. "People with this type of glaucoma generally lose most of their sight over time."

85. The nurse discusses glaucoma with Mr. Patterson. Which of the following topics is most important?

    1. Modification of his environment for safety
    2. Knowledge of signs and symptoms that require medical attention
    3. The need for strict compliance with his prescribed therapy
    4. Information on the relationship between increased eye pressures and vision

86. The nurse explains to Mr. Patterson that open-angle glaucoma is a chronic condition that will require lifelong treatment. Which of the following nursing interventions would best help Mr. Patterson to accept his condition?

    1. Schedule several appointments for follow-up health teaching
    2. Encourage him to express his feelings and concerns about the glaucoma
    3. Provide Internet resources for glaucoma information and support groups
    4. Involve his family in discussions about how he will manage his condition

END OF CASE 21

CASE 22

A registered nurse is the facilitator for a group of clients in a psychiatric facility. The purpose of the therapeutic group is to share experiences, gain peer support, and find effective stress-reduction strategies.

QUESTIONS 87 to 90 refer to this case.

87. The nurse meets with the group for the first time. What is the most appropriate initial statement by the nurse?

    1. "My name is Gabriel Frank. I am a registered nurse, and I will be your group leader."
    2. "Welcome to the group. Our purpose is to help you find stress-reduction strategies."
    3. "Hello. I hope you will be able to attend these meetings every morning from 9:00 to 10:00."
    4. "Let's start by sharing with each other a bit about ourselves."

88. The nurse would like the group members to begin to share their experiences. Which of the following statements would best help members to begin the dialogue?

    1. "Mr. Pao, tell the group about your problems."
    2. "Ms. Brankston, I believe you are here because you are addicted to heroin."
    3. "Ms. Halsey, could you start us off by describing what led you to being admitted to hospital?"
    4. "Who would like to start the conversation?"

89. After several meetings, the group becomes difficult for the nurse to manage. Clients arrive late, speak out of turn, and interrupt each other. What would be the best approach for the nurse to help the group to become functional?

    1. "Let's make some group rules for how we are going to show respect for each other."
    2. "I don't think the group is working well, and we need to do something about it."
    3. "For the group to function, we need to stop interrupting each other."
    4. "I am disappointed that we are not supporting each other in this group."

90. After group one day, a client with depression tells the nurse that she does not like the idea of taking medications for her depression and thinks she will start to take St. John's wort. What would be the best response by the nurse?

    1. "Your depression is chronic and serious and requires prescription medications."
    2. "I will certainly support you in your decision to use a herbal preparation."
    3. "I have heard St. John's wort is very effective in treating depression."
    4. "What have you heard about St. John's wort for the treatment of depression?"

END OF CASE 22

CASE 23

Mr. Desjardins, age 78, has been hospitalized for confirmation of a possible diagnosis of gastric cancer.

QUESTIONS 91 to 95 refer to this case.

91. Mr. Desjardins asks the nurse if his condition is "something like cancer." Which of the following responses by the nurse would be the most appropriate?

    1. "Do you think you have cancer?"
    2. "You are having tests to find out if you have cancer. Would you like to talk about it?"
    3. "This is really a discussion you should have with your doctor."
    4. "We are still waiting for a number of test results to come back, so don't worry about it now."

92. Mr. Desjardins has a surgical resection of his stomach. Because of his age, he may be at risk for which of the following postoperative complications?

    1. Hemorrhage
    2. Fluctuating blood glucose levels
    3. Renal failure
    4. Delayed wound healing

93. After Mr. Desjardins has surgery, which of the following factors would most influence his perception of pain?

    1. Age and sex
    2. Overall physical status
    3. Intelligence and economic status
    4. Previous experience and cultural values

94. Mr. Desjardins is to begin ambulating the morning after his surgery. His medications include morphine sulphate. When assisting him out of bed, the nurse initially has him sit on the edge of the bed, dangling his feet. Why is this action considered necessary?

    1. Because movement may temporarily increase his abdominal pain
    2. To restore adequate circulation to his legs and feet
    3. Because he may have some respiratory distress due to the abdominal incision

4. Because he may have postural hypotension from lying in bed

95. Two days after surgery, Mr. Desjardins tells the nurse that while walking he has pain in his right calf. What initial action should the nurse take?

1. Put Mr. Desjardins back in bed
2. Notify the physician
3. Apply warm soaks to the leg
4. Elevate his right leg

END OF CASE 23

CASE 24

Ms. Kovacs, age 84 years, has degenerative osteoarthritis. She lives by herself in a two-storey home. She is admitted to hospital for a total right-hip replacement.

QUESTIONS 96 to 100 refer to this case.

96. Which of the following statements is true regarding degenerative osteoarthritis?

1. It primarily affects weight-bearing joints and can be asymmetrical.
2. It primarily affects small joints and is symmetrical.
3. The rheumatoid factor is positive.
4. Joint effusion is common.

97. Ms. Kovacs has the hip-replacement surgery. Which of the following positions would be indicated for Ms. Kovacs after the surgery?

1. Dorsal recumbent
2. On the affected side

3. On the unaffected side
4. Low semi-Fowler position

98. The nurse plans nursing interventions to prevent circulatory complications postsurgery. Which of the following actions would best achieve this goal?

1. Turn from side to side every 3 hours
2. Exercise the ankles and other uninvolved joints
3. Ambulate as soon as the effects of anaesthesia are gone
4. Sit up in a low chair as soon as the effects of anaesthesia are gone

99. The nurse places Ms. Kovacs in the left side–lying position, with a firm pillow placed between the thighs so that the entire length of the upper leg is supported. Which of the following is the nurse's reason for this positioning?

1. To prevent strain on the operative site
2. To prevent thrombus formation in the leg
3. To prevent flexion contractures of the hip joint
4. To prevent skin surfaces rubbing together

100. The nurse discusses with Ms. Kovacs her discharge from hospital. Which would be the most appropriate plan for Ms. Kovacs to ensure appropriate postsurgical care and recuperation?

1. Home with biweekly community supports
2. Transfer to a long-term care facility
3. Remain an inpatient in the acute care hospital until she is able to walk
4. Discharge to a rehabilitation facility

END OF CASE 24

INDEPENDENT QUESTIONS

QUESTIONS 101 to 200 do not refer to a particular case.

101. Mr. Megadichan has five stage-four pressure ulcers that the wound care specialist has ordered to be cleansed and dressed daily. The dressings are complex and take over an hour to complete. Mr. Megadichan's nurse has a busy assignment and does not have the time to do the dressings. What would be the most appropriate action by the nurse?

   1. Leave the dressings to be done by the night-shift staff
   2. Delegate the dressing changes to the unregulated care provider (UCP)
   3. Document in Mr. Megadichan's health record the reason the dressings have not been done
   4. Consult with nursing colleagues to obtain assistance with the dressings

102. A student nurse taking Mr. Camponi's blood pressure wraps the cuff very loosely around his arm because she does not want to hurt him. Which of the following consequences may result from this action?

   1. A falsely low reading
   2. A falsely high reading
   3. An accurate systolic reading but inaccurate diastolic reading
   4. Only the first and last Korotkoff sounds will be heard

103. Which of the following statements about informed consent is true?

   1. The physician is responsible for obtaining written consent for procedures.
   2. Nurses must co-sign all consent for treatment forms.
   3. The person who is performing the procedure is responsible for obtaining verbal or written consent.
   4. Consent is always in a written form and signed by the client.

104. Ms. Karmally has poorly controlled type 1 diabetes. The nurse teaches her about the possible complications of diabetes. Which of the following statements indicates that Ms. Karmally has fully understood the teaching about possible diabetic complications?

   1. "I will book an appointment with an ophthalmologist."
   2. "I will test my blood with a glucose meter once a week."
   3. "I will test my urine for ketones every day."
   4. "I will cut back from full-time work to part-time work."

105. Ms. Walters, age 25 years, has just received a prognosis of terminal cancer. That evening, a nurse observes a female colleague holding Ms. Walters's hand in the client lounge. The nurse is aware that her colleague is a lesbian. What is the nurse's responsibility in this situation?

   1. Report her colleague's behaviour to the unit manager
   2. Discuss with her colleague her possible inappropriate behaviour
   3. Discuss the hand holding with Ms. Walters
   4. Accept this as therapeutic touch and take no action

106. A registered nurse (RN) who works full time in an acute care hospital and part time as a community nurse sustained a back injury. The RN claimed sick benefits from her full-time employer but continued to work part time at the community nursing agency. Evaluate this professional behaviour.

   1. Professional misconduct
   2. Professional incompetence
   3. Malpractice
   4. Lack of accountability

107. Cassandra, age 14 years, is to have surgical excision of a mole. Her parents did not accompany her to the appointment. Cassandra tells the nurse she will sign her own permission form for treatment. Which of the following statements is true?

1. The age of consent varies according to provincial legislation.
2. Cassandra is not able to make a mature or informed choice.
3. Cassandra is able to give voluntary consent when her parents are not available.
4. Cassandra will most likely be unable to choose between alternatives when asked to consent.

108. Which of the following infections, caused by the yeast *Candida albicans*, occurs often in infants and immunosuppressed persons?

   1. Thrush
   2. Dysentery
   3. Impetigo
   4. Scabies

109. A nurse who has been assigned to care for a client with acquired immune deficiency syndrome (AIDS) requests a change in assignment. She tells the charge nurse that she does not wish to care for clients with HIV (human immunodeficiency virus) or AIDS because they "bring the problem on themselves." Which of the following statements would be true in this situation?

   1. Nurses may not discriminate in the provision of nursing care.
   2. Because of the nurse's ethics, she should be assigned to another client.
   3. Nurses may refuse to care for clients whose lifestyle choices have caused illness and resulting expense to the health care system.
   4. The nurse should choose to work in an area where her personal ethics are not compromised.

110. Which of the following statements represents a major influence on the eating habits of the early-school-aged child?

   1. The availability of food selections
   2. The smell and appearance of food
   3. The example set by parents at mealtime
   4. Food preferences of the peer group

111. A 10-month-old infant has a gastrostomy tube and is receiving 240 mL of tube feeding every 4 hours. Which of the following actions is a primary nursing responsibility?

   1. Open the tube 1 hour before feeding
   2. Position the infant on the right side after feeding
   3. Give 10 mL of normal saline before and after feeding
   4. Elevate the tube 30 cm above the level of the mattress

112. A nurse in a pediatrician's office is reviewing the birth record of an infant brought into the office for a newborn assessment at 2 weeks of age. Which of the following data indicate that the infant may require special attention?

   1. A birth weight of 3000 g
   2. An Apgar score of 3 at birth
   3. A positive Babinski reflex
   4. A pulsating fontanelle

113. Samantha is a 10-year-old girl admitted to hospital for orthopedic surgery. Samantha's mother hands the nurse a bottle of capsules and says, "These are for Samantha's allergies. Would you make sure she takes one at 9 o'clock?" Which of the following responses would be the most appropriate by the nurse?

   1. "One capsule at 9 p.m.? Of course I will give it to her."
   2. "Did you ask the doctor if she should have this tonight?"
   3. "Samantha should not have this medication before her surgery."
   4. "I will speak with your daughter's doctor about the allergies and ask for an order to give her pills."

114. A client is ordered atropine 0.3 mg subcutaneously preoperatively. The vial reads, "atropine 0.4 mg/mL." What is the correct dosage to administer to the client?

   1. 0.12 mL
   2. 0.3 mL

Practice Exam 2

3. 0.75 mL
4. 1.2 mL

115. Which of the following precautions should the nurse take when administering a parenteral iron preparation?

1. Apply ice packs to the site after the injection
2. Rotate injections among the four extremities
3. Firmly massage the site after withdrawal of the needle
4. Change needles after drawing the drug into the syringe

116. One evening while making rounds in a long-term care facility for older adults, a nurse opens the door of a client's room and finds him engaged in sexual intercourse with a female resident. Which of the following actions would be the most appropriate by the nurse?

1. Quietly leave the room and close the door
2. Discuss this with the nursing team
3. Ask the two residents if they would like privacy
4. Counsel the residents about sexuality in the older adult

117. Which of the following steps is involved in making an occupied bed?

1. Ensure both side rails are in the raised position prior to turning the client.
2. Adjust the bed height to a comfortable working position.
3. Assemble equipment and place it on the bottom of the bed.
4. Remove soiled top sheets, then cover the client with a bath blanket.

118. Following a spontaneous abortion, the nurse notes that the client and her partner are visibly upset. The partner has tears in his eyes, and the woman has her face turned toward the wall and is sobbing quietly. Which of the following statements by the nurse would be the most therapeutic?

1. "I know that you are upset now, but hopefully you will become pregnant again very soon."
2. "I see that both of you are very upset. I brought you a cup of coffee and will be here if you want to talk."
3. "I know how you feel, but you should not be so upset now. It will make it more difficult for you to get well quickly."
4. "I can understand that you are upset, but be glad it happened early in your pregnancy and not after you carried the baby for the full term."

119. A woman experiencing the climacteric asks the nurse about the use of herbal supplements and soy products to decrease her symptoms. How should the nurse respond?

1. "These are not proven to work."
2. "You are better to take prescribed medications."
3. "I recommend that you take these natural supplements rather than medicines."
4. "Talk this over with your physician, and try the ones you find helpful."

120. Following extensive liposuction surgery, Ms. Samuels is extubated. What observation would indicate to the nurse that Ms. Samuels is starting to experience acute respiratory insufficiency?

1. Restlessness and confusion
2. Anxiety and constricted pupils
3. Decreased pulse and respirations
4. Cyanosis and dyspnea

121. Which of the following vitamins is not stored in the body and must be included in the daily diet?

1. A
2. C
3. D
4. K

122. A nurse working in a long-term care facility smells smoke as she makes her rounds. She opens the door to Mrs. Cummings's room and finds it

full of smoke. What should be the nurse's first priority action?

1. Dial the agency fire code number
2. Call out "Fire" to alert the residents and staff
3. Shut all the doors and windows
4. Get Mrs. Cummings to a safe place

123. A nurse receives a panicked phone call from her neighbour. She is screaming and crying that her 2-year-old daughter has just had a "fit." The nurse determines that the child has had a febrile seizure. What would be the best advice the nurse could give to her neighbour?

1. To call 9-1-1
2. To take the child to the emergency department or family physician immediately
3. To make an appointment with a neurologist as this is likely the start of epilepsy
4. To give the child liquid acetaminophen for the fever and monitor for any further seizures

124. A nurse working in a long-term care facility develops nausea and a headache within hours after the installation of a new carpet throughout the facility. Several clients in the facility voice similar complaints. The nurse believes that these manifestations are related to the new carpet and that he and the residents are exposed to a toxic environment. What would be the most appropriate initial action for the nurse to take?

1. Move the clients away from the new carpet
2. Research the toxic effects of environmental chemical exposure
3. Communicate to management his safety concerns
4. Document his concerns on the agency risk-management report

125. A young couple have just learned from the pediatric neurologist that their 2-year-old son, Charlie, has pervasive developmental disorder (PDD). They tearfully ask the nurse what will happen to Charlie for the rest of his life. What response by the nurse would be most appropriate?

1. "There is a wide range of severity and handicap with PDD, and at this stage, a prediction is not possible."
2. "Charlie will be mildly retarded but will be able to function within a normal school environment."
3. "Charlie will likely be severely cognitively impaired."
4. "This is a degenerative disorder, and Charlie's condition will likely deteriorate by about age 6 years."

126. The nurse is unable to read the physician's handwriting for the postoperative orders for a client. The physician has returned to his office. What should the nurse do?

1. Ask the client what his doctor ordered
2. Contact the doctor for clarification of the orders
3. Ask another nurse for clarification of the handwriting
4. Consult with another available physician regarding what the ordering physician likely wanted

127. A medical student has requested a nurse's computer password to access a client's chart. What should the nurse do?

1. Share the password; the medical student is part of the health care team
2. Ask the supervising doctor if she can share the password
3. Not share the password; have the medical student obtain access to the client chart via the medical team
4. Share the password; it is not confidential

128. A physician is admitted to the psychiatric unit of a hospital as a client. He is restless, loud, and aggressive during the admission procedure and states, "I will take my own blood pressure." What is the most therapeutic response by the nurse?

1. "I am sorry, Doctor, but right now you are not capable of taking blood pressure."
2. "It is my responsibility to take your blood pressure."

3. "Certainly, Doctor. I'm sure you will do it okay."
4. "You must cooperate, or I will need assistance to take your blood pressure."

129. Majid, age 5 years, has a history of being physically and sexually abused. Which of the following therapies would be most appropriate for him?

1. Play therapy
2. Group therapy
3. Individual counselling
4. Role play

130. A female client tells the nurse that she takes one "coated baby aspirin" every day. Which of the following adverse effects would be of greatest concern to the nurse?

1. Urinary calculi
2. Atrophy of the liver
3. Prolonged bleeding time
4. Premature erythrocyte destruction

131. Ms. Buchwold has type 2 diabetes. Recently her blood sugars have been unstable. She tells the nurse, "I know I can tell you, but I don't want to tell the doctor. I have been drinking a fair bit of gin every evening." Which of the following responses by the nurse would be most appropriate?

1. "I won't mention this to the doctor, but I want you to assure me you will not continue with the drinking because we must get your blood sugars more stable."
2. "Your drinking is affecting your health, and you must tell the doctor about it."
3. "We must let the doctor know because this is affecting your health. I will be with you while you explain it to him."
4. "I am not allowed to keep important information from the doctor."

132. Tom, age 11, has had surgery. He sees the pulse oximeter on his finger and asks the nurse why he has it. Which of the following responses by the nurse would provide the best answer?

1. "It is a noninvasive method of measuring the percentage of oxygen in your circulating blood."
2. "It measures how well your blood is carrying oxygen to all of your body. Anything over 95% is good."
3. "It measures how red your blood is."
4. "It tells us how well you are breathing."

133. Mr. Clements, age 82, tells the nurse that he does not feel like eating because nothing tastes as good as the food he remembers eating when he was young. Which of the following explanations by the nurse would provide the most accurate response?

1. "As we age, our taste buds do lose their sensitivity."
2. "These days foods are sometimes not cooked the way you remember."
3. "Much of our food is processed, and we lose some taste in the process."
4. "Your appetite decreases as you age, and that affects the way you perceive the taste of the food."

134. Ms. Saunders, a client with a history of endometriosis, has just delivered a healthy baby boy. She tells the nurse that now that the pregnancy is over, she is concerned that the endometriosis will return. Which of the following responses by the nurse would be most accurate and appropriate?

1. "Pregnancy almost always cures endometriosis."
2. "Endometriosis will usually cause an early menopause."
3. "A hysterectomy will be necessary if the symptoms recur."
4. "Breastfeeding your baby will delay the return of symptoms."

135. Kayla Gibson is awake and alert following a bronchoscopy and biopsy for suspected esophageal cancer. Which of the following nursing interventions is the most appropriate initial action?

1. Provide ice chips to reduce swelling
2. Advise her to cough frequently

3. Evaluate for the presence of a gag reflex
4. Advise her to stay flat for 2 hours

136. Ecstasy (*3,4*-methylenedioxymethamphetamine) is an illegal street drug. What is the drug classification of Ecstasy?

1. An opiate
2. A depressant
3. A hallucinogen
4. An angiotensin-converting enzyme inhibitor

137. Ms. Kovicki has had a partial gastrectomy. Immediately after the surgery, her nasogastric tube drains light red liquid. How long after gastric surgery does sanguinous drainage usually continue?

1. 1 to 2 hours
2. 3 to 4 hours
3. 10 to 12 hours
4. 24 to 48 hours

138. A nurse is obtaining a health history from a client who has peptic ulcer disease. Which of the following statements by the client might indicate a possible contributing factor for the peptic ulcer?

1. "My blood sugars are a little high."
2. "I smoke two packs of cigarettes a day."
3. "I have been overweight most of my life."
4. "My blood pressure has been high lately."

139. Mr. Peterkin has congestive heart failure. He admits to the nurse that he has not followed a salt-restricted diet. He is now experiencing ankle edema, orthopnea, and dyspnea on exertion. What additional signs of fluid retention may be manifested by Mr. Peterkin?

1. Dizziness on rising
2. Rhinitis
3. A weak and thready pulse
4. A decreased hemoglobin and hematocrit

140. Which of the following components is the most important aspect of hand hygiene?

1. Time
2. Soap
3. Water
4. Friction

141. A nurse takes a picture of a sleeping Ms. Tang with his cellphone camera. What may the nurse do with this picture?

1. Show it to Ms. Tang, and then save it
2. Show it to Ms. Tang's family, and then delete it
3. Show it to his colleagues, and then save it
4. Show it to no one, and then delete it

142. A registered nurse is a manager of a home health care company. Mr. Eigo contracts with the company to provide a companion for his wife, who has Alzheimer's disease. Mrs. Eigo is physically well but is forgetful and sometimes wanders out of the house. What would be the most appropriate category of caregiver for the nurse to assign to Mrs. Eigo?

1. A registered nurse (RN)
2. A registered or licensed practical nurse (RPN or LPN)
3. A geriatric activation therapist
4. A personal support worker or unregulated care provider (PSW or UCP)

143. Maude Grant has been on prolonged antibiotic therapy for a persistent abdominal infection. Which of the following diseases can arise from normal microbial flora, especially after prolonged antibiotic therapy?

1. Q fever
2. Candidiasis
3. Scarlet fever
4. Herpes zoster

144. Following a total hysterectomy, Ms. Mengal asks the nurse if it would be wise for her to take hormone replacement therapy (HRT) right away to prevent symptoms of menopause. Which of the following responses by the nurse would be most appropriate?

1. "It is best to wait; you may not have any symptoms at all."
2. "You should wait until symptoms are severe, as the hormones are dangerous."
3. "It would be best for you to take herbal supplements rather than hormones."
4. "You should discuss with your physician since there are risks associated with taking HRT."

145. Which of the following tests would be used to determine a diagnosis of benign prostatic hyperplasia?

1. Rectal exam
2. Biopsy of prostatic tissue
3. Cystoscopic exam
4. Prostate-specific antigen (PSA) levels

146. Which of the following nursing actions is correct when caring for a client with continuous bladder irrigation?

1. Monitor urinary-specific gravity
2. Record urinary output every hour
3. Subtract irrigating fluid from output to determine the urine volume
4. Include irrigating solution in any 24-hour urine tests ordered

147. Following abdominal surgery, Ms. Roark is encouraged to ambulate. Her wound is still draining a moderate amount of serosanguineous fluid. What type of dressing should the nurse use for Ms. Roark prior to ambulation?

1. A dressing with gauze reinforcing the suture line
2. A dressing with additional gauze at the base
3. A dressing with additional gauze over the site of drainage
4. A pressure dressing covering the abdomen

148. Which of the following is true concerning the use of evidence-informed practice in nursing?

1. It was recommended by physicians who were using evidence-informed medicine.

2. It was designed by hospitals to reduce client care delivery costs.
3. It grew out of the demand for high-quality, cost-effective care and the availability of rapidly expanding knowledge.
4. It developed as a result of nurses' sharing information on the Internet.

149. A nurse must perform perineal care on a male client. Which of the following actions is the correct procedure for cleansing his penis?

1. Using a circular motion, first cleanse the tip of the penis at the urethral meatus.
2. With gentle but firm downward strokes, cleanse the shaft of the penis first.
3. Initially, retract the foreskin and then cleanse around the base of the glans penis.
4. First, grasp the shaft of the penis and cleanse in upward strokes toward the meatus.

150. The mother of a preschool child asks the nurse how she can best ensure that her child always wears his bicycle helmet. Which of the following suggestions from the nurse would be the most effective?

1. She should buy him one that he chooses.
2. She should tell him the importance of wearing a helmet.
3. She should reward him each time he puts the helmet on.
4. She should role-model by always wearing a helmet when she rides her bicycle.

151. A palliative care nurse is caring for a client who has chosen to die in his home. The nurse assesses he is experiencing significant pain and requires an increase in his narcotic analgesic. What should the nurse do?

1. Administer the increased dose and have the physician sign the order at a later date
2. Contact the physician to obtain a telephone order for the increased dose of narcotic
3. Advise the family to administer the increased dose of narcotic
4. Provide non-narcotic pain relief therapies

152. Parents of 12-month-old Ava take her to a clinic for her scheduled immunizations. What vaccine will Ava receive?

    1. Diphtheria, tetanus, pertussis (DTaP)
    2. Measles, mumps, rubella (MMR)
    3. *Haemophilus influenzae* (Hib)
    4. None because she does not require any immunizations at 12 months

153. Three-month-old baby Jason has Down syndrome. His parents ask the nurse if the soft spot on his head is related to this disorder. What might the nurse respond?

    1. "This is called the fontanelle and is normal in all infants."
    2. "The soft spot is bigger in Jason because with Down syndrome he needs more room for his brain to grow."
    3. "Children with Down syndrome have incomplete closure of the bones in their head, and this is the soft spot."
    4. "One of the defects in Down syndrome is a premature closure of the fontanelle, so his soft spot is smaller than normal."

154. The nurse is caring for an Asian client after abdominal surgery. When performing a pain assessment, which of the following statements reflects a correct inference?

    1. All Asian clients are stoic about pain.
    2. Asian clients have a high pain threshold.
    3. Asian clients prefer herbal therapies for pain control.
    4. All clients are individual in their response to pain.

155. A nurse realizes on his day off that he forgot to sign off administration of ampicillin from the previous evening. There are no agency policies concerning this type of situation. Which of the following actions by the nurse would be most appropriate?

    1. Sign the medication record on his next shift, in two days' time

    2. Return to the unit to sign the medication record
    3. Call the nursing supervisor to report the incident and consult regarding the appropriate action
    4. Call the charge nurse and ask her to document that he administered the medication

156. A young female, Ms. Holly, has a blood pressure of 160/90 mm Hg. She tells the nurse that she would prefer to take a herbal preparation rather than the prescribed antihypertensive. What would be the nurse's best action?

    1. Discuss with Ms. Holly the health risks and benefits of the herbal therapy
    2. Tell Ms. Holly that she must not use herbal therapy
    3. Advise Ms. Holly that her prescribed antihypertensive is the necessary treatment
    4. Support Ms. Holly in her choice of the herbal preparation

157. Which of the following clients should be referred to a physician for further assessment?

    1. A 45-year-old woman with tenderness in both breasts three days prior to her menstrual period
    2. A 31-year-old woman in her third trimester of pregnancy with increased breast size and a yellow fluid discharge from her nipples
    3. A 26-year-old male with a fixed mass that is 2 cm × 2 cm in the upper outer quadrant of his left breast
    4. A 4-day-old male child with bilateral enlargement of the breasts and a white discharge from both nipples

158. Mr. MacDonald, age 32 years, returned from Afghanistan several months ago. As part of an armed forces unit engaging in military action, he witnessed many atrocities, including the deaths of several comrades. Mr. MacDonald has been diagnosed by physicians as having post-traumatic stress disorder and has been admitted to a

psychiatric unit. What is the priority consideration for his treatment?

1. Provide a positive, nonjudgemental attitude toward Mr. MacDonald
2. Encourage Mr. MacDonald to express his grief and guilt
3. Provide for group therapy with other soldiers with similar experiences
4. Maintain observation for suicidal thoughts or violent behaviour

159. A nurse working in a long-term care facility includes a spiritual assessment as a regular part of the admission process for new clients. Which of the following questions would be most appropriate when initiating a spiritual assessment?

1. "What is your religion?"
2. "Would you like to have the chaplain visit you?"
3. "What is your source of strength when you face challenging situations?"
4. "Do you participate in any spiritual practices we should know about?"

160. Candace, age 17 years, is brought to the emergency department by her parents, who tell the nurse that Candace has been raped. Which of the following actions should be the nurse's first priority?

1. Contact the sexual assault team
2. Ask if Candace would like the morning-after pill
3. Ask Candace for a brief history of the event
4. Perform a vaginal exam

161. A prenatal client voices apprehension to the nurse about the coming delivery of her baby. Which of the following responses is the most therapeutic?

1. "If you have had an uneventful pregnancy, there will be no problem."
2. "What in particular are you worried about?"
3. "Your prenatal classes should have reviewed the stages of labour."
4. "Do you feel your partner will not be here to support you during labour?"

162. The nurse notes that the premature newborn's core temperature is 35.0°C. What would be the most appropriate nursing action?

1. Place a stockinette cap on the baby's head
2. Take the infant to the mother for transfer of body heat
3. Place the infant under a radiant heater or in a warmed Isolette
4. Give the baby a bath in warm water

163. Which of the following parents might be at most risk for abusing their child?

1. Mr. Couture, who is unemployed and living in subsidized housing with his family
2. Ms. Patrick, who was abused as a child
3. Ms. Steele, a high school dropout who is depressed with her factory job
4. Mr. Miyagi, a socially isolated recent immigrant from South America

164. Mrs. Cooke, age 87 years, has mild dementia related to Alzheimer's disease. Her husband assists her with activities of daily living as necessary. A community care nurse performs a home assessment. What would be the most important safety assessment related to bathing?

1. Need for bathing devices, such as a hand-held shower
2. Solutions used by Mr. Cooke for his wife's bathing and skin care
3. Need for devices such as grab bars in the tub and shower area
4. Cognitive and musculoskeletal function of Mrs. Cooke

165. Mehmet, age 4, is diagnosed with chicken pox while he is an inpatient on a pediatric unit. Which of the following medications administered to other children on the unit would put them at increased risk for chicken pox?

1. Insulin
2. Steroids
3. Antibiotics
4. Anticonvulsants

166. Mr. and Mrs. Pappandreaou bring their 1-week-old infant son into the clinic. The infant is receiving formula, and they are concerned because he regurgitates with each feeding. What should the nurse instruct them to do?

    1. Keep him prone following feedings
    2. Prevent him from crying for prolonged periods
    3. Administer a minimum of 240 mL of formula at each feeding
    4. Keep him in a semi-sitting position, particularly after feedings

167. Which of the following statements is most accurate when describing depression during pregnancy?

    1. Estrogen and progesterone levels associated with pregnancy protect against depression.
    2. Signs and symptoms of antenatal depression are different from those in depression at other stages of life.
    3. Depression in pregnancy is most frequent during the first trimester.
    4. Antenatal depression is a risk factor for postpartum depression.

168. A newly graduated RN is employed in an adult medical-surgical setting. Most of her previous clinical experience has been in mental health and pediatrics, so she is not familiar with adult medications. She asks her preceptor many questions about the medications. The preceptor is surprised at her knowledge gap and is not receptive to the new nurse's questions. What should the new nurse do to practise safely?

    1. Change her employment to a pediatric setting
    2. Continue to ask the preceptor for support and teaching
    3. Tell the preceptor that if she makes a mistake, it will be the preceptor's responsibility
    4. Study a medications text so that she can learn about unfamiliar adult medications

169. A toddler has ingested some of his mother's medications. He is brought to the urgent care clinic, where he is administered ipecac syrup.

Which of the following actions suggested by the nurse will enhance the effect of ipecac syrup?

    1. Stimulating the gag reflex
    2. Having the child rest until vomiting occurs
    3. Having the child drink two to three glasses of water
    4. Encouraging normal activity until vomiting occurs

170. The physician orders meperidine hydrochloride (Demerol) 20 mg IM for a 9-year-old child. The container reads, "50 mg/mL." What dose should the nurse administer?

    1. 0.4 mL
    2. 0.6 mL
    3. 0.8 mL
    4. 1.0 mL

171. Ms. Clarke is in active labour and complains of low back pain. To increase her comfort, what would the nurse recommend to Ms. Clarke's partner?

    1. "Instruct her to flex her knees."
    2. "Place her in the supine position."
    3. "Apply back pressure during contractions."
    4. "Help her perform abdominal breathing."

172. Mr. Parsons tells the nurse at his workplace that he is tired all day and that his snoring keeps his wife awake at night. What should the nurse recommend?

    1. That he try to have naps during the day
    2. That his wife sleep in another room so that he does not wake her
    3. That he see a physician as he may have sleep apnea
    4. That he take a herbal sleep aid, such as melatonin

173. A blood test has revealed that Ms. Clarisse has iron-deficiency anemia. Which of the following menus would be best to treat her anemia?

1. Salmon steak, rice, and asparagus
2. Liver, spinach salad, and lima beans
3. Pork chops, cauliflower, and raw carrots
4. Cheeseburger, french fries, and a milkshake

174. Mr. Firth has told his nurse that he wishes to try acupuncture for his chronic pain. What would be the best response by the nurse?

1. "Acupuncture is not recommended for pain."
2. "Acupuncture is not an approved therapy in Canada."
3. "I will help you find an acupuncture practitioner."
4. "You probably need some help taking your pain medication."

175. An agency nurse is working her first shift in a long-term care facility. She must administer digoxin (Lanoxin) to Mr. Masters. What is the safest action to ensure that she is administering the digoxin to the correct client?

1. Check Mr. Masters's armband
2. Ask Mr. Masters his name
3. Ask the roommate if this is Mr. Masters
4. Ask the other nurses which client is Mr. Masters

176. The father of a child who is dying of cancer asks the nurse if he should tell his 7-year-old son that his sister is dying. Which of the following answers would be the nurse's best response?

1. "A child his age cannot comprehend the real meaning of death, so don't tell him until the last moment."
2. "Your son probably fears separation most and wants to know that you will care for him, rather than what will happen to his sister."
3. "Why don't you talk this over with your doctor, who probably knows best what is happening in terms of your daughter's prognosis."
4. "Your son probably doesn't understand death as we do but fears it just the same. He should be told the truth to let him prepare for his sister's death."

177. A client in her fourth month of pregnancy tells the nurse that her husband just admitted he has genital herpes. What should the nurse teach this client regarding sexual activity?

1. "It will be necessary to refrain from all sexual contact with him during pregnancy."
2. "You will need to use spermicides during sexual activity."
3. "You and your husband should use a condom for sexual activity."
4. "Meticulous cleaning of the vaginal area after intercourse is essential."

178. Ms. Gentile, a frail 86-year-old woman, begins to fall while she is ambulating with her nurse. What should be the initial action by the nurse?

1. Call for assistance
2. Assume a wide stance, bend the knees, and gently lower Ms. Gentile to the floor
3. Prevent her from falling to the floor by supporting her under her arms
4. Support Ms. Gentile against her body as she regains her strength

179. An RN hears an unregulated care provider introduce herself as a nurse to a client. Which of the following actions by the nurse would be most appropriate?

1. Tell the UCP that she is not allowed to call herself a nurse and she will be reported to the manager
2. Take the UCP aside and explain the title "nurse" is protected and may be used only by registered and practical nurses.
3. Tell the client that she is the nurse and the UCP is employed just to provide non-nursing care
4. Ask the nurse educator to hold an in-service for the staff to explain various levels of nursing care

180. Which of the following statements regarding drug abuse and older adults is correct?

1. Nurses are less likely to recognize drug abuse in older adults than in younger adults.

2. It involves a small percentage of older adults, and the abuse is primarily limited to over-the-counter medications.
3. Alcohol is the most common substance abused and is abused by over 50% of people over 60 years of age.
4. Older adults are more likely to be willing to discuss the issue than are younger people.

181. Ms. Marie, age 26 years, is scheduled for surgical removal of a small, benign cyst on her neck. She is concerned that she will form an "ugly" keloid scar since keloids run in her family. Which of the following statements by the nurse would be most therapeutic?

1. "It is unlikely that you will form a keloid just because your mother and sister did."
2. "This surgery is necessary. The scar will be very small, and I am sure no one will notice it."
3. "I understand your concern. Would you like to talk to the surgeon about the possibility of scar formation?"
4. "I know you are concerned, but the doctor will make sure that a keloid will not form."

182. Which of the following facts about the use of the female condom is correct?

1. Because the female condom is a polyurethane sheath, it may be washed and reused.
2. Only water-soluble lubricants should be used with these condoms.
3. A male condom should always be used at the same time as a female condom.
4. The condom may not be used for anal intercourse.

183. Ms. Evelyn Grant is scheduled to have a tracheotomy. The tracheotomy tube will have an inflated cuff. She asks her nurse if she will be able to talk with the tube in place. Which of the following would be the nurse's best response?

1. "The tube does not allow for speech, but we will be able to communicate in other ways."
2. "We will remove the tube when you wish to say something."

3. "Sometimes you can make yourself understood, but your speech will be slurred."
4. "Your throat will be too sore for you to want to talk, so it will not be a concern."

184. Sally lives in a youth shelter. She has come to a street health clinic with a persistent, productive cough. She asks the nurse if she has contracted tuberculosis (TB). Which of the following responses would be most therapeutic?

1. "TB has been pretty well eradicated in Canada, so I imagine it is just a cold."
2. "There is a risk you have contracted TB. We will do some tests, and if they are positive, you can be treated."
3. "Most cases of TB in Canada are among people who have come from another country."
4. "You seem to have a good immune system, so it is unlikely."

185. Ms. Pargeter, age 29, has hypertension. Ms. Pargeter has a history of poor compliance with her prescribed antihypertensive medication, having stated that the medications make her tired. The nurse determines Ms. Pargeter's blood pressure to be 165/100 mm Hg. What is the nurse's best approach to this situation?

1. Tell Ms. Pargeter her blood pressure is too high and that she must take her medications as prescribed
2. Suggest to Ms. Pargeter she make an appointment with the physician to discuss possible modifications to her medication plan
3. Tell Ms. Pargeter if she is not going to be compliant with her medication regime, then there is nothing to be done for her
4. Discuss with Ms. Pargeter what she can do to rest and reduce the stress in her life

186. A nurse has made an entry in the hard copy of the wrong client's health record. What should be the corrective action?

1. Remove the entry from the wrong chart
2. Draw a line through the entry, write "wrong chart," and date and sign it

3. Use whiteout to eliminate the entry
4. Complete an incident report and place a copy in both client charts

187. Ms. Leonard calls the telephone nursing consultation service. She tells the nurse that her husband has suddenly experienced dizziness, headache, and weakness in his left side and is having difficulty speaking. What is the most important directive the nurse should give to Ms. Leonard?

1. "Call 9-1-1."
2. "Take your husband to the family physician immediately."
3. "Give your husband an aspirin."
4. "Place him in a head-down position, and call the doctor."

188. Jeanine, age 6 years, has a severe allergy to peanuts. She carries a commercial preloaded epinephrine injection kit (EpiPen) in her school bag as she has experienced previous anaphylactic reactions. One day, the school nurse is called to the playground because Jeanine has collapsed after accidentally eating some peanut butter. Which is the most important initial action of the nurse in the emergency care of Jeanine?

1. Call Jeanine's parents
2. Administer the epinephrine injection
3. Take Jeanine's vital signs
4. Administer diphenhydramine hydrochloride (Benadryl) after ensuring a patent airway

189. Ms. Cameron has a history of urinary tract infections (UTIs). What would the nurse recommend to help prevent the incidence of her infections?

1. Drink cranberry juice regularly
2. Use commercially available perineal wipes
3. Limit her fluid intake to reduce urine production
4. Take a urinary antiseptic prophylactically

190. Mrs. Gingras is experiencing anorexia and cachexia as an adverse effect of her chemotherapy. Which of the following measures would the nurse recommend to help her increase her protein and calories?

1. Eat more food at each meal
2. Plan menus that include her favourite foods
3. Add high-calorie sauces and condiments to foods
4. Consume nutritional supplement drinks such as Ensure between meals

191. Mr. Michener died at 1830 hours. His family is at the bedside. It is now 1845 hours, and the registered nurse feels she should prepare the body before the night-shift staff arrives at 1915 hours. What should the nurse do?

1. Begin to prepare the body but encourage the family to stay at the bedside
2. Ask the family if they would leave because she has to prepare the body
3. Allow the family to stay as long as they need but request overtime pay for staying to prepare the body
4. Provide support to the family and offer the night staff assistance in preparing the body

192. Ms. Spinosa, RN, asks Ms. Millar, an RN colleague, to co-sign for a heparin injection, as per their agency policy. What does Ms. Millar need to do?

1. Ensure that she has witnessed all the rights of medication administration
2. Refuse to co-sign, as she cannot accept responsibility for the medication administration
3. Double-check the physician order for the heparin
4. Confirm that the dose in the syringe is correct, and then sign her name on the medication record

193. A nurse is working for the second day in a first aid clinic at a charity marathon race. What is the nurse's priority action when he arrives to work his shift at the event?

1. Check the equipment and supplies
2. Read the communication report about clients discharged on the previous shift
3. Perform a head-to-toe assessment on any clients awaiting care
4. Ensure medical directives (standing orders) are in place

194. Mr. Frost is recovering from an acute exacerbation of colitis. For what reason would he be placed on a high-protein diet?

1. To repair tissue
2. To slow peristalsis
3. To correct anemia
4. To improve smooth muscle tone in the colon

195. Mr. Sanderson, age 18 years, sustained a severance of the spinal cord during a gymnastics competition. The physician explained to him that he is now a paraplegic. Three weeks later, Kyle asks when he can leave hospital to practise for an upcoming tournament. Which of the following defence mechanisms is Mr. Sanderson using?

1. Denial
2. Verbalization of a fantasy
3. Inability to adapt
4. Extreme motivation to get well

196. Ms. Mills, age 30 years, is starting an estrogen–progestin oral contraceptive. Ms. Mills smokes approximately one pack of cigarettes a day. What potential adverse effect would the nurse advise her to report?

1. Nausea
2. Weight gain
3. Calf tenderness
4. Lighter than normal menstrual flow

197. Ms. Kirk has had a thrombotic cerebrovascular accident in the left hemisphere of her brain. She is conscious. What manifestations would the nurse expect Ms. Kirk to exhibit?

1. Left-sided paralysis and increased diaphoresis
2. Increased deep-tendon reflexes and rigidity
3. Urinary retention with dribbling
4. Anxiety, communication, and mobility difficulties

198. A nurse is visited in her home by her neighbour, who tearfully confesses to the nurse that she has been beating her children for many months. She begs the nurse to help her but not to tell anyone. What action must the nurse take?

1. Examine the neighbour's children to assess the seriousness of their injuries
2. Discuss with the neighbour community services that are available to help her
3. Ask the neighbour what she can do to help her
4. Tell the neighbour she will have to contact the local child welfare authorities

199. Ms. Carlyle, a 91-year-old client in a long-term care facility, is dehydrated. The physician orders hypodermoclysis with normal saline to run over 12 hours during the night. Where would be the best place for the nurse to insert a butterfly catheter?

1. Into a vein on the dorsal surface of the hand
2. Into the abdomen or upper thigh
3. Into the brachial vein in the antecubital fossa
4. Into a vein in Ms. Carlyle's pedal circulation

200. Which of the following is the greatest risk factor for a woman to develop peripheral arterial disease?

1. Her sex
2. Smoking a pack of cigarettes a day
3. An intake of 200 mL of wine daily
4. A diet high in saturated fats

END OF PRACTICE EXAM 2

Practice Exam 2

Answers and Rationales for Practice Exam 2

CASE–BASED QUESTIONS ANSWERS AND RATIONALES

CASE 1

1.   1. This teaching technique may be more effective with a group that is cohesive and familiar with one another. As part of a newly formed group, many members might be reluctant to volunteer answers because of fear of others viewing them as lacking in knowledge.

   2. This teaching technique, particularly when paired with visuals, is an efficient and effective method to impart knowledge.

   3. Pamphlets would provide an effective follow-up to the presentation as they would help the group members to recall the information at home.
   4. Role-playing allows participants to actively apply knowledge in a controlled situation, but the participants must first have the knowledge of the pathophysiology of MIs. Role-playing may not be the best strategy to teach pathophysiology.

CLASSIFICATION

Competency:
Professional Practice

Taxonomy:
Critical Thinking

2.   **1. All of these methods can be used to evaluate for obesity; however, waist-to-hip ratio is recommended, particularly with cardiac clients.**

   2. This measurement will be taken and used to compute the body mass index (BMI).
   3. Although there are standard weight and height charts for adults, they are not generally used to determine adult obesity. Pediatric growth charts may be used to determine obesity in children.
   4. Hydrostatic weight provides the most accurate measure of lean body weight; however, it is not considered to be practical in most clinical settings.

CLASSIFICATION

Competency:
Health and Wellness

Taxonomy:
Critical Thinking

3.   1. *Canada's Food Guide* recommends five to ten servings.

   2. These portions help promote a heart-healthy diet that is well balanced with protein and complex carbohydrates in the form of vegetables and that is also low in fat.

   3. Fat should make up approximately 25% of total calories.
   4. Complex carbohydrates are healthier than simple carbohydrates.

CLASSIFICATION

Competency:
Health and Wellness

Taxonomy:
Application

4.   1. This option will reduce sodium intake, but the group members may still eat foods that have high sodium content.

   2. Many foods, especially purchased fast foods, have high sodium content. The men will be best able to monitor their sodium intake if they are aware of the actual amount of salt in the foods. Reading labels will also help educate them about high-sodium and low-sodium foods.

CLASSIFICATION

Competency:
Health and Wellness

Taxonomy:
Critical Thinking

3. This option will reduce salt intake but will not help the men avoid the high sodium content in many prepared foods.

4. This option may reduce salt intake, but "reduced sodium" does not necessarily mean low sodium.

---

5. 1. **Salmon is a low-calorie and -sodium fish with omega 6 and omega 3 fats; a baked sweet potato contains carbohydrates and vitamins; a green salad is low-calorie vegetables containing fibre; vinegar dressing is low in calories and sodium.**

2. 250 g is far too large a quantity of pasta. Also, a low-calorie dressing may not be low in sodium.

3. Breaded fish may be high in calories. Baked beans may be high in sodium and calories.

4. Eggs, ham, and cheese are high in calories. Avocados, although a good fat, are also high in calories. Chicken broth is high in sodium.

CLASSIFICATION
Competency:
Health and Wellness
Taxonomy:
Application

CASE 2

6. 1. **All of the options must be performed by the nurse; however, he must wash his hands first to prevent transmission of microorganisms.**

2. Same as answer 1.

3. Same as answer 1.

4. Same as answer 1.

CLASSIFICATION
Competency:
Changes in Health
Taxonomy:
Application

---

7. 1. This action is not necessary. The pharmacist would have prepared the medications according to the physician order. The scope of practice for pharmacists allows them to prepare and dispense medications.

2. Nurses may administer medications that pharmacists have prepared provided they have performed the rights of medication administration. Nurses may not administer medications another nurse has prepared.

3. **Nurses must perform the rights of medication administration (variably documented as 5, 6, 7, or 8) before administering any medication.**

4. This step is included in the rights.

CLASSIFICATION
Competency:
Professional Practice
Taxonomy:
Application

---

8. 1. Cold compresses will not provide comfort although they may help to reduce the swelling. If used, they should be cool rather than cold.

2. **Moist heat provides comfort, increases circulation to the area, and cleanses the exudates.**

3. This measure will not help with the swelling and exudate.

4. Patching may provide some comfort, but the patch should be removed at intervals to cleanse the area and assess the eye.

CLASSIFICATION
Competency:
Changes in Health
Taxonomy:
Application

9.   1. This question may receive a yes or no answer, which will not
      provide the nurse with sufficient information to assess how he is
      managing.
      2. Same as answer 1.
      3. Same as answer 1.

      4. **This question is open ended and will be more likely to elicit
      information about how Mr. Poulos is managing with his daily
      activities and meal preparation.**

CLASSIFICATION
Competency:
Nurse–Client Partnership
Taxonomy:
Critical Thinking

10.   1. **The vancomycin levels must be ordered by a physician. It is the
      nurse's responsibility to ensure client safety and advocate for
      the client, so the nurse must ensure that the physician orders
      the levels.**

      2. The nurse cannot draw blood for vancomycin levels without an
      order unless a medical directive is in place.
      3. Mr. Poulos needs a requisition signed by a physician in order to
      have his blood drawn for the levels.
      4. The nurse has a professional responsibility and accountability
      for the client, Mr. Poulos. Consultation with another nurse is
      not required.

CLASSIFICATION
Competency:
Professional Practice
Taxonomy:
Application

11.   1. This action may be necessary depending on the observations after
      the site is assessed.
      2. The nurse should research drug references after assessing the site.
      3. This action should have occurred prior to the infusion of the
      antibiotics.

      4. **All options could be correct and may occur, but remember
      the nursing process: the first action needs to be an assessment
      of the insertion site to look for signs of infiltration or tissue
      irritation.**

CLASSIFICATION
Competency:
Professional Practice
Taxonomy:
Critical Thinking

12.   1. This option is not safe because it could lead to a needle-stick injury by
      anyone handling the garbage.
      2. Medications should not be disposed of into the public water supply.

      3. **The appropriate method of disposal is through the pharmacy.
      Pharmacies encourage the public to bring in unused medications
      for safe disposal.**

      4. The medication is the property of Mr. Poulos, and it is his
      responsibility to dispose of it. If the client asks the nurse to take
      the drugs because he is not able to dispose of them, the nurse
      can document this request and take the medication to the
      pharmacy.

CLASSIFICATION
Competency:
Professional Practice
Taxonomy:
Application

CASE 3

13.   1. Ms. Patel would not be able to pass stool into a specimen container.

2. **Ms. Patel may have limited mobility due to being day 1 postsurgery, and with this type of diarrhea, she would be unable to get to a bathroom quickly enough. If there are sufficient warning signs, the stool may be collected in a bedpan. If not, the stool may be scraped from an incontinence pad.**

CLASSIFICATION
Competency:
Changes in Health
Taxonomy:
Application

3. It is not likely that a nurse would be able to collect a specimen from a toilet.
4. This action may embarrass Ms. Patel and be disrespectful.

14.   1. **All options are a concern. Ms. Patel is losing fluid and necessary electrolytes in the diarrhea, and these losses must be closely monitored and corrected to prevent dehydration and circulatory collapse.**

CLASSIFICATION
Competency:
Changes in Health
Taxonomy:
Critical Thinking

2. This situation is a possibility, but the fluids are the first concern.
3. This situation may occur but is not the initial concern.
4. This situation may occur if Ms. Patel becomes dehydrated.

15.   1. **The nurse respects Ms. Patel's cultural preferences by consulting with her about appropriate practice for personal hygiene.**

CLASSIFICATION
Competency:
Professional Practice
Taxonomy:
Application

2. Ms. Patel is day 1 postoperative and weak. She may not be able to cleanse herself adequately.
3. The right hand is considered to be clean and would become unclean by touching the bedpan. The left hand should be used for both the bedpan and the cleansing.
4. This action is expected of all nurses with all clients regardless of cultural practices.

CASE 4

16.   1. Recommended weight gain during pregnancy depends on the mother's prepregnancy weight. If the client is an appropriate weight prepregnancy, a weight gain of 7 to 8 kg is not sufficient.
2. Low-calorie diets may be harmful to the developing fetus.
3. This response closes off communication; it does not allow the client to ask more questions about weight gain.

CLASSIFICATION
Competency:
Health and Wellness
Taxonomy:
Application

4. **This response is factual and answers Mrs. Corrigan's question.**

17.   1. This point in the labour is too early. She likely still has a great deal of time and may feel more comfortable at home.

CLASSIFICATION
Competency:
Health and Wellness

2. A bloody show and back pressure may be early signs of labour or signs of posterior fetal position. She should notify the physician or midwife, but it is too early to go to the birthing centre.

Taxonomy:
Application

3. **When the membranes rupture, the potential for infection is increased, and when the contractions are 5 to 8 minutes apart, they are usually of sufficient force to warrant skilled observation. Therefore, for the safety of the mother and fetus, the mother should go to the birthing centre.**

4. This time between contractions is indicative of advanced labour, and the client may have difficulty getting to the birthing centre at this point.

---

18.   1. **Progressive dilation of the cervix is the most accurate indication of true labour.**

2. Contractions may not begin until 24 to 48 hours afterward.
3. This statement is untrue; contractions will increase with activity.
4. Contractions of true labour persist in any position.

CLASSIFICATION
Competency:
Health and Wellness
Taxonomy:
Application

---

19.   1. This response is untrue: successful breastfeeding requires mastery, and some women have difficulty.
2. This response presumes Mrs. Corrigan has issues with breastfeeding and may be interpreted negatively by Mrs. Corrigan.

CLASSIFICATION
Competency:
Health and Wellness
Taxonomy:
Application

3. **This response offers correct information and would be reassuring to Mrs. Corrigan.**

4. The baby's sucking and emptying of the breasts, not the amount of fat and glandular tissue, determine the amount of milk produced.

CASE 5

20.   1. Rubella is not a severe disease in childhood.

2. **Rubella in a pregnant woman may cause teratogenic effects in the fetus. Thus, children are immunized to prevent them from transmitting the disease to a pregnant woman.**

CLASSIFICATION
Competency:
Health and Wellness
Taxonomy:
Application

3. Canadian law does not require children to be vaccinated against rubella.
4. Rubeola and chicken pox may cause severe sequelae, but rubella generally does not.

---

21.   1. **The Hib, *Haemophilus influenzae* type B, vaccine has greatly reduced the incidence of infant meningitis, a disease with high mortality and morbidity.**

CLASSIFICATION
Competency:
Health and Wellness
Taxonomy:
Knowledge/Comprehension

2. The Hib vaccine does not protect against various strains of influenza. It specifically protects against *H. influenzae* type B, which causes meningitis.

3. The Hib vaccine does not prevent hepatitis. Hepatitis is prevented by the hepatitis B vaccine.

4. The Hib vaccine does not increase general immunity.

---

22. 1. This blood pressure is normal for a newborn.

2. This blood pressure is normal for a 1-year-old.

3. This blood pressure is normal for a 12-year-old.

4. This blood pressure is normal for an adult.

CLASSIFICATION

Competency:

Health and Wellness

Taxonomy:

Knowledge/Comprehension

---

23. 1. Fevers in children normally subside within several days. It is not necessary for the parents to take Ravi to the doctor with a temperature of 38°C.

2. No liquids other than room-temperature water should be sponged on a child.

3. Because fever is not an illness, parents do not necessarily have to "fight" the fever. If the child is more than 3 months old and is feeling uncomfortable, the parents can administer acetaminophen in liquid form. It is important to follow the directions on the box for the correct dosage based on the child's weight.

4. The parents should consult a physician if the fever lasts longer than 3 days.

CLASSIFICATION

Competency:

Changes in Health

Taxonomy:

Application

---

24. 1. Milk is a poor source of iron.

2. Lamb contains iron in small amounts and is not as easily digested as cereal.

3. Orange juice does not contain iron.

4. Fortified cereal is a rich source of iron that is easily digested by children.

CLASSIFICATION

Competency:

Health and Wellness

Taxonomy:

Application

CASE 6

25. 1. This response dismisses the client's concerns.

2. The client has made no reference to wanting to speak to any member of the clergy.

3. This response addresses the client's concern and also provides a practical solution.

4. Same as answer 1.

CLASSIFICATION

Competency:

Nurse–Client Partnership

Taxonomy:

Application

Answers Exam 2

26.   1. Most people with this type of multiple sclerosis live for approximately 25 years after diagnosis.

       2. This response offers hope without false reassurance.

       3. This response is neither therapeutic nor professional.
       4. This response is glib and does not answer the client's concerns.

CLASSIFICATION
Competency:
Nurse–Client Partnership
Taxonomy:
Application

27.   1. This response does not address the issue of eating fast food because of Ms. Blackhawk's fatigue.

       2. This response addresses the client's concerns and offers practical help.

       3. This response is not helpful and trivializes the importance of a balanced diet.
       4. It is true that fast foods offer little nutrition, but this does not mean they may not be occasionally enjoyed.

CLASSIFICATION
Competency:
Nurse–Client Partnership
Taxonomy:
Critical Thinking

CASE 7

28.   **1. The extensive growth of lymphoblasts suppresses the normal growth of red cells, white cells, and platelets. Neutropenia is a low level of white cells, specifically neutrophils, which are part of the immune system and are required to prevent infection.**

       2. Internal bleeding would be the result of thrombocytopenia.
       3. Anemia would be the result of decreased red blood cells and hemoglobin.
       4. Anorexia may occur with leukemia and neutropenia but is not a specific risk.

CLASSIFICATION
Competency:
Changes in Health
Taxonomy:
Application

29.   1. Alopecia does not result from steroid therapy.
       2. An increased appetite, not anorexia, results from steroid therapy.
       3. Weight gain, not weight loss, results from steroid therapy.

       4. Euphoria and mood swings may result from steroid therapy.

CLASSIFICATION
Competency:
Changes in Health
Taxonomy:
Knowledge/Comprehension

30.   1. An improved quality of life is not the primary reason for the treatment. Radiation is a curative measure.
       2. Reducing the risk of systemic infection is not the reason for cranial radiation.
       3. Leukemia is a cancer of the lymphatic system and bone marrow; it is not a metastasis.

       4. Radiation destroys leukemic cells in the brain because chemotherapeutic agents are poorly absorbed through the blood–brain barrier.

CLASSIFICATION
Competency:
Changes in Health
Taxonomy:
Application

31.   1. This intervention may irritate the oral mucosa; mouthwash should
          always be diluted.

       2. Foam is soft and will not damage the oral mucosa.

       3. This intervention will injure the oral mucosa.
       4. This intervention has an offensive taste and will irritate the mucosa.

CLASSIFICATION

Competency:

Changes in Health

Taxonomy:

Application

CASE 8

32.   1. Clients fear this therapy because of the expected pain. If they are
          reassured that they will be asleep and will feel no pain, there will be
          less anxiety and more cooperation.

       2. Permanent memory loss should not occur.
       3. While electroconvulsive therapy (ECT) may be frightening to
          Mr. Ahmed, this statement cuts off future communication.
       4. No treatment requiring anaesthesia is totally safe.

CLASSIFICATION

Competency:

Nurse–Client Partnership

Taxonomy:

Application

33.   1. This statement may be false reassurance.

       2. The staff's presence will provide continued emotional support and
          help relieve anxiety.

       3. Not all clients experience amnesia, and the amnesia passes; placing
          emphasis on amnesia will increase fear.
       4. The nurse should not place focus on Mr. Ahmed's fear. It is more
          reassuring for him to know that someone will be with him.

CLASSIFICATION

Competency:

Nurse–Client Partnership

Taxonomy:

Application

34.   1. This intervention would come later if the client asked for food.

       2. Clients are confused when they awaken after ECT. They may
          experience temporary disorientation, so it is important to orient
          them to time, place, and situation.

       3. This intervention would not be appropriate for a client who has just
          awakened after a treatment.
       4. This intervention is not necessary. Routine postoperative vital signs are
          adequate.

CLASSIFICATION

Competency:

Changes in Health

Taxonomy:

Application

CASE 9

35.   1. These tests, which include tidal volume, airway resistance, peak
          expiratory volume, and others, would provide the most useful
          information.

CLASSIFICATION

Competency:

Changes in Health

Taxonomy:

Critical Thinking

2. This test may be indicated but is not conclusive in diagnosing chronic obstructive pulmonary disorder (COPD).

3. This test would be done but is not diagnostic for COPD.

4. This test would be ordered but would not be conclusive.

---

36.   1. Oxygen saturations are lower in older-adult clients. Ms. Da Costa, however, is only 64 years old.

2. Hypoxemia is a common finding for clients with COPD.

3. Oxygen therapy may or may not be indicated for clients with COPD and is sometimes contraindicated since it may suppress the respiratory centre.

4. Dyspnea is not always accompanied by low oxygen saturation.

CLASSIFICATION

Competency:

Changes in Health

Taxonomy:

Critical Thinking

---

37.   1. This action should be done but may not be the most effective way of decreasing anxiety.

2. This action is also recommended but, again, would not reduce anxiety.

3. This action would give the nurse an opportunity to observe as well as to set an appropriate pace.

4. This action would not generally be necessary at this time.

CLASSIFICATION

Competency:

Changes in Health

Taxonomy:

Critical Thinking

CASE 10

38.   1. These manifestations are signs of the progressive, or intermediate, stage of shock.

2. These manifestations are early signs of shock.

3. Bradycardia occurs in the refractory, or late, stage. An increased respiratory rate occurs in the progressive stage.

4. These manifestations are signs of the progressive, or intermediate, stage of shock.

CLASSIFICATION

Competency:

Changes in Health

Taxonomy:

Knowledge/Comprehension

---

39.   **1. All of these actions are necessary and important in the emergency treatment of shock, regardless of the cause. The most immediate need, however, is for a high concentration of oxygen to be available for tissue perfusion. Administration of oxygen is a quick task that can be accomplished before undertaking the other actions.**

2. A secondary IV line may be required for infusion of medications and fluid resuscitation.

3. This action will be done at some time during the treatment but is not a priority. The decrease in blood volume will make accessing an artery difficult.

CLASSIFICATION

Competency:

Changes in Health

Taxonomy:

Critical Thinking

4. It is possible that Ms. Jansen will need assistance maintaining a patent airway, but this is not yet indicated and is not the initial intervention.

40. 1. These manifestations are signs of a reaction to the infusion of blood products. They also may appear due to the septic component of her shock.
   2. This manifestation is unlikely with the large infusion of fluids; however, the client's blood pressure will need to be monitored.

   3. With septic shock, large amounts of fluids will be infused, and there is a danger of fluid overload. The signs the nurse should watch for include tachycardia, an increased respiratory rate, and crackles in the lungs.

   4. Anuria may occur if the perfusion to the kidneys is compromised. Fluid overload is the more common happening.

CLASSIFICATION
Competency:
Changes in Health
Taxonomy:
Critical Thinking

41. 1. This situation could possibly occur, but of greater importance is monitoring the urine output.
   2. Same as answer 1.
   3. Same as answer 1.

   4. The urine output needs to be monitored accurately to determine fluid balance.

CLASSIFICATION
Competency:
Changes in Health
Taxonomy:
Critical Thinking

CASE 11

42. 1. The nurse's priority responsibility is to the client. The police and the team leader do not have authority in this case to prevent the nurse from obtaining informed consent and reassuring Mr. Donny about his condition.

   2. The priority responsibility is to the client. The nurse must ensure the nurse–client partnership is maintained and must ensure Mr. Donny understands his treatment plan.

   3. There is no reason to consult agency policies, as the duty to the client is clear.
   4. This action is inappropriate as Mr. Donny does not understand English.

CLASSIFICATION
Competency:
Nurse–Client Partnership
Taxonomy:
Critical Thinking

43. 1. In some situations, a nurse may be the spokesperson for the agency to the media.

   2. This consideration addresses confidentiality. A nurse is not allowed to share client information with others unless the client's consent is obtained.

   3. With the client's permission, agency spokespeople can confirm the client has been admitted to the facility. A status report may also be released with client permission.

CLASSIFICATION
Competency:
Professional Practice
Taxonomy:
Critical Thinking

Answers Exam 2

4. In some situations, the police may legally restrict what is divulged to the media; however, the nurse's first priority is the confidentiality of the client.

44. 1. It may not be safe to remove both of Mr. Donny's handcuffs.
2. The nurse will not likely be able to provide complete skin care while the handcuffs are in place.

3. This option provides safety for the nurse and enables the nurse to provide care for the skin.

4. Mr. Donny has a right to appropriate care. Skin care must be provided to prevent further injury and infection.

CLASSIFICATION

Competency:
Professional Practice
Taxonomy:
Application

CASE 12

45. 1. Same-gender roommates at this age are desirable for companionship and to maintain privacy needs.
2. An 8-year-old boy would be too young to provide companionship for Neville.
3. Same as answer 1.

4. Ten is closer in age to Neville. He will prefer the company of someone of the same gender and age group.

CLASSIFICATION

Competency:
Professional Practice
Taxonomy:
Application

46. **1. This calculation is correct:**

Desired dose ÷ Dose on hand × Volume
Desired dose: 20 units
Dose on hand: 1 mL = 100 units
Volume: 1 mL
20 units ÷ 100 units × 1 mL = 0.2 mL

2. This dose is too large.
3. Same as answer 2.
4. Same as answer 2.

CLASSIFICATION

Competency:
Professional Practice
Taxonomy:
Application

47. 1. With increased growth and the associated dietary intake, the need for insulin increases.
2. An infectious process, if severe enough, may require increased insulin.
3. An emotional upset is a stress that increases the need for insulin.

4. Exercise reduces the body's need for insulin. Increased muscle activity accelerates the transport of glucose into the muscle cells, thus producing an insulinlike effect.

CLASSIFICATION

Competency:
Changes in Health
Taxonomy:
Application

48.   1. **With type 1 diabetes, particularly in younger children, blood glucose levels may fluctuate. Neville is admitted to hospital because his blood sugar levels have been unstable. At the first sign of hypoglycemia, Neville needs to have a quick, concentrated source of glucose to immediately raise his blood sugar.**

      2. This action may be advisable for some people with diabetes but is generally not necessary.
      3. This statement is not completely true, and telling Neville he is not allowed treats may cause him to rebel against his disease and the diet.
      4. These items should be eaten once his blood sugar has been raised by quick-acting glucose.

CLASSIFICATION
Competency:
Changes in Health
Taxonomy:
Application

CASE 13

49.   1. An illusion would be a misinterpretation of a sensory stimulus.

      2. **A delusion is a fixed, false personal belief that is not founded in reality.**

      3. Autistic thinking is a distortion in the thought process associated with schizophrenic disorders.
      4. A hallucination is a perceived experience that occurs in the absence of an actual sensory stimulus.

CLASSIFICATION
Competency:
Changes in Health
Taxonomy:
Knowledge/Comprehension

50.   1. This intervention would be a form of entering into the client's delusions. The client may feel that only a particular part of the food was free of poison.
      2. This suggestion may reinforce the delusion that the hospital food is poisoned.

      3. **Clients cannot be argued out of delusions, so the best approach is a simple statement of reality.**

      4. Threats are always poor nursing interventions, no matter how exasperated the nurse feels.

CLASSIFICATION
Competency:
Changes in Health
Taxonomy:
Application

51.   1. This question is close ended and may not encourage Mr. Gordon to explore his fears.

      2. **This statement is the only one that helps Mr. Gordon to focus and explore his feelings.**

      3. Although this statement is true, it is not something Mr. Gordon is ready to understand; it is a closed statement.
      4. This statement offers false reassurance and is not realistic; Mr. Gordon will still have concerns as to what will happen when the nurse is not there.

CLASSIFICATION
Competency:
Changes in Health
Taxonomy:
Application

Answers Exam 2

CASE 14

52.   **1. All history is potentially important. However, clients with peripheral vascular disease are at risk for infection, foot ulceration, and poor wound healing. They may require a physician order for nail cutting.**

2. This information may have significance but is not the most important information.
3. This information will have relevance to wound healing and maintenance of skin integrity but is not the most important information.
4. This information has significance for ability to perform foot care and respond to health teaching but is not the most important initial information.

CLASSIFICATION
Competency:
Changes in Health
Taxonomy:
Critical Thinking

---

53.   1. While it is a comfort measure, this is not the most important reason for the foot soaks.

2. Warm water softens nails and thickened epidermal cells and allows for easier removal of the nails and dead skin.

3. Soaking will increase circulation to the area, which is therapeutic. However, assessment of circulation to the feet is best done prior to the foot soaks.
4. While it will decrease odour, this is not the most important reason for the foot soaks.

CLASSIFICATION
Competency:
Health and Wellness
Taxonomy:
Critical Thinking

---

54.   **1. Cutting the nails straight across prevents splitting of nail margins and formation of sharp nail spikes that can irritate lateral nail margins.**

2. Filing the nails with an emery board is not an efficient method for shortening them; however, an emery board may be used to smooth rough nail edges after clipping.
3. Nails should be cut straight across.
4. Nail clippers are preferable since they are designed for the thickness of toenails. Using sharpened scissors presents more of a risk for accidentally injuring the toes and may not be safe.

CLASSIFICATION
Competency:
Changes in Health
Taxonomy:
Knowledge/Comprehension

---

55.   1. It is a best practice, but this does not adequately answer Mr. Marsh's question.
2. This response does not answer the question.
3. This response may be true, but the nurse should change gloves to prevent transmission of possible fungal infections, not because it makes her more comfortable to do so.

CLASSIFICATION
Competency:
Nurse–Client Partnership
Taxonomy:
Application

4. This response correctly answers Mr. Marsh's question, providing the reason for the change of gloves between clients.

56.   1. **The nurse must keep her salaried and private work completely separate. The only action that could not be perceived as a conflict of interest is receiving permission from the director of care.**

2. This action is a conflict of interest and would not be professional behaviour.
3. Same as answer 2.
4. Same as answer 2.

CLASSIFICATION
Competency:
Professional Practice
Taxonomy:
Application

CASE 15

57.   1. Impaled objects should be stabilized; they should never be removed since removal could cause a large influx of air into the chest cavity.
2. This action is important but is not the first step.

3. **In an emergency situation, the priority is airway and breathing. Sam is cyanotic and has dyspnea, indicating that he requires oxygen. This can be administered quickly, and then other interventions can be initiated.**

4. This action is important but is not the first step.

CLASSIFICATION
Competency:
Changes in Health
Taxonomy:
Critical Thinking

58.   1. **There would be diminished or no breath sounds over the affected left side since there is accumulated air in this area.**

2. This finding is seen more frequently in cardiac tamponade.
3. These findings are symptoms of asthma and fluid in the airways.
4. The nonaffected side does not have the ability to increase air entry. Because Sam is in pain, it is likely he is breathing shallowly, and air entry may be decreased.

CLASSIFICATION
Competency:
Changes in Health
Taxonomy:
Application

59.   1. Without the local anaesthetic, the knife may hurt just as much as or possibly more than the spike because of the anticipated pain. This statement would not be reassuring to Sam.
2. This statement may provide some comfort but is unlikely to completely calm Sam's fears.
3. It is obvious what he is afraid of. This response is not helpful.

4. **Before chest tube insertion, the area is prepared with a local anaesthetic. If Sam is aware that there will be no pain from the scalpel, he may be less afraid of "that knife."**

CLASSIFICATION
Competency:
Nurse–Client Partnership
Taxonomy:
Application

60.   1. Bubbling should be gentle. Vigorous bubbling only causes increased evaporation.

2. **All connections must be taped to prevent any air leaks or disconnection.**

CLASSIFICATION
Competency:
Changes in Health
Taxonomy:
Application

3. Stripping the chest tubes is not recommended because it increases pleural pressures. With newer chest tubes, blood clots are not likely to form.
4. Tubes must be kept below the level of the chest.

CASE 16

61.   1. **These words constitute a threat. A threat is a type of assault that is an intentional tort.**

2. Isolation is considered to be a restraint. It may be ordered by a physician when the client is assessed to be a danger to others. It is unnecessary at this time.
3. Mr. Stein's behaviour may be expected but should be dealt with directly. Behaviour should never be ignored.
4. This generalization draws a conclusion that may not be true.

CLASSIFICATION
Competency:
Professional Practice
Taxonomy:
Application

62.   1. This response does not show acceptance of the client, nor does it help Mr. Stein control his behaviour.
2. It is not appropriate at this stage to involve the other clients. The nurse needs to take responsibility for actions to decrease Mr. Stein's inappropriate behaviour.
3. This response does not deal with the problem directly and may confuse Mr. Stein because he may not be aware of why the nurse is refusing to talk to him.

CLASSIFICATION
Competency:
Nurse–Client Partnership
Taxonomy:
Application

4. **This response sets appropriate limits for Mr. Stein, who cannot set self-limits; it rejects the behaviour but accepts the client.**

63.   1. It would be unrealistic, not therapeutic, and not indicated to keep Mr. Stein sedated at all times.
2. This precaution is not necessary unless the client commits repeated acts of violence, in which case, a physician may order the client to be placed in four-point restraints.
3. There had been no previous history of violence that would warrant a secure, segregated unit.

CLASSIFICATION
Competency:
Professional Practice
Taxonomy:
Critical Thinking

4. **The nursing staff, knowing the client was disruptive and volatile, was negligent in not providing close supervision. Mr. Stein should have been closely observed to protect him against self-imposed injury as well as to protect others.**

64.   1. This response is true but shows no consideration of how Mr. Stein may feel.
2. It may be true that Mr. Stein must ask the physician for a change in his involuntary status, but this response implies that the nurse simply does not wish to deal with his request and is putting him off.

CLASSIFICATION
Competency:
Nurse–Client Partnership
Taxonomy:
Critical Thinking

3. This response implies Mr. Stein may be able to go shopping later when there is a staff member available, yet this may not be the case.

4. **This response clearly states that Mr. Stein is not allowed to leave and may decrease his anxiety by taking the time to find out what he thinks he needs.**

CASE 17

65.   **1. This situation is an emergency. The nurse will need help with a possible delivery and should delegate someone to call 9-1-1.**

2. This action is important but is not the first action.
3. Same as answer 2.
4. Same as answer 2.

CLASSIFICATION
Competency:
Health and Wellness
Taxonomy:
Critical Thinking

66.   1. If the woman is asking, then further explanation is necessary.
2. Registered nurses have a duty to provide complete and accurate explanation, regardless of the situation. A complete explanation would likely reassure the woman, rather than make her more anxious.
3. Same as answer 2.

CLASSIFICATION
Competency:
Nurse–Client Partnership
Taxonomy:
Application

4. **Registered nurses have a duty to provide complete and accurate explanation, regardless of the situation.**

67.   **1. An open airway is the priority action.**

2. This action is not the priority at present; the uterus still contains the placenta and will not contract.
3. There is no need for haste in cutting the cord; a clear airway is the priority.
4. The infant's airway is the priority. Hemorrhaging, if it occurs, will be evident.

CLASSIFICATION
Competency:
Health and Wellness
Taxonomy:
Critical Thinking

68.   1. Heart rates below 120 beats per minute are considered bradycardia; above 180 beats per minute is considered tachycardia.
2. The normal heart rate is between 120 and 160 beats per minute.

CLASSIFICATION
Competency:
Health and Wellness
Taxonomy:
Knowledge/Comprehension

3. **The heart rate varies with activity; crying will increase the rate, whereas deep sleep will lower it. A rate between 120 and 160 beats per minute is within the normal range.**

4. A heart rate below 120 beats per minute is considered bradycardia.

69.   1. This response offers false reassurance and closes off communication with the mother.

CLASSIFICATION
Competency:
Nurse–Client Partnership

2. Crying is not indicative of the absence of congenital defects. A strong cry does not ensure "normalcy."
3. The "normalcy" of the mother's delivery does not always bear a relationship to the "normalcy" of the infant.

4. Mothers need to explore their infants visually and tactilely to assure themselves that the infant is normal in all respects.

Taxonomy:
Application

---

70.   1. In most jurisdictions in Canada, if they have the knowledge, skill, and competency, registered nurses (RNs) are allowed to start IVs if the infusion is 0.9% normal saline. This explanation to the paramedic is inadequate.

2. Paramedics function under medical directives but do not have prescribing authority. RNs are not permitted to take orders from health care providers who do not have the authority to prescribe medications.

3. This situation is not an emergency.
4. This statement may be true, but, primarily, the nurse is not allowed to accept orders from a paramedic.

CLASSIFICATION
Competency:
Professional Practice
Taxonomy:
Critical Thinking

CASE 18

71.   **1. These manifestations, along with malaise, are the most common manifestations of hepatitis A.**

2. Anorexia is more likely with these manifestations, and flank pain is associated with renal problems.
3. Hypertension is more usual than hypotension in the case of hepatitis A, and bradycardia is not a manifestation.
4. The client is more likely to have a fever than hypothermia, and no confusion.

CLASSIFICATION
Competency:
Changes in Health
Taxonomy:
Knowledge/Comprehension

---

72.   1. Hospitalization is not usually required for hepatitis A, and isolation is only for clients incontinent of stool.
2. There is no reason for quarantine.
3. Incontinence of stool is not an indication for hospitalization. It is not likely that Ms. Connor will be unable to care for herself because of the infection. If, however, this does occur, there are care options other than hospitalization.

4. Appropriate infection control and enteric precautions are sufficient.

CLASSIFICATION
Competency:
Changes in Health
Taxonomy:
Application

---

73.   **1. Long-term damage is rare with hepatitis A.**

2. This statement is untrue.

CLASSIFICATION
Competency:
Changes in Health
Taxonomy:
Application

3. The client should not consume alcohol until there is no remaining trace of infection.
4. No medication will protect the liver.

---

74. 1. A high-carbohydrate diet may not be palatable, and protein will be required for healing.
2. There is no requirement for supplementation.

> 3. **The most successful approach is to recommend eating appetizing foods in small quantities.**

4. Ms. Connor will more likely be most nauseated in the morning.

CLASSIFICATION
Competency:
Changes in Health
Taxonomy:
Application

---

75. 1. This measure is necessary but not the most effective.
2. Same as answer 1.

> 3. **Immunization is the most successful method since it provides complete protection.**

4. Same as answer 1.

CLASSIFICATION
Competency:
Health and Wellness
Taxonomy:
Critical Thinking

CASE 19

76. 1. This calculation is incorrect. Also, infusion pumps are not regulated in drops.
2. Same as answer 1.

> 3. **This calculation is correct:**
> **Amount of fluid = 3000 mL**
> **÷ 12 hrs**
> **= 250 mL/hr**

4. Same as answer 1.

CLASSIFICATION
Competency:
Professional Practice
Taxonomy:
Application

---

77. 1. Kofi may feel he is being punished by having to make the bed. Also, he is likely in pain and likely has an IV line, which would make assisting with the bed making difficult.
2. This action would embarrass Kofi and make him feel worse.
3. This action would be demeaning to Kofi as he would view the incontinence pants as diapers.

> 4. **Kofi will have received a large amount of fluids to provide hemodilution. With the excess fluids and the expected regression that occurs with hospitalization of children, urinary incontinence happens frequently. The nurse can best help Kofi handle this embarrassment by helping him into dry clothing and back into a dry bed.**

CLASSIFICATION
Competency:
Nurse–Client Partnership
Taxonomy:
Application

78.   1. This response validates the parents' feelings of distress.

2. Sickle-cell disease is genetically transmitted, so the parents may legitimately feel it is their fault.
3. The nurse does not know how the parents feel.
4. This response changes the subject and does not provide support to the parents' feelings.

CLASSIFICATION
Competency:
Nurse–Client Partnership
Taxonomy:
Application

---

79.   1. Immediate physical safety takes priority over further assessment.

2. The child's immediate physical safety takes priority. The child must sit down to avoid falling.

3. The subjective symptom of dizziness alone does not warrant calling for help at this time.
4. Immediate physical safety takes priority; walking at this time would be unsafe.

CLASSIFICATION
Competency:
Changes in Health
Taxonomy:
Critical Thinking

CASE 20

80.   1. At this point, Mr. Wogan is most likely unable to think beyond the present, much less deal with future plans; this question is too general.
2. This action is inappropriate and a violation of confidentiality.
3. The family would be one resource, but it is best to approach Mr. Wogan directly.

4. Directness is the best approach at the first interview because the nurse can thereby set the focus and concern and also determine how serious Mr. Wogan is about suicide.

CLASSIFICATION
Competency:
Changes in Health
Taxonomy:
Application

---

81.   1. This statement could be true but is an unlikely motivation for the behaviour.
2. Same as answer 1.
3. This statement may be true, but, more important, the client is seeking help and protection.

4. Clients frequently report suicidal feelings so that staff will have the chance to stop them. They are really asking, "Do you care enough to stop me?"

CLASSIFICATION
Competency:
Changes in Health
Taxonomy:
Application

---

82.   1. This measure would be punishment for the client, and he still may find a way to carry out a suicide attempt in the room.
2. This measure would be routinely taken. By itself, it is not necessarily therapeutic.
3. This measure is not a suicide precaution.

CLASSIFICATION
Competency:
Changes in Health
Taxonomy:
Critical Thinking

4. **Emotional support and close surveillance can demonstrate to Mr. Wogan that the staff cares and is attempting to prevent his acting out of suicidal ideation.**

83. 1. This response would place the client on the defensive.
     2. This response is inappropriate in a rather obvious situation.

     3. **This response helps the client realize that staff members care and believe that the client is worthy of care.**

     4. This response is an evasive tactic by the nurse.

CLASSIFICATION
Competency:
Nurse–Client Partnership
Taxonomy:
Application

CASE 21

84. 1. **This response is accurate. This type of glaucoma does have a strong familial component, but with appropriate treatment, Mr. Patterson should experience no further deterioration in his vision.**

     2. It is true that night vision can be affected, but this response is not therapeutic.
     3. This response is untrue. With appropriate treatments, the prognosis may be determined.
     4. This response is not therapeutic and is also untrue.

CLASSIFICATION
Competency:
Changes in Health
Taxonomy:
Application

85. 1. This action may be necessary, but if the intraocular pressure is controlled, there should be no deterioration in Mr. Patterson's vision.
     2. This knowledge could be important; however, there are often no symptoms of increased pressure.

     3. **The client must understand that strict compliance with his prescribed therapy is essential. Routine administration of eye drops can prevent further increases in intraocular pressure and prevent loss of vision.**

     4. This information is important but not as necessary as information about the importance of compliance.

CLASSIFICATION
Competency:
Changes in Health
Taxonomy:
Critical Thinking

86. 1. Follow-up appointments will be scheduled and will help him to feel supported. They will likely help with compliance. However, they are not likely to be the most effective intervention for assisting Mr. Patterson to accept the glaucoma.

     2. **Encouraging Mr. Patterson to discuss his condition and express his concerns will help to decrease his anxiety and help him to deal with the diagnosis of a chronic illness.**

CLASSIFICATION
Competency:
Nurse–Client Partnership
Taxonomy:
Critical Thinking

Answers Exam 2

3. This intervention will provide Mr. Patterson with additional information to assist him to manage his glaucoma but is not likely to be as effective as discussing his feelings and concerns.
4. The family may need to be involved with the treatment regimen and will provide support, but that will not help him to accept his condition as much as being able to verbalize his feelings.

CASE 22

87.   **1. In the initial stage of group process, the leader's responsibility is to create an atmosphere of respect and trust. He can demonstrate respect through common manners of introducing himself and his role.**

CLASSIFICATION
Competency:
Nurse–Client Partnership
Taxonomy:
Critical Thinking

2. This statement may be the next most important one as it states the purpose of the group (i.e., what goals the group aims to accomplish).
3. Although it is important to provide timing for the group, this initial statement may not be perceived as welcoming.
4. While a group task is to get to know each other, this is best left until after the initial "housekeeping" activities have occurred.

88.   1. Mr. Pao may view this approach as an authoritative statement that does not demonstrate respect.
2. This statement is a breach of confidentiality.

CLASSIFICATION
Competency:
Nurse–Client Partnership
Taxonomy:
Critical Thinking

3. It is often helpful with a new group to start the dialogue with a specific person since many will not want to be the first to speak. This question invites Ms. Halsey to describe her experiences rather than label her with a diagnosis.

4. This statement is not likely to elicit volunteers to begin the conversation.

89.   **1. This statement applies principles of effective group process by involving all members in establishing group norms.**

CLASSIFICATION
Competency:
Nurse–Client Partnership
Taxonomy:
Critical Thinking

2. While this statement may be true, the nurse's saying the group is not working may make the clients anxious and may be perceived to be punitive.
3. While this statement may be true, the problem is not just that the group members are interrupting each other. This statement does not seek a solution.
4. While the nurse may be disappointed and may share this feeling with the group, it does not seek a solution to the dysfunction.

90.   1. This response does not respect the client's choice to use alternative therapies.
2. While the nurse should support the client's choice, he needs to first find out if she has made an informed choice.

CLASSIFICATION
Competency:
Health and Wellness
Taxonomy:
Critical Thinking

3. While this response is supportive of the client's choice, there has been controversy about the effectiveness of St. John's wort. Also, the nurse needs to find out if the client has made an informed choice.

4. **This open-ended question enables the nurse to find out if the client is making an informed choice regarding St. John's wort.**

CASE 23

91. 1. This response may elicit only a "yes" or "no" from Mr. Desjardins, and it may make him feel defensive.

2. **The nurse should demonstrate to Mr. Desjardins recognition of his verbalized concern and a willingness to listen.**

CLASSIFICATION
Competency:
Nurse–Client Partnership
Taxonomy:
Application

3. Avoiding the question indicates that the nurse is unwilling to listen.
4. This response could increase anxiety rather than reduce worry; furthermore, it cuts off communication and denies Mr. Desjardins's feelings.

92. 1. Postoperative hemorrhage is a danger with liver disease and use of anticoagulants, not age.
2. Fluctuating blood glucose levels are a concern for people with diabetes, not people of advanced age.
3. Renal failure is associated with dehydration and an electrolyte imbalance, not age.

CLASSIFICATION
Competency:
Changes in Health
Taxonomy:
Application

4. **Older adults are at increased risk for delayed wound healing and decreased tolerance to anaesthesia.**

93. 1. Age and sex affect pain perception only indirectly.
2. Overall physical condition may affect one's ability to cope with stress, but it would not greatly affect pain perception.
3. Intelligence is a factor in understanding pain, but it does not affect the perception of pain intensity; economic status has no effect on pain perception.

CLASSIFICATION
Competency:
Health and Wellness
Taxonomy:
Critical Thinking

4. **Interpretation of pain sensations is highly individual and is based on past experiences, which include cultural values.**

94. 1. Abdominal pain will not be prevented by sitting on the edge of the bed.
2. There should be no circulation problems with his legs and feet by the morning after surgery.
3. He may experience shallow breathing due to the abdominal incision, but this is not respiratory distress and is not prevented by sitting on the side of the bed.

CLASSIFICATION
Competency:
Changes in Health
Taxonomy:
Critical Thinking

Answers Exam 2

4. Following the administration of narcotics, the client's neurocirculatory reflexes may have some difficulty adjusting to the force of gravity when an upright position is assumed. Postural or orthostatic hypotension occurs, and the blood supply to the brain is temporarily decreased.

---

95. 1. Pain in the calf may be a sign of thrombophlebitis, a possible postoperative complication. If the thrombus becomes dislodged, it may lead to pulmonary embolism. Any client with this complaint should immediately be confined to bed.

CLASSIFICATION
Competency:
Changes in Health
Taxonomy:
Application

2. The physician needs to be notified, but this is not the first action.
3. The application of heat may be contraindicated if a thrombus has developed.
4. The leg should not be elevated above heart level without a physician's order; gravity may dislodge the thrombus, creating an embolism.

CASE 24

96. 1. Degenerative osteoarthritis affects the weight-bearing joints, such as knees, hips, and spine, and is not usually symmetrical.

CLASSIFICATION
Competency:
Changes in Health
Taxonomy:
Knowledge/Comprehension

2. This finding is true of rheumatoid arthritis.
3. Same as answer 2.
4. Same as answer 2.

---

97. 1. This position is unacceptable because the knees must be bent; this position would cause hip flexion, stressing the joint.
2. Pressure on the operative site may cause unnecessary pain and impair circulation necessary for healing.

CLASSIFICATION
Competency:
Changes in Health
Taxonomy:
Application

3. Supine or on the unaffected side is the position of choice; however, a wedge, thigh spreader, or pillows must be used to maintain abduction of the affected thigh. Adduction can result in displacement of the prosthesis.

4. A low semi-Fowler position would cause flexion of the hip and put stress on the prosthesis, possibly causing it to become loose.

---

98. 1. The client must be turned at least every 2 hours to help prevent the complications of immobility. Three hours is too long to keep a client in one position.

CLASSIFICATION
Competency:
Changes in Health
Taxonomy:
Application

2. Ankle movement, particularly dorsiflexion of the foot, allows muscle contraction, which compresses veins, reducing venous stasis and the risk of thrombus formation.

3. It is too soon for this action.

4. It is too soon for this action, and sitting in a low chair is contraindicated because hip flexion can cause displacement of the prosthesis.

---

99. 1. **This position supports the operative site; the involved leg must be maintained in alignment, avoiding adduction.**

2. The pillow will not affect venous return, which relates to thrombus formation.
3. Adduction, not flexion, contractures are of most concern after surgery.
4. Although friction is decreased when skin does not interface with skin, this is not the reason for separating the thighs and lower limbs.

CLASSIFICATION
Competency:
Changes in Health
Taxonomy:
Application

---

100. 1. Ms. Kovacs will need initial intensive physiotherapy that would not be able to be provided at home with biweekly community supports. Her living arrangements, living alone in a two-storey house, are not appropriate for rehabilitation care.
2. Ms. Kovacs does not require this level of care.
3. This plan is not the best use of limited acute care facilities.

4. **Ms. Kovacs will require intensive physiotherapy to enable her to regain mobility. This can best be achieved at a rehabilitation centre.**

CLASSIFICATION
Competency:
Professional Practice
Taxonomy:
Critical Thinking

INDEPENDENT QUESTIONS ANSWERS AND RATIONALES

101. 1. The night shift may not have time to do the dressings either. Leaving the care to the night shift demonstrates a lack of accountability and will also cause a delay in Mr. Megadichan receiving care.
2. This delegation is inappropriate. The dressings are complex and require skills and knowledge beyond those of an unregulated care provider.
3. Documenting does not solve the problem of the wounds requiring care by the nurse.

4. **This option is the only one that involves a possible solution to the need to complete the dressing changes and provide safe care to Mr. Megadichan.**

CLASSIFICATION
Competency:
Professional Practice
Taxonomy:
Critical Thinking

102. 1. This consequence will result if the cuff is too wide.

2. **This consequence will result from a loosely or unevenly wrapped cuff.**

3. This consequence will result if multiple caregivers use different interpretations of Korotkoff sounds.
4. This consequence will result from too rapid deflation of the cuff.

CLASSIFICATION
Competency:
Health and Wellness
Taxonomy:
Application

103. 1. The physician is responsible for obtaining consent for only those procedures that she is performing.
2. A nurse may sign a written consent as a witness to a client signature; however, the witness does not have to be a nurse.

3. **If a nurse is performing a procedure, it is she who must obtain consent.**

4. Consent may be written, verbal, or implied.

CLASSIFICATION
Competency:
Professional Practice
Taxonomy:
Knowledge/Comprehension

104. 1. **Diabetic retinopathy is a common complication of poorly controlled diabetes. People with diabetes need to have their eyes examined on a routine basis by an ophthalmologist or optometrist.**

2. It is important to test the blood, but it should be done daily rather than weekly.
3. This action is not necessary unless blood sugar levels are very high.
4. There is no need to reduce the number of hours worked unless Ms. Karmally's lifestyle is interfering with her management of the diabetes.

CLASSIFICATION
Competency:
Changes in Health
Taxonomy:
Application

105. 1. This action is not appropriate. There is no cause for a report.
2. There is no evidence of inappropriate behaviour.

CLASSIFICATION
Competency:
Professional Practice

3. It would be inappropriate to approach Ms. Walters; it would likely upset her and could lead to legal and professional sanctions against the nurse.

Taxonomy:
Application

4. **There is no indication that the nurse's action was anything other than therapeutic touch. It is prejudicial to assume sexual behaviour just because the nurse is a lesbian.**

---

106. 1. **Professional misconduct is behaviour that would be considered a fundamental breach of nursing ethics, conduct that discredits the profession. Falsely claiming sick benefits is professional misconduct.**

2. Incompetence relates to a lack of knowledge, skills, or judgement required to provide safe comprehensive care.
3. Malpractice is negligence performed in professional practice, an unreasonable lack of skill, or illegal or immoral conduct that results in the injury of a client.
4. Accountability is being responsible for one's actions and the consequences of those actions. There is no indication that the nurse accepts or does not accept responsibility for her actions.

CLASSIFICATION
Competency:
Professional Practice
Taxonomy:
Application

---

107. 1. **The age of consent varies from province to province. In some provinces, it is 16 years. In Ontario, there is no minimum age of consent.**

2. An adolescent may be capable of mature and informed decisions, but it is the legality that is at issue.
3. Cassandra's ability to give consent depends on the provincial legislation regarding age of consent, and not whether her parents are available.
4. Adolescents have the capacity to choose between alternatives but may not have the legal right in this situation, depending on provincial legislation.

CLASSIFICATION
Competency:
Professional Practice
Taxonomy:
Application

---

108. 1. **Thrush, also called moniliasis and candidiasis, usually affects the mucous membranes of the oral cavity, causing painful white patches. Individuals with immunological deficiencies, those receiving prolonged antibiotic therapy, and infants are particularly susceptible to this organism.**

2. Dysentery is usually caused by an amoeba or a bacterium; it is not common in infants.
3. Impetigo is a bacterial infection of the skin caused by streptococci or staphylococci.
4. This infectious condition of the skin is a result of infestation by mites.

CLASSIFICATION
Competency:
Changes in Health
Taxonomy:
Knowledge/Comprehension

---

109. 1. **Nurses may not discriminate on cultural, socioeconomic, or health status grounds.**

CLASSIFICATION
Competency:
Professional Practice

2. This action allows the nurse to choose clients based on her biases, not professional ethics.
3. This action is not ethically permitted in Canada.
4. This possible solution to the problem does not change this particular situation. As well, it is unlikely that the nurse will find an area of practice that meets the criteria for her personal ethics.

Taxonomy:
Application

---

110. 1. Selection does not have a major influence on eating habits.
    2. Food's smell and appearance certainly have some influence, though not major, on eating habits at this age.

    3. **The early-school-aged child has become a cooperative member of the family and will mimic parents' attitudes and food habits readily.**

    4. The peer group does not become highly influential until a later school age and adolescence.

CLASSIFICATION
Competency:
Health and Wellness
Taxonomy:
Knowledge/Comprehension

---

111. 1. Feeding may proceed immediately after opening the tube.

    2. **Positioning the infant on the right side after feeding facilitates digestion because the pyloric sphincter is on this side and gravity aids in emptying the stomach.**

    3. It is standard procedure to flush the tube with water, not normal saline, after the feeding to ensure that all the formula gets into the stomach; it is not necessary before the feeding.
    4. The usual height for the elevation of the gastrostomy tube when feeding an infant is 15 to 20 cm.

CLASSIFICATION
Competency:
Changes in Health
Taxonomy:
Application

---

112. 1. This weight is within the normal range. The average birth weight is about 3200 g.

    2. **An Apgar score of 3 indicates neonatal distress and should signal to the nurse that the infant requires close supervision and support.**

    3. A positive Babinski reflex is normal through the age of 2 years.
    4. It is normal to detect the pulse of cerebrospinal fluid in the fontanelle of an infant.

CLASSIFICATION
Competency:
Changes in Health
Taxonomy:
Application

---

113. 1. The nurse cannot administer medication without authorization from a registered prescriber.
    2. The nurse must get a physician's order for the medication and cannot accept the parent's information alone.
    3. The nurse does not know if Samantha should have the medication and must consult with the physician.

CLASSIFICATION
Competency:
Professional Practice
Taxonomy:
Knowledge/Comprehension

4. A nurse should not administer these medications without a prescription. The nurse should also ensure that the doctor is aware of Samantha's allergies before the surgery.

---

114. 1. This calculation is incorrect.
     2. Same as answer 1.

     3. This calculation is correct:
        0.4 mg = 1 mL
        0.3 mg = 1 mL ÷ 0.4 × 0.3 = 0.75 mL

     4. Same as answer 1.

CLASSIFICATION
Competency:
Professional Practice
Taxonomy:
Application

---

115. 1. This action would constrict blood vessels and impair absorption.
     2. Deep penetration is necessary; only the ventral gluteal muscles should be used because of their size and the decreased visibility of staining.
     3. This action should be avoided. It might cause seepage of the drug into the muscle, with subsequent tissue irritation and staining.

     4. Residual medication on the needle may stain and irritate the tissues during penetration.

CLASSIFICATION
Competency:
Professional Practice
Taxonomy:
Application

---

116. 1. Humans are sexual from birth to death. Consenting older adults engaging in intercourse are no different from younger adults and must be afforded the same respect. Resident rooms in a long-term care facility are considered the clients' homes. The nurse should not have entered the room without knocking and asking permission to enter.

     2. This action is not appropriate. The nurse witnessed a private relationship and does not need to share what she saw with the nursing team.
     3. To ask would be an interruption. The couple should already have privacy in his room. At another time, the nurse could discuss with the resident the possibility of changing rooms to one that may offer more privacy.
     4. This action is not appropriate or, obviously, necessary.

CLASSIFICATION
Competency:
Professional Practice
Taxonomy:
Critical Thinking

---

117. 1. While side rails are considered a restraint, when making an occupied bed, the nurse may raise one rail at a time for safety, but not both.

     2. This action minimizes strain on the back. It is easier to remove and apply linen evenly when the bed is in a flat position, and a comfortable height provides easy access to the bed and linen.

     3. The equipment is assembled before starting the procedure, but it should be placed on a clean chair or overbed table. Placing it on the bottom of the bed puts it on the soiled linen and interferes with the making of the bed.

CLASSIFICATION
Competency:
Professional Practice
Taxonomy:
Knowledge/Comprehension

Answers Exam 2

4. The client is covered with the bath blanket, and then the soiled top sheet is removed. This provides for client warmth and comfort.

---

118. 1. This statement makes an assumption that another pregnancy will ensue; it also cuts off further communication.

2. This statement allows both partners to comfort each other and lets them know the nurse is available; it also allows them to recognize and accept their feelings of loss.

CLASSIFICATION
Competency:
Nurse–Client Partnership
Taxonomy:
Application

3. Telling clients not to be upset cuts off communication and wrongly implies that sadness prolongs recovery.
4. Grieving for the unborn child will and should occur during any period of pregnancy.

---

119. 1. This response closes off discussion and is not necessarily true.
2. This response is not necessarily true, and there are some established risks in taking hormone replacement therapy.
3. The nurse should avoid recommendations based on personal beliefs. It is up to the client to decide.

CLASSIFICATION
Competency:
Professional Practice
Taxonomy:
Application

4. The woman is best to discuss treatment options with her physician to get full information. The physician should be aware of any herbal supplements the woman is taking. After the discussion, if the woman chooses, she can safely try alternative therapies for symptom relief.

---

120. **1. Inadequate oxygenation of the brain may produce restlessness or behavioural changes. The pulse and respiration rates increase as a compensatory mechanism for hypoxia.**

CLASSIFICATION
Competency:
Changes in Health
Taxonomy:
Application

2. The pupils dilate with cerebral hypoxia.
3. The pulse and respiration rates increase with hypoxia.
4. There will be cyanosis at a later stage. Dyspnea may or may not be present.

---

121. 1. This vitamin is fat soluble and stored in the body.

2. Vitamin C is water soluble and not stored in the body.

CLASSIFICATION
Competency:
Health and Wellness
Taxonomy:
Knowledge/Comprehension

3. Same as answer 1.
4. Same as answer 1.

---

122. 1. This action needs to be done but is not the first priority.
2. The nurse does need to immediately alert the other staff, but not by yelling, "Fire," which may cause residents to panic.

CLASSIFICATION
Competency:
Professional Practice
Taxonomy:
Critical Thinking

3. This action should be done as soon as possible, but removing Mrs. Cummings is the priority.

4. Client safety is the nurse's first priority. Mrs. Cummings must be removed from danger.

---

123. 1. This action is not necessary. Febrile seizures are generally not a medical emergency.

   2. Febrile seizures are frightening but generally harmless and usually stop by themselves. The child should be seen by a physician immediately to check on her condition, monitor for other seizures, and advise on temperature control.

   3. Febrile seizures are not related to epilepsy.
   4. The child should be examined by a physician.

CLASSIFICATION
Competency:
Changes in Health
Taxonomy:
Application

---

124. 1. This action would be a wise initial action if there were a safe place to take the residents. However, the carpet has been installed throughout the facility.
   2. This action is beneficial, but the most immediate concern is to inform management of the possible dangers of the chemical exposure.

   3. Management needs to be made aware of the situation so that corrective action may be taken and staff and clients protected.

   4. This action will need to be done but is not the initial action.

CLASSIFICATION
Competency:
Professional Practice
Taxonomy:
Critical Thinking

---

125. **1. Pervasive developmental disorder (PDD) and autistic spectrum disorder have a wide range in severity of clinical manifestations and cognitive and behavioural outcomes. Early recognition and early interventions help to manage the disorder. It is not possible at the time of diagnosis to predict eventual functioning.**

   2. It is not possible to predict this outcome when the child is 2 years old.
   3. Same as answer 2.
   4. PDD is not a degenerative disorder.

CLASSIFICATION
Competency:
Changes in Health
Taxonomy:
Knowledge/Comprehension

---

126. 1. It is not up to the client to determine the orders of the physician.

   2. The nurse is legally responsible for ensuring that he implements the physician orders correctly. The only way to do this is to speak directly with the physician.

   3. The physician, not another nurse, must clarify the physician's orders.
   4. It is the responsibility of the ordering physician to clarify his orders.

CLASSIFICATION
Competency:
Professional Practice
Taxonomy:
Application

Answers Exam 2

127.   1. Same as answer 3.
    2. Same as answer 3.

CLASSIFICATION
Competency:
Professional Practice
Taxonomy:
Application

    3. Passwords should never be shared. Passwords protect client confidentiality. The medical student should have her own password if allowed access to the chart.

    4. Same as answer 3.

128.   1. Being a doctor may be a big part of this client's self-esteem, and this remark threatens that self-esteem.

CLASSIFICATION
Competency:
Nurse–Client Partnership
Taxonomy:
Application

    2. This response simply states facts without getting involved in role conflict.

    3. Firm, consistent limits need to be set so that the nurse–client role is established.
    4. This response could be viewed as a threat and is more about the nurse's need than the client's behaviour.

129.   1. The most effective therapy method is for the child to play out his feelings; when feelings are allowed to surface, the child can then learn to face them by controlling, accepting, or abandoning them. Through this process, the child can experience growth.

CLASSIFICATION
Competency:
Changes in Health
Taxonomy:
Application

    2. This therapy is not child specific and, generally, is more suited for adolescents, young adults, and adults.
    3. Same as answer 2.
    4. Same as answer 2.

130.   1. Urate excretion is enhanced by high doses of aspirin.
    2. Aspirin is readily broken down in the gastrointestinal tract and liver.

CLASSIFICATION
Competency:
Changes in Health
Taxonomy:
Application

    3. Aspirin interferes with platelet aggregation, thereby lengthening bleeding time.

    4. Aspirin inhibits platelet aggregation; it does not destroy erythrocytes.

131.   1. This response does not present a therapeutic solution to the situation. The nurse is aiding the client.
    2. This response places the responsibility on the client, but she may not be compliant with the nurse's advice.

CLASSIFICATION
Competency:
Nurse–Client Partnership
Taxonomy:
Critical Thinking

    3. This response supports the client and also ensures that the physician will be informed of the client's drinking.

    4. This response implies the nurse is functioning by rules, not by nursing standards.

132. 1. This response is too technical and would not be understood by an 11-year-old.

2. **This response provides accurate information in a manner easily understood.**

CLASSIFICATION
Competency:
Changes in Health
Taxonomy:
Critical Thinking

3. This response is partly true but is not a complete answer and is too simplistic for an 11-year-old.
4. Same as answer 3.

133. 1. **With aging, the taste buds become less sensitive.**

CLASSIFICATION
Competency:
Health and Wellness
Taxonomy:
Critical Thinking

2. This response may be true but is not the most accurate explanation.
3. Same as answer 2.
4. Same as answer 2.

134. 1. Pregnancy temporarily suppresses ovarian function; the aberrant endometrial tissue is still present.
2. Endometriosis may lead to sterility; it does not cause menopause.
3. Conservative medical therapy will be used first; a hysterectomy is a last resort.

CLASSIFICATION
Competency:
Changes in Health
Taxonomy:
Application

4. **Lactation delays ovarian function after delivery. It also therefore delays the symptoms of endometriosis.**

135. 1. Ice chips must not be given until the gag reflex returns.
2. Coughing should not be encouraged; it might initiate bleeding from the site of the biopsy.

CLASSIFICATION
Competency:
Changes in Health
Taxonomy:
Application

3. **After administration of a local anaesthetic during a bronchoscopy, fluids and food should be withheld until the gag reflex returns.**

4. To allow drainage and minimize the possibility of aspiration, the client should be kept in a semi-Fowler position.

136. 1. It is not an opiate.
2. It is not a depressant.

CLASSIFICATION
Competency:
Health and Wellness
Taxonomy:
Knowledge/Comprehension

3. **Ecstasy is a hallucinogenic that produces a heightened sense of awareness, distortions of time, and hallucinations. It is taken to heighten the individual's response to noise, music, and bright lights.**

4. It is not an antihypertensive.

137. 1. The trauma of surgery will result in some blood loss, which will continue until coagulation takes place; this time range is too short for coagulation to occur.

CLASSIFICATION
Competency:
Changes in Health

2. Same as answer 1.

3. **The trauma of surgery normally results in some seeping or oozing of blood into the remaining gastric area for approximately 12 hours. This blood is immediately suctioned out of the body via the nasogastric tube.**

Taxonomy:
Application

4. It is abnormal for the light red liquid to still be draining 24 to 48 hours after surgery; the physician should be notified.

---

138. 1. There is no correlation between high blood sugars and peptic ulcers.

2. **Smoking increases the acidity of gastrointestinal secretions, which damages the mucosal barrier.**

3. Weight is unrelated to peptic ulcer disease.
4. High blood pressure is not directly related to peptic ulcer disease.

CLASSIFICATION
Competency:
Changes in Health
Taxonomy:
Knowledge/Comprehension

---

139. 1. This manifestation occurs when the pooling of blood in the peripheral vessels causes hypotension; it rarely occurs with hypervolemia.
2. Rhinitis would not be a manifestation of congestive heart failure.
3. An increased fluid volume in the intravascular compartment (overhydration) will cause the pulse to feel full and bounding.

4. **An increase in the extracellular fluid volume can cause a relative decrease in the hemoglobin and hematocrit by dilution of the blood.**

CLASSIFICATION
Competency:
Changes in Health
Taxonomy:
Application

---

140. 1. Although this aspect of hand hygiene is important, without friction it has minimal value.
2. Although soap reduces surface tension, without friction it has minimal value.
3. Although water flushes some microorganisms from the skin, without friction it has minimal value.

4. **Friction is necessary for the removal of microorganisms.**

CLASSIFICATION
Competency:
Professional Practice
Taxonomy:
Critical Thinking

---

141. 1. Ms. Tang has not provided consent for the picture to be taken. For confidentiality reasons, the photo must not be saved.
2. Ms. Tang may not wish her family to see the photo. There is no indication Ms. Tang has provided consent for the photo to be shown.
3. Same as answer 1.

4. **Taking the picture in itself is a breach of confidentiality. The photo must be immediately deleted.**

CLASSIFICATION
Competency:
Professional Practice
Taxonomy:
Application

142. 1. For the level of care she needs, Mrs. Eigo does not require an RN.
2. For the level of care she needs, Mrs. Eigo does not require a registered or licensed practical nurse.
3. Mrs. Eigo does not require the services of a geriatric activation therapist.

4. A personal support worker (PSW) or unregulated care provider (UCP) is most suitable for Mrs. Eigo. The PSW or UCP has the education and skills to assist a client with the activities of daily living.

CLASSIFICATION
Competency:
Professional Practice
Taxonomy:
Critical Thinking

143. 1. *Coxiella burnetii*, a *Rickettsia*, is not part of the normal flora; it is spread by contact with infected animals, drinking of contaminated milk, or the bite of a vector tick.

2. Candidiasis (a *Candida* infection) arises in certain individuals when local resistance is decreased through prolonged antibiotic therapy or with certain diseases (e.g., diabetes) and debilitating conditions (e.g., drug addiction).

CLASSIFICATION
Competency:
Changes in Health
Taxonomy:
Knowledge/Comprehension

3. *Streptococci* would be responsive to antibiotic therapy and are not considered part of the normal flora.
4. The varicella zoster virus is not part of the normal flora.

144. 1. This response is evasive; the client is left without direction.
2. There are concerns with taking hormone replacement therapy (HRT), but this response would alarm Ms. Mengal.
3. Herbal supplements are not always the best option for treating the symptoms of surgical menopause.

4. The use of hormones is controversial and needs to be discussed with a physician.

CLASSIFICATION
Competency:
Health and Wellness
Taxonomy:
Application

145. 1. Palpation of the prostate gland is not a definitive diagnosis; it reveals only size and configuration.
2. This test is not done unless prostatic cancer is suspected.

3. A definitive diagnosis relies on a cluster of symptoms of prostatism, a decrease in flow, and a cystoscopic exam.

CLASSIFICATION
Competency:
Changes in Health
Taxonomy:
Application

4. An elevated prostate-specific antigen (PSA) level indicates a prostate condition but not the pathophysiology of the condition.

146. 1. An accurate specific gravity cannot be obtained when irrigating solutions are being instilled into the bladder.
2. Hourly outputs are indicated only if there is concern about renal failure or oliguria.

CLASSIFICATION
Competency:
Changes in Health
Taxonomy:
Application

3. **The total amount of irrigation solution instilled into the bladder is eliminated with the urine and, therefore, must be subtracted from the total output to determine the volume of urine excreted.**

4. Twenty-four-hour urine tests would not be accurate if the client were receiving continuous irrigation.

---

147. 1. Gauze dressing would not reinforce the suture line.

2. **Additional gauze at the base would ensure that drainage resulting from gravity would be absorbed.**

3. Gravity during ambulation would cause the drainage to flow downward.
4. A pressure dressing is not necessary.

CLASSIFICATION
Competency:
Changes in Health
Taxonomy:
Application

---

148. 1. Both physicians and nurses mutually accepted the practice.
2. Hospitals appreciate cost cutting, but evidence-informed practice was not a hospital initiative.

3. **This statement accurately reflects the origin of the concept.**

4. Although much information is shared over the Internet, this statement does not describe the origin of the concept.

CLASSIFICATION
Competency:
Professional Practice
Taxonomy:
Application

---

149. 1. **This action is the correct procedure. The direction of cleansing moves from the area of least contamination to the area of most contamination, preventing microorganisms from entering the urethra.**

2. The tip around the meatus is cleansed first.
3. The foreskin will need to be retracted, but the meatus is cleansed first.
4. Cleansing in upward strokes would move microorganisms toward the urethra.

CLASSIFICATION
Competency:
Health and Wellness
Taxonomy:
Application

---

150. 1. He might not choose a safe helmet.
2. A preschool child may not be able to understand the safety implications.
3. Rewards may work but will not be effective if the child is riding a bike when the parent is not there to provide the reward.

4. **Children learn best from effective role models.**

CLASSIFICATION
Competency:
Health and Wellness
Taxonomy:
Application

---

151. 1. The nurse is not permitted to change an ordered dose of medication unless there has been a previous medical directive.

2. **This is the most professional and legally acceptable choice. It enables the nurse to provide pain medication to the client in a timely fashion.**

CLASSIFICATION
Competency:
Professional Practice
Taxonomy:
Application

3. This action is not professional.

4. These therapies are unlikely to provide the required level of pain relief.

---

152. 1. Diphtheria, tetanus, pertussis (DtaP) is given at ages 2 months, 4 months, 6 months, and 18 months.

2. **Measles, mumps, rubella (MMR) is given at 12 months.**

3. Hib is most often administered before 6 months of age.

4. Ava requires her MMR.

CLASSIFICATION
Competency:
Health and Wellness
Taxonomy:
Knowledge/Comprehension

---

153. 1. **This response is factual.**

2. The fontanelle is not typically larger in children with Down syndrome.

3. All infants have incomplete closure of the bones in their skulls at birth.

4. Children with Down syndrome typically do not have premature closure of the fontanelle.

CLASSIFICATION
Competency:
Changes in Health
Taxonomy:
Application

---

154. 1. This inference is a stereotype.

2. Same as answer 1.

3. Same as answer 1.

4. **This inference recognizes that, above and beyond any cultural health practices, clients are individuals.**

CLASSIFICATION
Competency:
Professional Practice
Taxonomy:
Application

---

155. 1. Two days' time is too late. It will be assumed that the ampicillin was not administered.

2. This action is not necessary unless made so by an agency policy.

3. **Since there is no policy, the nurse must consult with a supervisor to determine the appropriate action.**

4. This action may be appropriate if determined so after consultation with the nursing supervisor.

CLASSIFICATION
Competency:
Professional Practice
Taxonomy:
Application

---

156. 1. **The nurse is responsible for providing the client with knowledge about all treatment options. As a first step, the nurse must assess and discuss the effectiveness of the herbal preparation.**

2. The nurse does not decide for clients what choices they should make about treatment.

3. This action can be done, but the client has already stated a preference for the herbal preparation. This response by the nurse indicates a bias for her own treatment preferences.

CLASSIFICATION
Competency:
Professional Practice
Taxonomy:
Application

4. The nurse should support Ms. Holly's decision but only after the client is given all the information about the herbal preparation and the antihypertensive.

---

157. 1. This finding is normal and is related to premenstrual syndrome.
2. These findings are normal in the third trimester of pregnancy. The yellowish fluid is colostrum.

CLASSIFICATION

Competency:

Changes in Health

Taxonomy:

Critical Thinking

3. **Although men do not have the same incidence of breast cancer as women, the finding of a lump in the breast area is of concern as it may be cancerous.**

4. These findings happen occasionally in newborn males as a result of hormones from the mother and will subside in several days.

---

158. 1. This consideration is important but not the priority.
2. Same as answer 1.
3. Same as answer 1.

CLASSIFICATION

Competency:

Changes in Health

Taxonomy:

Critical Thinking

4. **Clients with post-traumatic stress disorder may experience aggressive outbursts, use violence to solve problems, and display suicidal thoughts. The safety of the client and others is a priority.**

---

159. 1. Formal religion does not necessarily relate to spirituality. This question may be asked later in the interview.
2. This question should be asked but is not necessarily part of a spiritual assessment nor an initial question.

CLASSIFICATION

Competency:

Professional Practice

Taxonomy:

Critical Thinking

3. **Spirituality is unique to each adult. All people are considered to be spiritual whether or not they have a religious affiliation. This question would be appropriate as an initial question that could lead to gathering more specific information about the client's belief system.**

4. This question is important to ask but is not the best initial question when exploring spirituality with a client.

---

160. 1. This action is appropriate after a history has been taken.
2. This offer will definitely be made to Candace at some point in her care but is not the first action.

CLASSIFICATION

Competency:

Health and Wellness

Taxonomy:

Critical Thinking

3. **This action is the nurse's priority. The nurse needs more information to be able to determine the next action and to provide necessary information to the sexual assault team.**

4. This action will need to be done but is not the first action. It would be traumatic to Candace for a vaginal exam to happen first. If the hospital has a sexual assault team, they will perform the exam.

161.   1. This statement is not necessarily true and does not allow the client to voice her concerns.

   2. This response is open ended and allows the client to voice her concerns.

   3. This response assumes the woman's concerns are related to stages of labour and closes discussion.
   4. This response makes an assumption that may not be correct.

CLASSIFICATION
Competency:
Changes in Health
Taxonomy:
Application

162.   1. This action will help the infant not to lose heat from the head but is not the most effective action to reduce heat loss and warm the baby.
   2. This action will help warm the infant through body heat but is not the most effective method.

   3. This action is the most effective to prevent further heat loss and to warm the infant. Hypothermia is a danger for premature infants and places them at risk for other complications.

   4. This action is not the most effective for raising the body temperature of a premature infant and may cause further cooling due to loss of heat from evaporating water on the skin.

CLASSIFICATION
Competency:
Changes in Health
Taxonomy:
Critical Thinking

163.   1. This parent's situation is a stressor but does not necessarily predispose the parent to child abuse.

   2. A risk factor for abusing a child is having experienced previous abuse.

   3. Same as answer 1.
   4. Same as answer 1.

CLASSIFICATION
Competency:
Changes in Health
Taxonomy:
Critical Thinking

164.   1. Such devices may likely be needed and are important to recommend to Mr. and Mrs. Cooke, but this is not the most important assessment.
   2. This assessment is important to ensure that Mr. Cooke uses mild moisturizers that do not dry out sensitive skin.
   3. The need for assistive devices should be determined once Mrs. Cooke's cognitive and musculoskeletal functions have been determined, but this is not the most important assessment.

   4. Because Mrs. Cooke is in the early stages of Alzheimer's disease, she is likely able to manage many of her own hygiene needs. The nurse's primary responsibility is to determine if Mrs. Cooke has the cognitive ability and the coordination to bathe herself.

CLASSIFICATION
Competency:
Health and Wellness
Taxonomy:
Critical Thinking

165.   1. There is no known correlation between chicken pox and insulin.

   2. Steroids have an anti-inflammatory effect. It is believed that resistance to certain viral diseases, including chicken pox, is greatly decreased when a child is taking steroids regularly.

CLASSIFICATION
Competency:
Health and Wellness
Taxonomy:
Application

3. Since chicken pox is viral, antibiotics would have no effect.
4. There is no known correlation between chicken pox and anticonvulsants.

166.
1. This action will promote regurgitation.
2. This action will probably have little effect on reflux.
3. This action will promote vomiting since it is too much formula for a week-old infant.

4. Some mild reflux is common in newborn infants. Reflux results from an incompetent cardiac sphincter, which allows a reflux of gastric contents into the esophagus and eventual regurgitation. Although there is some research that finds positioning of the infant has no effect on regurgitation, the general practice is to place the infant in an upright position, which uses gravity to help keep the gastric contents in the stomach and also limits the pressure against the cardiac sphincter.

CLASSIFICATION

Competency:

Changes in Health

Taxonomy:

Application

167.
1. During the 1970s, elevated estrogen and progesterone levels associated with pregnancy were viewed as protective against depression. This hypothesis is now known to be untrue.
2. Signs and symptoms of depression in pregnancy do not differ from depression at any other time of life.
3. Antenatal depression occurs most frequently in the last two trimesters.

4. Women who have antenatal depression have a 6.5-fold increased risk of postpartum depression.

CLASSIFICATION

Competency:

Changes in Health

Taxonomy:

Knowledge/Comprehension

168.
1. This option is probably not realistic.

2. A preceptor should assist with a learning plan, and the nurse should feel comfortable asking for learning resources and feedback on performance. The preceptor should assess the progress of the nurse and not intimidate her.

CLASSIFICATION

Competency:

Professional Practice

Taxonomy:

Application

3. This action does not aid in forming a supportive relationship, nor is it true.
4. It would be unrealistic to assume that the nurse could learn about all the medications. The preceptor, however, would be able to suggest a learning plan.

169.
1. Stimulating the gag reflex will have no effect on the action of ipecac and may frighten the child.
2. Resting has no effect on drug efficacy.

3. Ipecac syrup exerts its effect through direct stimulation of the vomiting control centre and local irritation of the gastric mucosa; ipecac syrup's effects are enhanced through dilution of the drug in large quantities of fluid.

CLASSIFICATION

Competency:

Changes in Health

Taxonomy:

Application

4. The child should be kept calm and quiet.

170.   1. This calculation is correct:

$20 \text{ mg} = x \text{ mL}$

$50 \text{ mg} = 1 \text{ mL}$

$50x = 20 \text{ mg}$

$x = 20 \div 50 = 0.4 \text{ mL}$

CLASSIFICATION

Competency:

Professional Practice

Taxonomy:

Application

2. This calculation is incorrect; the dose is too high.
3. Same as answer 2.
4. Same as answer 2.

---

171.   1. Although this position may be comfortable for some individuals, rubbing the back and alternating positions are more universally effective.
2. The supine position places increased pressure on the back and often aggravates the pain.

CLASSIFICATION

Competency:

Health and Wellness

Taxonomy:

Application

3. **The application of back pressure, combined with frequent positional changes, will help alleviate Ms. Clarke's discomfort.**

4. Abdominal breathing is used to teach relaxation in labour; it will not relieve back pain.

---

172.   1. This recommendation will not solve the problem; besides, he cannot nap at work.
2. This recommendation does not solve the client's problem.

CLASSIFICATION

Competency:

Health and Wellness

Taxonomy:

Application

3. **These signs suggest sleep apnea, which needs to be investigated by a physician.**

4. The client has not stated that he has a problem with insomnia.

---

173.   1. These foods are not rich sources of iron.

CLASSIFICATION

Competency:

Changes in Health

Taxonomy:

Application

2. **Organ meats, green vegetables, and legumes are rich sources of iron.**

3. Pork is a rich source of iron, but these vegetables are not.
4. Meat and potatoes are rich sources of iron, but milk is not.

---

174.   1. This response is not true. Acupuncture does help some clients with chronic pain.
2. Acupuncture is approved in some provinces.

CLASSIFICATION

Competency:

Nurse–Client Partnership

Taxonomy:

Application

3. **The nurse is functioning as a client advocate in assisting the client to act on his decision.**

4. This response ignores what the client has requested and assumes that he is not taking his pain medication correctly.

Answers Exam 2

175. 1. **This action is the most professional and safest for determining the correct client.**

2. The nurse does not know the clients. Mr. Masters may be confused or may not know his name.
3. It is not the responsibility of another client to provide client identification.
4. The individual nurse is responsible for ensuring that she has the correct client. Advice should be asked from other nurses if there is no other means of identification.

CLASSIFICATION
Competency:
Professional Practice
Taxonomy:
Application

176. 1. A child this age needs to know the seriousness of the illness and that recovery may not be possible.
2. Children of this age interpret death as separation and punishment. This response indicates the son will not care what happens to his sister.
3. This response only avoids the question.

4. **Children at early school age are not yet able to comprehend death's universality and inevitability, but they do fear it, often personifying death as a monster or dark angel. They need an opportunity to prepare for this situation.**

CLASSIFICATION
Competency:
Nurse–Client Partnership
Taxonomy:
Critical Thinking

177. 1. It is unrealistic for the couple to refrain from sexual intercourse for the entire pregnancy.
2. Spermicides are of limited effectiveness with the herpes virus.

3. **There is evidence that the herpes virus is shed even when there are no symptoms. In case the client has not already contracted the virus from her husband, the couple should use a condom. The client will likely deliver the child through a Caesarean section.**

4. Washing is not enough to prevent contraction of this virus; contact has already been made.

CLASSIFICATION
Competency:
Changes in Health
Taxonomy:
Application

178. 1. The immediate priority is to prevent harm to the client. Calling for assistance may or may not be indicated later.

2. **This action will provide stability as the nurse lowers the client to the floor.**

3. This action puts an unnecessary strain on the nurse and may cause injury to her.
4. This action may not be feasible and may be a strain for the nurse, causing injury to her.

CLASSIFICATION
Competency:
Professional Practice
Taxonomy:
Application

179. 1. This approach is threatening and nonprofessional.

CLASSIFICATION
Competency:
Professional Practice

2. **This approach is professional. The UCP may not be aware that she is not allowed to use the title "nurse."**

Taxonomy:
Application

3. This action is not professional because it is not supportive of the role of the UCP and may confuse the client.
4. The situation involves only one UCP, and it is likely other caregivers are aware of "nurse" being a protected title.

---

180.   1. **It is often more difficult to detect substance abuse in older adults since it may be masked by chronic disease.**

CLASSIFICATION
Competency:
Health and Wellness
Taxonomy:
Application

2. This statement is not true; abuse also involves alcohol and prescription medications.
3. Alcohol abuse is found in approximately 20% of the general population, not just older adults.
4. Older adults are generally reluctant to discuss the problem.

---

181.   1. There is a strong familial link with keloid formation.
2. This statement offers false reassurance and dismisses Ms. Marie's concern.

CLASSIFICATION
Competency:
Nurse–Client Partnership
Taxonomy:
Application

3. **This statement supports Ms. Marie's concern and provides an option for her to discuss her worry about a scar with the physician.**

4. This outcome cannot be guaranteed.

---

182.   1. These condoms should never be reused as they may retain traces of sperm or microorganisms and may sustain small tears.

CLASSIFICATION
Competency:
Health and Wellness
Taxonomy:
Application

2. **Only water-soluble lubricants should be used for body orifices.**

3. Male and female condoms should not be used together. It may promote tearing, and they do not work smoothly during intercourse.
4. It may be used for this purpose with the inner ring not placed inside.

---

183.   1. **This response is best because it is truthful and provides reassurance about postoperative communication.**

CLASSIFICATION
Competency:
Changes in Health
Taxonomy:
Application

2. This option is not possible.
3. There will be no voice production with a tracheotomy tube with an inflated cuff in place.
4. This response dismisses Ms. Grant's concerns.

---

184.   1. This response is untrue. About 1600 new cases are diagnosed each year.

CLASSIFICATION
Competency:
Nurse–Client Partnership

2. This response is best. It answers Sally's concern and suggests a course of action toward determining if she has TB.

Taxonomy:
Application

3. This response is true but does not answer Sally's concern.
4. This response is not therapeutic, and the immune system cannot be assessed visually.

---

185. 1. This approach is unhelpful and states the obvious.

2. There may be other medications with fewer adverse effects that Ms. Pargeter could take. The situation must be evaluated and discussed with her physician.

CLASSIFICATION
Competency:
Nurse–Client Partnership
Taxonomy:
Critical Thinking

3. This approach is a threat to abandon care.
4. Ms. Pargeter has not mentioned stress, just that she was tired.

---

186. 1. Chart entries must never be removed or deleted.

2. This action is the legally accepted correction.

CLASSIFICATION
Competency:
Professional Practice
Taxonomy:
Knowledge/Comprehension

3. Same as answer 1.
4. This action is not necessary. Incident reports are generally required by agencies when a client's safety is at risk.

---

187. 1. These signs are indicative of a cerebrovascular accident (stroke) and require emergency treatment. Immediate transportation to the nearest hospital is vital. If tissue plasminogen activator (tPA) is assessed to be the appropriate treatment, it must be administered within 3 hours of the stroke to prevent permanent cerebral damage.

CLASSIFICATION
Competency:
Changes in Health
Taxonomy:
Critical Thinking

2. Mr. Leonard requires quick transport to services that only a hospital can provide.
3. This directive is not wise until it is established whether the stroke is hemolytic or thrombotic.
4. Same as answer 2.

---

188. 1. This action will need to be done but not until treatment has been initiated. This task should be delegated to the school officials.

2. This action is the correct emergency treatment. With anaphylactic responses, death can occur very quickly, even in minutes. The epinephrine should be given at the same time that 9-1-1 is called.

CLASSIFICATION
Competency:
Changes in Health
Taxonomy:
Critical Thinking

3. This action is important, but the epinephrine is life-saving.
4. Diphenhydramine hydrochloride is an antihistamine that is used to treat less critical allergies. It is not appropriate in this case.

189.   1. **Regular consumption of cranberry juice is believed to prevent bacteria from adhering to the lining of the urinary tract. Blueberry juice is also helpful.**

2. These products may actually increase the incidence of UTIs.
3. This suggestion is the opposite of what is recommended. Increased fluids help to flush the bladder of bacteria.
4. This treatment is prescribed only in the case of chronic, serious UTIs (e.g., in clients with neurogenic bladders). The antiseptic must be ordered by a physician, not a nurse.

CLASSIFICATION
Competency:
Changes in Health
Taxonomy:
Application

---

190.   1. This option may not be possible if Mrs. Gingras is anorexic.
2. This option is possible; however, with anorexia, sometimes even favourite foods are not appealing or tolerated.
3. This option is possible but does not address the need for more protein.

4. **This strategy is the easiest and most consistent way to achieve a high-calorie, high-protein intake. Nutritional supplements come in a variety of flavours, and serving them over ice may help improve acceptance.**

CLASSIFICATION
Competency:
Changes in Health
Taxonomy:
Critical Thinking

---

191.   1. It is not appropriate to prepare the body in view of the family. Only 15 minutes have passed: the family needs more time with their loved one.
2. This action is not respectful of the family's needs.
3. The family should be allowed to stay for as long as they require; however, it is not appropriate use of nursing financial resources to stay overtime for pay prior to consulting with the night staff.

4. **This action allows the family the necessary time with their loved one and uses nursing resources appropriately.**

CLASSIFICATION
Competency:
Professional Practice
Taxonomy:
Critical Thinking

---

192.   1. **When a nurse co-signs a medication record, she is equally responsible for all aspects of the administration.**

2. Unless the nurse is not able to take the time to co-sign, she should not refuse.
3. This action covers only one aspect of ensuring the medication is administered correctly.
4. Same as answer 3.

CLASSIFICATION
Competency:
Professional Practice
Taxonomy:
Application

---

193.   1. **This action is the priority because the nurse must ensure he has the necessary equipment and supplies to treat clients, who may arrive at any time.**

2. While the nurse should have an idea of what types of clients have been treated on the previous shift, it is not a priority.

CLASSIFICATION
Competency:
Professional Practice
Taxonomy:
Critical Thinking

3. Unless there is a client requiring urgent care, head-to-toe assessments may not be necessary in this setting. If one is required, the nurse will need to take the time for a proper assessment.
4. This action is necessary; however, the medical directives are not likely to have changed since the nurse's previous shift.

---

194.   **1. The affected areas of the intestines are in need of repair. Protein is required in the building and repairing of tissues.**

2. Increased protein will not significantly affect peristalsis.
3. Anemia may result from chronic bleeding; it usually is corrected, however, with an increased iron intake and a normal intake of protein.
4. Protein is given to promote healing; once tissues are repaired, muscle tone may improve.

CLASSIFICATION
Competency:
Changes in Health
Taxonomy:
Application

---

195.   **1. Denial is a pattern of defence often demonstrated in the self-protective stage of adaptation to illness. Thoughts and feelings are so painful and provoke such anxiety that the client rejects the existence of the paraplegia.**

2. From the information available, it cannot be assumed that the client is fantasizing; a fantasy is the transformation of undesirable experiences into imagined events to fulfill an unconscious wish or need.
3. Denial is a method of psychological adaptation.
4. Motivation involves the setting of realistic goals; this client is in denial.

CLASSIFICATION
Competency:
Nurse–Client Partnership
Taxonomy:
Knowledge/Comprehension

---

196.   1. Nausea may occur but is not common with the low-dose formula of estrogen–progestin. It is not a critical adverse effect.
2. Weight gain may occur but is not a critical adverse effect.

3. Thrombophlebitis (calf pain) has been associated with contraceptives, especially in women who smoke.

4. This effect generally occurs with oral contraceptives and may, in fact, be a desired side effect.

CLASSIFICATION
Competency:
Health and Wellness
Taxonomy:
Critical Thinking

---

197.   1. With a left-sided thrombus, right-sided weakness would be expected.
2. A decrease in tendon response would be the normal manifestation.
3. Urinary incontinence would be expected.

4. Anxiety and difficulty communicating are common physical findings since the primary speech centre is located in the left hemisphere.

CLASSIFICATION
Competency:
Changes in Health
Taxonomy:
Application

---

198.   1. This action may be warranted if a recent beating had occurred, but the neighbour has said this is a chronic situation occurring over many

CLASSIFICATION
Competency:
Professional Practice

months. This action is not the most important unless the neighbour indicates to the nurse that the children have been severely injured.

2. This action could be taken by the nurse but is not the most important action.
3. This action is a helpful and therapeutic response but not the most important action.

4. **By law, all nurses must report any actual or suspected cases of child abuse.**

Taxonomy:
Critical Thinking

---

199. 1. Insertion into a vein would be intravenous therapy.

2. **Hypodermoclysis catheters are inserted into the abdomen or upper thigh to allow for slow absorption through the tissue.**

3. Same as answer 1.
4. Inserting a catheter into the pedal circulation may be harmful and is intravenous therapy.

CLASSIFICATION
Competency:
Changes in Health
Taxonomy:
Application

---

200. 1. There is no sex-related difference.

2. **Nicotine is a powerful vasoconstrictor, which can lead to peripheral arterial disease.**

3. This quantity of alcohol intake is a recommended allowance for women.
4. A high-fat diet may cause coronary rather than peripheral arterial problems.

CLASSIFICATION
Competency:
Changes in Health
Taxonomy:
Application

END OF ANSWERS AND RATIONALES TO PRACTICE EXAM 2

Answers Exam 2

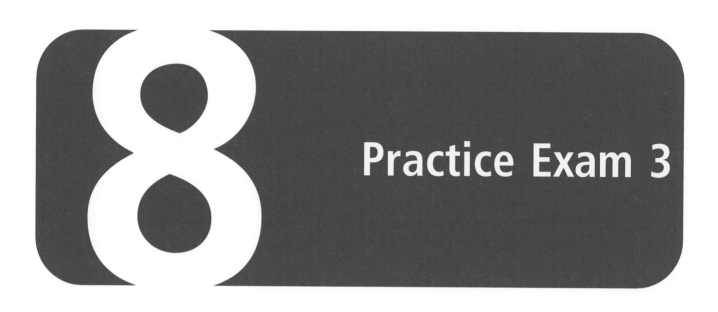

8

Practice Exam 3

INSTRUCTIONS FOR PRACTICE EXAM 3

You will have 4 hours to complete the exam. The questions are presented as nursing cases or as independent questions. Read each question carefully, and then choose the answer that you think is the best of the four options presented. If you cannot decide on an answer to a question, proceed to the next question and return to this question later if you have time. Try to answer all the questions. Marks are not subtracted for wrong answers. If you are unsure of an answer, it will be to your advantage to guess.

Circle each answer in the exam book, and then transfer your answer to the scoring sheet found on p. 268. Be sure that the pencil mark completely fills the oval, but do not press so heavily that you cannot erase it if you decide to change the answer. Ensure that you are marking the question number that corresponds to the question you are answering. Make sure you do not fill in more than one oval for a question. Erase completely any answer you wish to change, and mark your new choice in the corresponding oval.

Answers to Practice Exam 3 appear on p. 214.

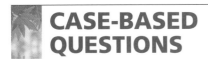

CASE-BASED QUESTIONS

CASE 1

Mr. Tolea, age 65, is in the terminal stage of liver failure resulting from hepatitis C. He has been unemployed for many years and lives below the poverty line in a low-income rooming house that has inadequate cooking and sanitation facilities. He is estranged from his former wife and two children.

QUESTIONS 1 to 4 refer to this case.

1. Mr. Tolea is seen by a nurse who coordinates a regional hepatitis C clinic. The nurse is aware that most new cases of hepatitis C are a result of which of the following?

    1. Unprotected sexual activity
    2. Blood transfusions
    3. Co-infection with human immunodeficiency virus (HIV)
    4. Intravenous drug abuse

2. The nurse is aware that Mr. Tolea has not been receiving the nutritional support he requires to manage his disease. How would the nurse best facilitate quality nutritional intake for him?

    1. Encourage him to purchase liquid nutritional supplements

    2. Suggest he add fresh fruit and vegetables to his diet
    3. Consult with the clinic social worker to find a resource for a charitable meal service
    4. Contact his family to persuade them to help provide him with nutritious food

3. Mr. Tolea's condition deteriorates, and he decides to be admitted to a palliative care hospice. What is the most important aspect of care for the palliative care nurse to provide to Mr. Tolea?

    1. Ensuring he has adequate sedation
    2. Enabling him to make choices about his care
    3. Managing symptoms related to pruritus
    4. Preventing pressure ulcers

4. The palliative care nurses are concerned that many people are not aware of the services the hospice provides for dying clients and their families. What would be the most effective method of providing information to this target population?

    1. Communicating with health care providers in the community
    2. Lobby   to promote the se
    3. Consu
    4. Encou   lient families to spr

END OF CASE 1

CASE 2

A registered nurse works in a pediatric obesity clinic. Rickhelm, age 11 years, is a new client in the clinic.

QUESTIONS 5 to 11 refer to this case.

5. What causes obesity?

   1. Eating high-calorie foods
   2. Lack of physical exercise
   3. Caloric intake that exceeds caloric requirements
   4. Sedentary lifestyle

6. Which of the following factors would be the most predictive etiology for Rickhelm's obesity?

   1. A birth weight of 5.5 kg
   2. Obese parents
   3. A culture that considers fat children to be healthy children
   4. A parenting style that provides food as a reward for good behaviour

7. Rickhelm has screening tests relating to his obesity. Which of the following results would be of most concern to the nurse?

   1. Total cholesterol: 4.4 mmol/L
   2. Fasting blood sugar: 7.8 mmol/L
   3. Blood pressure: 105/63 mm Hg
   4. Spirometry: 85% of predicted values

8. The nurse calculates Rickhelm's body mass index (BMI). The formula for calculating BMI is weight in kilograms divided by height in centimetres squared times 10,000. Rickhelm is 132 cm tall and weighs 58 kg. What is Rickhelm's BMI?

   1. 29
   2. 31
   3. 33
   4. 35

9. The nurse begins a therapeutic plan for managing Rickhelm's obesity and goal of losing weight.

What approach would likely have the most positive results?

   1. Behaviour modification
   2. A calorie-reduced diet
   3. Appetite-suppressant drugs
   4. Gastric bypass surgery

10. Rickhelm asks the nurse if he can still go to fast-food restaurants after school with his friends. What should the nurse recommend?

    1. "Yes, I'll give you a list of low-calorie options from fast-food restaurants."
    2. "Yes, you can go, but limit what you eat to just one hamburger and a small fries."
    3. "It is probably not wise for you to go because you will be tempted to eat fatty foods."
    4. "Fast-food restaurants serve high-fat, high-calorie foods, so you should never eat there."

11. Knowing that obese children are often teased by other children and may suffer low self-esteem, the nurse performs a psychosocial assessment of Rickhelm. Which question asked of Rickhelm would best approach this topic?

    1. "Who are your friends?"
    2. "Do you find that you are teased because you are overweight?"
    3. "Do you feel bad about yourself because you are overweight?"
    4. "Tell me how you feel about being overweight."

END OF CASE 2

CASE 3

Mr. Jason, age 79 years, is admitted to hospital to have a tumour on his neck removed. The surgery has been explained to him in detail by the surgeon, but he remains very anxious.

QUESTIONS 12 to 16 refer to this case.

12. Which of the following approaches by the nurse would help to reduce Mr. Jason's anxiety?

Practice Exam 3

1. Talk with him to discover his specific concerns
2. Explain, in simple terms, what the surgeon has already told him
3. Demonstrate the suction equipment and teach him how to use it before the surgery
4. Include Mr. Jason in developing a plan for postsurgery communication

13. Following his surgery, the nurse places Mr. Jason in a high Fowler position. Which of the following reasons would be the most important for the nurse's choosing this position?

    1. To prevent strain on the incision
    2. To promote drainage from the wound
    3. To provide stimulation to Mr. Jason
    4. To limit the amount of edema at the operative site

14. Mr. Jason required a tracheotomy and is receiving humidified oxygen via the tracheotomy. What would be the initial action for the nurse to take when preparing to change the tracheotomy dressing and perform inner cannula care?

    1. Perform suctioning on Mr. Jason before removing the old dressing
    2. Open the sterile tracheotomy kit and set up the supplies
    3. Remove the inner cannula for cleaning
    4. Cut the correct lengths of twill tape to replace the present ties

15. Which of the following nursing actions would the nurse take when performing tracheal suctioning on Mr. Jason?

    1. Preoxygenate before suctioning
    2. Apply negative pressure as the catheter is being inserted
    3. Ensure the catheter reaches well beyond the base of the tube
    4. Instill acetylcysteine (Mucomyst) into the tracheotomy prior to suctioning to loosen secretions

16. Mr. Jason communicates to the nurse that his neck dressing is too tight and is choking him.

Which of the following initial actions by the nurse would be most appropriate?

1. Assess Mr. Jason's neck for signs of constriction
2. Observe the dressing for bleeding
3. Explain to Mr. Jason that the tight dressing is necessary
4. Remove the dressing to relieve the pressure

END OF CASE 3

CASE 4

An Aboriginal nurse begins employment at a community health clinic in the northern reserve where she grew up.

QUESTIONS 17 to 20 refer to this case.

17. The nurse understands that the objective of Aboriginal health care is to bring balance to the body, mind, emotions, and spirit. Which of the following terms is used to describe this type of health care?

    1. Holistic health care
    2. Primary health care
    3. Spiritual health care
    4. Socioenvironmental health care

18. Shortly after the nurse begins work on the reserve, an outbreak of respiratory syncytial virus (RSV) occurs. Why is there a high incidence of RSV in northern Aboriginal communities?

    1. There is a lack of adequate housing, and the resulting overcrowding contributes to the disease's spread.
    2. Aboriginal infants are particularly susceptible to the virus.
    3. The cold weather in the north favours the spread of the virus.
    4. Members of the population have a depressed immune system related to poor diet.

19. The nurse is concerned that several members of the community have a poor diet, consuming many foods that have little nutritional value.

Which of the following is the underlying reason for the poor diet?

1.   Aboriginal people do not like the taste of fruits and vegetables.
2.   Genetic makeup causes Aboriginal people to crave foods with a high sugar content.
3.   In northern Canada, sugar-filled foods and soft drinks are less expensive than foods that have a higher nutritional value.
4.   There has been inadequate education regarding the dangers of poor nutrition.

20.   On the reserve, many of the people are related. The nurse's 14-year-old niece comes to the community clinic for advice on birth control because she is sexually active. The other nurse who works in the clinic will not be on duty for another week. The nurse is concerned about confidentiality issues in treating a relative. What should she do?

1.   Advise her niece to return to the clinic when the other nurse is on duty
2.   Tell her niece that because she is a relative, she is not allowed to provide care to her
3.   Attempt to arrange a physician consultation in a nearby community via a telehealth link
4.   Provide the necessary health teaching to her niece while ensuring confidentiality and professional boundaries

END OF CASE 4

CASE 5

Ms. Bennett, a resident of a group home for young adults, has a history of bipolar disorder. One day, she tells the registered nurse (RN) she has a date with a counsellor who works at the group home. Ms. Bennett says she has bought the counsellor a gold ring and they will go to an expensive restaurant because she is "very wealthy" and appreciates the help the counsellor has given her.

QUESTIONS 21 to 22 refer to this case.

21.   Following the conversation with Ms. Bennett, what would be the most appropriate initial response by the nurse?

1.   Set boundaries for Ms. Bennett by telling her that it is not appropriate to engage in social activities with her counsellor
2.   Advise Ms. Bennett that the counsellor is not allowed to accept any type of gift from a client
3.   Report the counsellor to his immediate supervisor and regulatory body
4.   Document the conversation and clarify her perceptions with the counsellor directly

22.   Which of the following statements would reflect the nurse's immediate concerns relating to the conversation with Ms. Bennett?

1.   An inappropriate relationship has developed between Ms. Bennett and the counsellor.
2.   Ms. Bennett is potentially displaying the manic phase of her mental health disorder.
3.   The counsellor will be placed in an awkward, unprofessional position by Ms. Bennett.
4.   The nurse will have no immediate concerns since she will understand that there is no truth in Ms. Bennett's claim.

END OF CASE 5

CASE 6

Mr. Braun, age 47 years, is brought to the hospital by ambulance after his wife found him unconscious. Following a computed tomography (CT) scan, he is diagnosed as having experienced a ruptured aneurysm with a prognosis of no hope of recovery. He is on full life support in the intensive care unit (ICU).

QUESTIONS 23 to 27 refer to this case.

23.   Mr. Braun's nurse has recently started work in the ICU and has never experienced the death of a client. What is his priority action to facilitate his competence to care for Mr. Braun and his family?

1.   Reflect on his own beliefs and feelings about death
2.   Research recent publications about death and dying
3.   Talk with his co-workers about caring for a dying client
4.   Ask for assistance with care for Mr. Braun

24. There is nothing written in Mr. Braun's health record concerning resuscitation. The nurse does not know what to do if Mr. Braun should "code." What should be the first step in determining action by the nursing staff in this situation?

    1. Have the physician write a do-not-resuscitate order (DNR)
    2. Ensure that all staff members are prepared to resuscitate Mr. Braun
    3. Speak with the family regarding Mr. Braun's previously stated wishes or advance directive concerning end-of-life care
    4. Research directives from the Canadian Nurses Association's *Code of Ethics for Registered Nurses* regarding end-of-life decision making

25. The physician has spoken with Mrs. Braun regarding the fact that her husband will most likely die within 48 hours. The nurse overhears Mrs. Braun telling her young-adult children in the family waiting room, "The doctors and nurses are doing everything they can. I know he is going to be okay, so don't worry." When the nurse speaks with Mrs. Braun, what would be an appropriate question to ask?

    1. "Why did you tell your family that your husband is going to get better?"
    2. "Tell me about your discussion with the physician."
    3. "Would you like me to explain to you what the physician told you about your husband?"
    4. "Have you told your children that their father is going to die?"

26. Mr. Braun is removed from life support and, shortly afterward, pronounced dead. What does the nurse need to document in the health record after his death?

    1. Whether an autopsy will be conducted
    2. Time of death and who pronounced the death
    3. All specific hygiene care provided to the body
    4. What time the family left the bedside

27. The nurse is having difficulty managing the grief he feels upon the death of Mr. Braun, and he has lingering feelings of inadequacy with regard to his support of the family. What should be the nurse's initial action to work through his grief?

    1. Transfer out of the ICU to a unit where there are few deaths
    2. Discuss his feelings with colleagues
    3. Recognize the feelings of inadequacy as normal grieving
    4. Ask the unit manager how he could have done a better job of supporting the Braun family

END OF CASE 6

CASE 7

Ms. Hudson brings her 2-week-old infant, Jeremy, to the well-baby clinic. She requests help with breastfeeding from the nurse.

QUESTIONS 28 to 34 refer to this case.

28. Ms. Hudson does not think she is providing enough milk for Jeremy because she has small breasts. The nurse tells her that there are only very few reasons why a woman cannot successfully breastfeed. Which of the following maternal conditions is a contraindication to breastfeeding?

    1. Substance abuse
    2. Inverted nipples
    3. Mastitis
    4. A diagnosis of cancer

29. Ms. Hudson is worried about Jeremy because she says her girlfriend's baby, who is bottle-fed, is putting on much more weight than Jeremy. What explanation should the nurse provide to Ms. Hudson?

    1. Babies who are fed formula are generally overfed, and that is why they gain more weight.
    2. Although breast milk is better for the baby's immune system, it lacks enough fat for adequate growth during the first 6 months.
    3. Breastfed infants tend to be leaner and have less body fat, but this is not an indication of inadequate nutritional status.

4. Infant formulas have more calories per millilitre, so infants who are bottle-fed gain more weight.

30. What suggestion should the nurse provide to Ms. Hudson to increase her milk supply?

   1. "Give more frequent feedings."
   2. "Drink at least 15 glasses of water per day."
   3. "Massage your breasts prior to feeding."
   4. "Use oxytocin nasal spray to induce milk production."

31. How will Ms. Hudson best evaluate whether Jeremy is receiving adequate breast milk and fluids?

   1. He will have six to eight wet diapers per day.
   2. He will have good skin turgor.
   3. She will weigh him before and after she breastfeeds him to determine how much he drinks at each feeding.
   4. Jeremy will have at least one stool per day.

32. Ms. Hudson reports that sometimes Jeremy wakes up crying and cannot focus on feeding because he is so fussy. What should the nurse recommend in this situation?

   1. "Change his diaper before feeding."
   2. "Apply a cool cloth to his face."
   3. "Increase the lighting to focus his attention on you."
   4. "Swaddle him and have him suck on your finger."

33. Ms. Hudson wonders if there is any point in continuing with breastfeeding because she wants to return to work in a few months. What is the most appropriate action for the nurse to suggest?

   1. "After 2 months, you should gradually decrease breastfeeding so that your milk supply will have dried up when you return to work."
   2. "Discuss with your partner the possibility of not returning to work."

   3. "Feed Jeremy formula during the day and breastfeed at night so that this feeding pattern will be established when you return to work."
   4. "I'll arrange a meeting with the lactation consultant for strategies to enable you to continue breastfeeding when you return to work."

34. Which of the following organizations has as its primary function the provision of support and education to breastfeeding women?

   1. La Leche League International
   2. Lamaze International
   3. Public Health Agency of Canada
   4. Victorian Order of Nurses (VON)

END OF CASE 7

CASE 8

Ms. Loates, age 67 years, has a subtotal gastrectomy for cancer of the stomach. After surgery, she returns to the unit with an IV and a nasogastric tube set to low suction (a Gomco pump).

QUESTIONS 35 TO 37 refer to this case.

35. Two hours after the subtotal gastrectomy, the nurse observes a small amount of bright red drainage from Ms. Loates's nasogastric tube. What should the nurse do?

   1. Notify the physician immediately
   2. Clamp the nasogastric tube for 1 hour
   3. Recognize that this is an expected finding
   4. Irrigate the nasogastric tube with iced saline

36. The nurse notes that there has been no nasogastric drainage for 30 minutes. There is an order to irrigate the nasogastric tube prn. How should the nurse irrigate the nasogastric tube?

   1. Instill 30 mL of normal saline and withdraw slowly
   2. Instill 20 mL of air and clamp off the suction for 1 hour
   3. Instill 50 mL of saline and increase the pressure of the suction

4.   Instill 15 mL of distilled water and disconnect the suction for 30 minutes

37.   After a subtotal gastrectomy, pulmonary complications may occur. During the first 24 hours postoperatively, how would the nurse help to prevent pulmonary complications in Ms. Loates?

1.   Frequent oral suctioning
2.   Maintaining a consistent oxygen flow rate
3.   Ambulating Ms. Loates to increase respiratory exchange
4.   Promoting frequent turning, moving, and deep breathing

END OF CASE 8

CASE 9

Juanita is a 17-year-old woman who was diagnosed with a rare type of cancer at age 4 years. Although there have been several remissions, she has lived most of her life with pain and repeated hospitalizations. She experienced a terminal relapse and while in hospital decides she wishes no further treatment.

QUESTIONS 38 to 42 refer to this case.

38.   The nurse needs to ensure Juanita is making an informed decision regarding refusal of treatment. What should the nurse say to best confirm Juanita is making an informed decision?

1.   "Are you aware of what will happen if you refuse treatment?"
2.   "Describe what will happen if treatment is stopped."
3.   "This is a very hard decision for you to make, isn't it?"
4.   "I will make arrangements for you to speak with a client advocate so you are aware of the information you need to know before you make this decision."

39.   Juanita's parents disagree with her decision. The nurse, who has a daughter close to Juanita's age, disagrees as well. According to the Canadian Nurses Association's *Code of Ethics for Registered*

Nurses, what is the nurse's primary role in this situation?

1.   To be an advocate for Juanita after she has made an informed decision
2.   To provide counselling to Juanita's parents to help them persuade Juanita to change her decision
3.   To refrain from being Juanita's primary nurse because she has an ethical disagreement with her
4.   To call a meeting of the health care team, including Juanita and her parents, to discuss her decision

40.   Juanita's family is large and includes, in addition to her mother and father, five siblings. All of them visit and call requesting information about Juanita. At times the family becomes frustrated with the nurses and complains that they are receiving confusing information about Juanita. How should the nurse best manage this situation?

1.   Tell the family that only the parents will receive information about Juanita
2.   Request that Juanita and her family choose a designated person to communicate with health care staff
3.   Have Juanita be the person to provide all her family with relevant information
4.   Ask the family to choose one primary nurse to speak with for all information about Juanita

41.   Juanita is transferred to the palliative care service at her request. On the palliative unit, her family angrily tells the nurse that Juanita is receiving inadequate care. What would be the most helpful response from the nurse?

1.   "I know how you feel. It is difficult when a loved one is in pain."
2.   "I am sorry. We are understaffed and haven't been able to provide the best care."
3.   "I will discuss your concern with the other nurses, and we will change her plan of care."
4.   "Tell me what it is that is bothering you about your daughter's care."

42. Juanita has chosen a DNR status, which is documented on the health record. One night while the family is with Juanita, she stops breathing. Her mother screams at the nurse, "She's stopped breathing! Do something or I'll sue!" What should the nurse do?

    1. Shake Juanita, as per CPR sequence, to stimulate her to breathe
    2. Call a code
    3. Take Juanita's pulse
    4. Comfort her mother by reminding her this was Juanita's stated wishes and informed decision

END OF CASE 9

CASE 10

Mr. Partilucci, age 58 years, has type 2 diabetes. Several weeks ago, a pebble lodged in his shoe while he and his wife were hiking. He developed a large gangrenous area on his left foot and has been admitted to hospital.

QUESTIONS 43 to 45 refer to this case.

43. Mrs. Partilucci says that she cannot understand how this happened so rapidly. She asks the nurse what will happen to her husband's foot. Which of the following responses would provide her with the most accurate information?

    1. "The blackened areas of the foot indicate that the tissue in these areas has died. The physician will probably remove those areas to keep the rest of the foot healthy."
    2. "Your husband will likely have an amputation below the knee to ensure the disease does not progress any further."
    3. "The doctor will have to explain what he will do for your husband. I cannot say what he will decide."
    4. "It looks pretty serious. You probably should have sought medical attention before now."

44. Mrs. Partilucci would like to know more about diabetes and wants to be involved in her husband's care. How would the nurse best facilitate her learning at this time?

    1. Provide her with handouts and the address of the local diabetes association
    2. Arrange a meeting with Mrs. Partilucci and the diabetes nurse educator
    3. Encourage Mrs. Partilucci to assist with all aspects of his in-hospital diabetes management
    4. Tell Mrs. Partilucci that her husband will be able to manage his disease by himself after discharge, so she need not worry

45. Mr. Partilucci's son asks if he will get diabetes like his father. Which of the following responses by the nurse would best answer his question?

    1. "You will not develop diabetes. There is no increase in your risk because your father has it."
    2. "Yes, but probably not until you are over 40 years of age. The severity varies from person to person."
    3. "Diabetes tends to have a familial link. I will give you some information about some of the risk factors and preventive strategies."
    4. "Diabetes runs in families. Your mother does not have it, so your chance of developing diabetes is reduced by 50%."

END OF CASE 10

CASE 11

Mr. O'Morrissey works for a hydroelectric company and spends most of his time outdoors. He makes an appointment to see the nurse at the company health unit because he is concerned about a mole on his neck that has recently changed shape and colour. The nurse examines the lesion and finds it has an irregular border and looks very dark. She refers him to the company physician.

QUESTIONS 46 to 48 refer to this case.

46. The physician tells Mr. O'Morrissey he believes the mole may be malignant melanoma. Mr. O'Morrissey asks the nurse what this means. Which of the following responses by the nurse would be most accurate?

    1. "It is a cancerous tumour that starts in the cells that produce pigment."

2. "It is a rare type of superficial skin cancer."
3. "It is caused by radiation from the sun."
4. "It is a tumour that grows from a freckle."

47. Mr. O'Morrissey is referred to a cancer specialist, who will perform a surgical excision of the melanoma. Prior to surgery, Mr. O'Morrissey returns to the company health clinic to speak with the nurse. He asks her whether she thinks the surgery will cure him of the cancer. Which of the following responses by the nurse would be most accurate?

1. "Malignant melanoma can generally be cured by surgery with little chance of relapse."
2. "Surgical removal will take care of only that one lesion; others are likely to develop."
3. "It is possible to cure malignant melanoma with surgery; however, this type of cancer is known to spread rapidly."
4. "Chemotherapy or radiation will follow the surgery."

48. Mr. O'Morrissey's surgery is successful, and he receives follow-up care at the company health clinic. The nurse teaches him about prevention of further melanomas. Which of the following would be most important for the nurse to teach Mr. O'Morrissey?

1. To stay out of direct sunlight
2. To wear protective headgear when outside
3. To routinely monitor skin and moles for any changes
4. To wear sunscreen with a sun protection factor (SPF) of at least 20

END OF CASE 11

CASE 12

Mr. Nigel, age 26, has a history of moderate to severe asthma since childhood. He presents at the emergency department with chest tightness, dyspnea, and anxiety and states that he feels as though he is suffocating.

QUESTIONS 49 to 55 refer to this case.

49. What is the definition of asthma?

1. A genetic disorder that produces airway obstruction because of changes in glandular secretions
2. A condition characterized by destructive changes that result in a loss of lung elasticity
3. Chronic inflammation of the mucous membranes of the bronchi, causing excessive secretion of mucus
4. A chronic lung condition characterized by variable airflow obstruction as a result of airway hyper-responsiveness and airway inflammation

50. The nurse performs a chest assessment on Mr. Nigel. Which of the following manifestations would be of most concern to the nurse?

1. Wheezing on expiration
2. Wheezing on inspiration and expiration
3. Use of accessory muscles to breathe
4. Diminished or absent breath sounds

51. The nurse determines that Mr. Nigel is experiencing pulsus paradoxus. Which of the following vital signs indicates pulsus paradoxus?

1. A drop in his systolic pressure from 140 to 120 mm Hg during inspiration
2. A pulse of 92 in the upper limbs and 72 in the lower limbs
3. An apical heart rate that increases from 65 to 90 beats per minute on expiration
4. The difference between the systolic blood pressure of 150 mm Hg and the diastolic pressure of 70 mm Hg

52. The nurse evaluates Mr. Nigel to be in a state of status asthmaticus. What should be the nurse's initial action?

1. Administer the ordered bronchodilator
2. Place Mr. Nigel on a vital signs monitor
3. Notify the physician of an emergency situation
4. Provide a bolus of IV fluid, as per protocol

53. Blood gases readings are taken on Mr. Nigel. Evaluate the following arterial blood gases: partial pressure of oxygen (PaO_2) 72 mm Hg; partial pressure of carbon dioxide ($PaCO_2$) 50 mm Hg; pH 7.28.

    1. Hypoxia, hypercapnia, and acidosis
    2. Hypoxia, hypocapnia, and alkalosis
    3. Hyperoxia, hypercapnia, and acidosis
    4. Normal oxygen, hypocapnia, and alkalosis

54. Mr. Nigel is admitted to the intensive care unit for 12 hours. When his condition stabilizes, he is transferred to a medical unit, where he receives health teaching prior to discharge. According to best practice guidelines for the treatment of asthma, which of the following interventions is the most important component of Mr. Nigel's asthma management?

    1. Eliminating or avoiding triggers
    2. Education and the use of an action plan
    3. Appropriate pharmacotherapy
    4. Regular follow-up with a respirologist

55. The nurse demonstrates to Mr. Nigel the appropriate administration of his inhaled bronchodilator and inhaled steroid. Which of the following procedures is correct concerning the use of metered dose inhalers?

    1. Shake the inhaler vigorously twice; then give two quick puffs of the inhaler
    2. Put lips around the inhaler, and breathe out while depressing the canister
    3. Use a spacer, such as an AeroChamber, if coordination cannot be achieved
    4. Inhale as deeply as possible, and then depress the canister

END OF CASE 12

CASE 13

Ms. Wilmox, a 46-year-old mother of two adolescent children, has been admitted to an inpatient psychiatric unit. She is accompanied by her sister, who states that Ms. Wilmox has been using crack cocaine, alcohol, and possibly marijuana. The sister reports that Ms. Wilmox has a history of intermittent substance abuse but that she has been "clean" for almost 4 years. The nurse performs an admission assessment.

QUESTIONS 56 to 59 refer to this case.

56. What would be the nurse's primary concern with regard to Ms. Wilmox?

    1. History of self-harm
    2. Previous use of crack cocaine
    3. Current substance use
    4. Lack of support systems

57. During the assessment, Ms. Wilmox looks at the nurse intently and blinks her eyes in a rhythmic pattern. Ms. Wilmox states that she is answering his questions mentally and is projecting her responses directly into his mind. What would be the most appropriate action by the nurse?

    1. Remind Ms. Wilmox that this is impossible and that she should answer his questions verbally
    2. Advise Ms. Wilmox that she is suffering from the effects of drug use, and it would be better for her if she would answer questions appropriately
    3. Excuse himself from the assessment and seek clarification from Ms. Wilmox's sister
    4. Advise Ms. Wilmox that he is only able to understand spoken replies

58. The sister appears to know a significant amount of information relating to Ms. Wilmox's drug abuse history. Which of the following actions by the nurse would ensure he is able to obtain the sister's information?

    1. Ensure Ms. Wilmox is present when the sister is questioned
    2. Ask Ms. Wilmox's permission to seek information from her sister
    3. Speak to the sister separately without advising Ms. Wilmox, to avoid upsetting her
    4. Insist that Ms. Wilmox sign a "confidentiality disclosure" document before he speaks to the sister

59. Later that evening, Ms. Wilmox becomes verbally abusive toward the sister and the nurse. Which of the following interventions is the most appropriate?

    1. Place Ms. Wilmox in four-point restraints for the safety of herself and others
    2. Advise Ms. Wilmox that abusive behaviour is not appropriate and will not be tolerated
    3. Ignore the behaviour since it is most likely attention seeking
    4. Give Ms. Wilmox the maximum ordered anti-anxiety medication

END OF CASE 13

CASE 14

An occupational health nurse at a large manufacturing company conducts weekly educational sessions with employees regarding a wide variety of health and wellness topics.

QUESTIONS 60 to 64 refer to this case.

60. The nurse discusses smoking cessation with a group of employees who are heavily addicted to nicotine. What should the nurse recommend as the most effective method to quit smoking?

    1. Nicotine-replacement therapy
    2. Hypnosis combined with aversion therapy
    3. Group support programs and behavioural interventions
    4. Any method that individuals feel will be effective for them

61. Mr. Louis, an employee, asks the nurse why he should get the seasonal influenza vaccine this year when he already got one last year. How should the nurse respond?

    1. "The vaccine effect lasts for only 8 to 12 months."
    2. "Because, as with your childhood immunizations, with the flu vaccine, you need a booster."
    3. "The influenza viruses change into new strains every year, and there is a different vaccine for each specific strain."

    4. "Each year, the process for refining the vaccine improves so that you will have better immunity with this year's vaccine."

62. The nurse talks about the importance of sleep. Mr. Steele, who works 12-hour shifts, complains that he has chronic insomnia. What strategies should the nurse recommend to help Mr. Steele improve his sleep?

    1. A bedtime ritual combined with relaxation techniques
    2. Moderate exercise 1 hour before bedtime
    3. A mild over-the-counter sedative
    4. A spicy meal 2 hours before bedtime

63. The nurse conducts WHMIS training for all employees. What is WHMIS?

    1. Safety education to prevent accidents with manufacturing equipment
    2. Training in infection control
    3. Workplace Health Ministry Instructions for Safety
    4. A system to control hazardous substances in the workplace

64. Many of the men and women at the company complain about the stress in their lives. The nurse discusses how stress affects the health and wellness of individuals. Which of the following statements is true regarding stress?

    1. Men are more likely than women to experience stress.
    2. Stress-management techniques should be tailored to the individual's stressors.
    3. Stress is always harmful and causes physical and emotional illness.
    4. Stress is primarily an urban myth and is not as prevalent as portrayed by the media.

END OF CASE 14

CASE 15

Ms. Magnusson, age 69 years, has been admitted to a cardiac unit with atrial fibrillation.

QUESTIONS 65 to 66 refer to this case.

65. Ms. Magnusson is to have an electrocardiogram (ECG). As the nurse prepares the equipment, Ms. Magnusson asks if this test is really necessary because she does not want electricity going through her. Which of the following responses by the nurse would be most appropriate?

1. "The doctor has ordered this test, so you need to have it."
2. "The ECG provides necessary information about your heart's electrical patterns. It does not send electricity through you."
3. "Don't worry; only a small amount of electricity actually comes from the machine. The test is necessary so that there will be a baseline record of your heart's function."
4. "A lot of people ask about the electrical charge, but you will be fine and probably won't feel a thing."

66. Ms. Magnusson asks the nurse if her atrial fibrillation is a rare condition that can be prevented from recurring. Which of the following answers would be the nurse's best response?

1. "This is the most common heart rhythm disturbance in Canada. Reducing your alcohol and caffeine intake may help to prevent attacks."
2. "It is not rare. There are no lifestyle changes that can help to prevent it happening again."
3. "Many people have only one episode in their life. It is not really known why it happens."
4. "This is a rare condition caused by scarring in the heart, so it is uncertain whether it will recur."

END OF CASE 15

CASE 16

The Nursing Practice Committee at Mount Summit Hospital reviews medication policies and practice at its facility.

QUESTIONS 67 to 69 refer to this case.

67. At Mount Summit, nurses must complete an agency medication incident report when they discover a medication error. What is the intended and most important reason for medication incident reports?

1. Tracking errors and trends to improve client safety
2. Identifying nurses who require remediation in medication administration
3. Documentation of facts in case of future legal action
4. A record of client reaction and adverse effects of error

68. The committee would like to draft a policy concerning clients taking their own medication they have brought from home. What is the most important guiding principle when deciding if clients should administer their own medication?

1. Whether the physician has ordered the medication
2. Whether the medication interacts with any of the other ordered medications
3. Whether the drugs are considered to be high risk for error
4. Whether the client has the knowledge, skill, and judgement to self-administer

69. The committee discovers that many medication errors are caused by nurse fatigue. Which of the following has research shown to be the most effective strategy in decreasing nurse fatigue?

1. Limiting shift length to 8 hours
2. Prohibiting overtime shifts
3. Promoting equal day and night shifts
4. Providing choice of shift type and length

END OF CASE 16

CASE 17

Ms. LeBlanc, a 38-year-old primigravida, has been diagnosed with pre-eclampsia at 32 weeks' gestation.

QUESTIONS 70 to 74 refer to this case.

Practice Exam 3

70. In spite of treatment, Ms. LeBlanc develops severe eclampsia and is admitted to hospital at 36 weeks' gestation. What is the priority nursing care for a severely pre-eclamptic client?

   1. Isolating her in a dark room
   2. Maintaining her in a supine position
   3. Encouraging her to drink clear fluids
   4. Protecting her against extraneous stimuli

71. Ms. LeBlanc has a generalized seizure. Following the seizure, she has an elevated temperature of 39°C. What is the cause of the increased temperature?

   1. Excessive muscular activity
   2. Development of a systemic infection
   3. Dehydration caused by rapid fluid loss
   4. Disturbance of the cerebral thermal centre

72. Ms. LeBlanc develops severe abdominal pain and heavy vaginal bleeding and is showing signs of shock. What condition does the nurse suspect has developed?

   1. *Abruptio placentae*
   2. *Placenta previa*
   3. Disseminated intravascular coagulopathy
   4. HELLP syndrome

73. The nurse prepares Ms. LeBlanc for emergency treatment. Which of the following would be an expected intervention?

   1. A high forceps delivery
   2. The insertion of a fetal monitor
   3. An immediate Caesarean delivery
   4. The administration of oxytocin (Pitocin)

74. Ms. LeBlanc delivers a healthy 2600-g baby. At which point in the postpartum period will the danger of a seizure end for her?

   1. At the time of delivery
   2. 2 hours after delivery
   3. 24 hours postpartum
   4. 48 hours postpartum

END OF CASE 17

CASE 18

Charlie, age 9 months, is sent to the emergency department by his pediatrician because of diarrhea and dehydration related to gastroenteritis. He has been breastfed but has lost a great deal of fluid due to numerous watery stools. The triage nurse assesses Charlie.

QUESTIONS 75 to 78 refer to this case.

75. Which of the following organisms is the most common causative organism for infant gastroenteritis?

   1. *Escherichia coli* (*E. coli*)
   2. Shigella
   3. Rotavirus
   4. Salmonella

76. The nurse assesses Charlie for dehydration. Which of the following manifestations would be of most concern to the nurse?

   1. Poor skin turgor
   2. A sunken fontanelle
   3. Dry mucous membranes
   4. A rapid, thready pulse

77. Charlie needs intravenous rehydration. The physician orders a bolus of 0.9% sodium chloride, then IV + p.o. to equal 20 mL/kg per hour. Charlie weighs 9 kg. He drinks 120 mL of oral electrolyte solution and will be fed again in 3 hours. At what hourly rate should the IV be infused for the next 3 hours?

   1. 60 mL
   2. 120 mL
   3. 140 mL
   4. 220 mL

78. Charlie responds well to IV treatment, and his vital signs stabilize. He is discharged. What nutrition would be recommended for Charlie to maintain hydration?

   1. Breast milk and oral rehydration solutions
   2. Soy formula and glucose water

3. BRAT diet and breast milk
4. Half-strength lactose-free formula and apple juice

END OF CASE 18

CASE 19

Mr. Clarkson, age 40 years, has been brought to an emergency psychiatric facility by the police after he assaulted his neighbour. He has had numerous episodes of violent behaviour in the past. He is diagnosed as having an antisocial personality disorder. He is placed in the close observation unit.

QUESTIONS 79 to 82 refer to this case.

79. The nurse performs an admission assessment on Mr. Clarkson. Mr. Clarkson says he is concerned about confidentiality and does not want anyone listening to what he tells her. Where is the best setting for the nurse to conduct the interview?

1. In a private interview room, situated close to the rest of the clients but with the door closed
2. In an open area, where there are others to provide safety
3. In a room close to the nursing station, with the nurse seated between Mr. Clarkson and the door
4. In a room with a police officer beside her

80. Which concept about antisocial personality disorders should the nurse consider when planning care for Mr. Clarkson?

1. He may suffer from a great deal of anxiety.
2. He probably cannot postpone gratification.
3. He will rapidly learn by experience and punishment.
4. He will have a great sense of responsibility toward others.

81. Which of the following is characteristic of people who have an antisocial personality disorder?

1. They have a history of chronic depression.
2. They do not easily become frustrated.
3. They are motivated to change their behaviour.

4. They have a lifelong pattern of maladaptive behaviour.

82. Mr. Clarkson asks the nurse for her phone number so that he can call her for a date. How should the nurse respond?

1. "We are not permitted to date clients."
2. "No, you are the client, and I am the nurse."
3. "Thank you, but our relationship is professional."
4. "It is against my personal and professional ethics to date clients."

END OF CASE 19

CASE 20

A nurse is a preceptor for a recent nursing graduate, Ms. Baldassarian. He teaches the new graduate about the care of central venous access devices.

QUESTIONS 83 to 85 refer to this case.

83. A client has an implanted infusion port. Prior to accessing this type of device, which of the following preparatory steps is most important in preventing infection?

1. Donning an N-95 mask
2. Preparing a sterile field with appropriate supplies
3. Using antimicrobial swabs to prepare the client's skin overlying the access port
4. Wearing sterile gloves

84. The new graduate documents a dressing change in the client's health record. Which of the following examples is the most accurate documentation?

1. 10/29/11 1000 CVAD dressing changed, insertion site pale pink, skin intact, no signs of infection. S. Baldassarian, RN
2. 10/29/11 1000 CVAD site healthy, taught client care of dressing. S. Baldassarian, RN
3. 10/29/11 1000 CVAD dressing changed, new Tegaderm dressing applied as per Dr. Ogden's

orders, pt. tolerated procedure well.
S. Baldassarian, RN

4. 10/29/11 1000 CVAD dressing changed, catheter in place, Dacron cuff in correct position. S. Baldassarian, RN

85. As a learner, which of the following guidelines does the new graduate understand?

1. She must clarify her knowledge and limitations with her preceptor.
2. Her preceptor is co-responsible for the care she provides to clients.
3. Her preceptor has the responsibility to identify the need for supervision in client care situations.
4. She is solely accountable for all errors even if she is directed by the preceptor to provide care beyond her level of competency.

END OF CASE 20

CASE 21

Ms. Baverstock, age 94 years, is a resident in a long-term care facility. She is in the mid-stage of Alzheimer's disease and has dysphagia. Her nurse is the preceptor for a second-year RN student who is interested in the care of older adults.

QUESTIONS 86 to 89 refer to this case.

86. The nurse teaches the nursing student about dysphagia. Which of the following statements would be accurate information?

1. "Always give liquids with a straw so that the client can place them more accurately in the mouth."
2. "Dysphagic clients are best fed by gastrostomy tube."
3. "Spices and seasonings should be kept to a minimum as they may stimulate the gag reflex."
4. "Dysphagic assessment and teaching are usually performed by a trained speech therapist."

87. Ms. Baverstock has a pressure ulcer on her ankle. During the dressing change, the student asks the nurse why she is using a transparent film dressing. Which of the following explanations would provide the correct information?

1. It allows the nurses to see the wound without having to change the dressing.
2. It maintains a moist environment to promote wound healing.
3. It provides a surface that will resist the irritation of bed linens.
4. It is used on wounds that do not require debridement.

88. Ms. Baverstock's husband died many years ago. She tells the student that when her husband comes to take her home, she would like her to visit them for dinner. Which of the following approaches by the student would be most therapeutic?

1. Gently explain to Ms. Baverstock that her husband died and she now lives in a residence
2. Tell Ms. Baverstock that she is very kind, but it would be unethical for her to arrange a visit outside the facility
3. Ask Ms. Baverstock what her favourite foods are for dinner
4. Sit quietly with Ms. Baverstock and hold her hand

89. Ms. Baverstock often wanders at night, disturbing other clients. Which of the following nursing actions would be the safest approach to care for Ms. Baverstock when she wanders?

1. Request that a relative come in to sit with her at night
2. Repeat her nighttime sedation when she starts to walk around
3. Apply restraints to ensure that she remains in bed
4. Encourage her to stay near the nursing station rather than wander elsewhere

END OF CASE 21

CASE 22

A registered nurse works at a summer camp for children who have chronic illnesses.

QUESTIONS 90 to 94 refer to this case.

90. Several of the children begin experiencing fever and runny noses. What action should the nurse initially implement?

    1. Notify the parents of the affected children
    2. Arrange for the affected children to be treated with antipyretics and fluids
    3. Isolate the affected children in a separate cabin
    4. Examine the rest of the children in the camp for similar symptoms

91. A counsellor brings Hunter, age 9, to the first aid room because a wasp has stung him. What is the priority consideration by the nurse in this situation?

    1. Determine if Hunter has had any previous anaphylactic or allergic response to insect bites
    2. Give Hunter an antihistamine, as per medical directive
    3. Provide comfort and reassurance to Hunter
    4. Attempt to remove the stinger

92. The nurse realizes at 0830 hours that she has administered the 0800 furosemide (Lasix) to Madison instead of Meghan, for whom the Lasix was ordered. What is the priority action by the nurse?

    1. Notify the prescribing physician
    2. Document the error on the health forms of Madison and Meghan
    3. Assess and monitor Madison for any adverse reactions to the Lasix
    4. Administer the correct dose of Lasix to Meghan

93. The family of Fatima gives the nurse gift certificates from a local coffee shop for looking after their child. What is the most appropriate response by the nurse to Fatima's family?

    1. "I am not allowed to accept gifts."
    2. "You are very kind, and I will take good care of Fatima."

    3. "Why are you giving me a gift?"
    4. "I will share this gift with the rest of the health care staff."

94. After working at the camp for 2 weeks, a nurse discovers that he was exposed to chicken pox just prior to leaving home for the camp. He has never had chicken pox. What is the most appropriate action by the nurse?

    1. Withdraw from providing care to the children at the camp
    2. Contact his personal physician for advice
    3. Ensure appropriate infection control practices, such as an N-95 mask
    4. Obtain immunization for chicken pox from the camp physician

END OF CASE 22

CASE 23

Ms. Anderson, a postmenopausal woman, discovers a lump in her breast while bathing. She delays going to the doctor for several weeks until her husband insists that she have the lump examined. A fine-needle aspiration confirms that the lump is malignant.

QUESTIONS 95 to 97 refer to this case.

95. The physician suggests that Ms. Anderson have breast conservation surgery (a lumpectomy), followed by radiation therapy. Ms. Anderson asks the nurse if she should have a modified radical mastectomy instead of the lumpectomy in case there has been spread of the cancer to her lymph nodes. Which of the following responses by the nurse would provide the most accurate information?

    1. "Both surgical approaches remove lymph nodes."
    2. "Research indicates that both surgeries have similar results."
    3. "I think you require more information from your physician to clarify these options."
    4. "The decision is really up to you; I'm not sure what I would do."

96. Ms. Anderson states that she cannot think of anyone else in her family who has had breast cancer. She tells the nurse that she has been on hormone replacement therapy (HRT) and asks if this puts her at a higher risk for developing breast cancer. Which of the following responses by the nurse would be most accurate?

    1. "There is still a lot of controversy, but some studies indicate that long-term use may put a woman at greater risk."
    2. "Most women who develop breast cancer have no identifiable risk factors."
    3. "Estrogen is naturally occurring in your body, so I don't think it would be a cause."
    4. "It is probably genetic, and you could not have prevented it."

97. Ms. Anderson's husband asks if there are any observations he should be alert for while his wife receives treatment for her cancer. What would be the most appropriate response by the nurse?

    1. "Make sure she comes in for her scheduled treatment, and everything should be fine."
    2. "Your wife will know if she is experiencing serious problems and will seek medical attention."
    3. "There are a number of facts you should know about the surgery and chemotherapy. I will give you a complete list before she is discharged."
    4. "It is great that Ms. Anderson has someone who is concerned for her."

END OF CASE 23

CASE 24

Mr. Thompson, age 60 years, makes an appointment with his family physician because his dentist told him to have the sore on the undersurface of his tongue examined by a doctor. Mr. Thompson has not had regular dental care for many years.

QUESTIONS 98 to 100 refer to this case.

98. The physician diagnoses oral cancer, and Mr. Thompson has a hemiglossectomy. Which of the following assessments would be a priority when Mr. Thompson returns to the unit from the recovery room?

    1. Pulse oximetry
    2. Level of pain
    3. Airway clearance
    4. Level of consciousness

99. Postoperatively, which of the following positions would be most suitable for Mr. Thompson?

    1. Supine with his head immobilized
    2. A semi-Fowler position
    3. Sims position
    4. A left lateral position

100. Mr. Thompson asks the nurse what he can do in the future to reduce the risk of the cancer recurring. Which of the following points would the nurse cover in health teaching?

    1. Preventive dental care
    2. Eating a diet according to *Canada's Food Guide*
    3. Drinking plenty of fluid to keep well hydrated
    4. Exercising at least three times a week

END OF CASE 24

INDEPENDENT QUESTIONS

QUESTIONS 101 to 200 do not refer to a particular case.

101. Some competitive athletes have been known to abuse amphetamines such as methylphenidate hydrochloride (Ritalin). Which of the following effects do these drugs have on an athlete's performance?

1. Enhance muscle strength and performance
2. Improve fine and gross motor coordination
3. Increase the ability to manage the stress of competition
4. Increase alertness and provide relief from fatigue

102. An infant has torticollis. Which of the following therapeutic interventions would be recommended by the nurse to treat this condition?

1. Gentle stretching exercises in the neck
2. Range-of-motion exercises for the legs
3. Positioning of the infant in the supine position when asleep
4. Extra padding in the diapers to hold the hips in adduction

103. Carys, age 8 years, is brought to the pediatrician's office displaying manifestations of allergic rhinitis. What initial question should the nurse performing the health assessment ask of the parents?

1. "Do you have pets at home?"
2. "Does anyone in the household smoke cigarettes?"
3. "Is there a family history of allergies?"
4. "Can you tell me the history and pattern of her symptoms?"

104. The parents of a 10-year-old child have just been informed that their son's disease is terminal. They will need to learn some skills associated with his palliative care needs. What is the initial consideration for the nurse when she plans teaching with his parents?

1. Individualizing the teaching plan
2. Assessing their readiness to learn
3. Planning evaluation criteria
4. Determining their baseline knowledge

105. Which of the following clients would be at greatest risk for developing delirium when admitted to an acute care facility?

1. A 21-year-old male with renal colic and a history of drug abuse
2. An 87-year-old male with congestive heart failure
3. A 42-year-old male with appendicitis and depression
4. A 53-year-old female with ovarian cancer

106. Why do corticosteroids increase a client's risk for infections?

1. Corticosteroids increase the production of leukocytes.
2. Corticosteroids interfere with antibody production in the lymphatic tissues.
3. Corticosteroids promote the growth and spread of enteric viruses.
4. Corticosteroids suppress the inflammatory response of the body.

107. Ms. Pitre, age 35 years, tells the nurse she is very worried because her doctor has found a condyloma during her annual gynecological exam. She is waiting for biopsy results to see if it is cancerous. Which of the following statements by the nurse would be the most therapeutic?

1. "Sexually transmitted condylomas are a risk factor for developing cervical cancer."
2. "It is very upsetting to have to wait for a biopsy report."
3. "You probably don't have cancer because a condyloma is usually benign."
4. "Even if it's cervical cancer, you don't have to worry much because the cure rate is high."

108. When auscultating Ms. Gash's lungs, the RN hears a dry, grating sound on inspiration. She asks Ms. Gash to cough, but the sound persists and is loudest over the lower, lateral, anterior surface. Which of the following conditions would most likely explain what the nurse is hearing?

    1. A wheeze due to a narrowed bronchus
    2. A pericardial friction rub
    3. A pleural friction rub
    4. An atelectatic lobe

109. Ms. Chang has been diagnosed with gonorrhea. What is the most important action by the public health nurse?

    1. Asking Ms. Chang for a list of her sexual contacts
    2. Reporting the case of gonorrhea to public health officials
    3. Providing Ms. Chang with birth control information
    4. Discussing with Ms. Chang the dangers of unprotected sexual activity

110. Which of the following recordings is the most accurate and objective example of client documentation?

    1. "Mr. Tang has a history of alcohol abuse."
    2. "Ms. Gileppo has a large sacral pressure ulcer."
    3. "Ms. Lok's urine specific gravity is 1.030."
    4. "Mr. Halsey showed a high level of anxiety."

111. A nurse must prioritize client care when beginning a night shift at 1945 hours. Which of the following clients should be seen first?

    1. A client who was scheduled for turning every 2 hours, even hours
    2. A client who is receiving a continuous gastrostomy tube feeding by infusion pump
    3. A client who had a hypoglycemic episode at 1900 hours
    4. A client who was medicated for pain at 1930 hours

112. A registered nurse works at a community clinic where most of the clients are from countries other than Canada. In caring for these multi-ethnic clients, what is the most important principle that the nurse should follow?

    1. The client is the primary source of data.
    2. Family members should always be included in care.
    3. Health beliefs and practices of clients may be different from those of the nurse.
    4. Culturally sensitive care may be provided only if the nurse has knowledge of the culture.

113. Which of the following points about alcohol consumption would be included in health teaching for a client with newly diagnosed type 2 diabetes mellitus?

    1. No alcohol should be consumed while taking diabetic medications.
    2. Alcohol increases the ability of the pancreas to produce insulin.
    3. Both diabetics and nondiabetics should observe the same precautions about moderation of alcohol consumption.
    4. Alcohol may be consumed, but the client must monitor the effects on his blood sugar and incorporate the calories into his meal plan.

114. Ms. Davis has a urinary tract infection. Which of the following teaching points would the nurse review with her?

    1. "Take a daily shower, not a tub bath."
    2. "Increase your intake of apple juice."
    3. "Void every hour during the day."
    4. "Do not have intercourse until urine cultures are negative."

115. Prostate cancer is the most common cancer in Canadian men. Which of the following statements about prostate cancer is true?

    1. It is reliably diagnosed by the prostate-specific antigen (PSA).
    2. Surgical removal is the treatment of choice.

3. Cancer must be confirmed by a prostate biopsy.
4. Treatment causes impotence and incontinence.

116. Mr. Laszlo is a 21-year-old university student. He has been sent to student health services because he has been hearing voices. The nurse is concerned that this is a sign of schizophrenia. When considering Mr. Laszlo's manifestations, which of the following factors should the nurse take into consideration?

1. Substance abuse can mimic some of the symptoms of schizophrenia.
2. He should be assessed by a psychiatrist immediately.
3. The nurse needs to implement safety precautions because the client may be violent.
4. He is too young to display any type of first-episode psychosis.

117. Ms. Dougherty, age 76 years, has aphasia. The nurse did not obtain a signed consent before inserting an indwelling urinary catheter. Which of the following statements accurately reflects this situation?

1. The catheter was necessary, so written consent was not required.
2. This treatment requires a specific written consent form.
3. This situation is an example of treatment without consent, which is contrary to Canadian laws.
4. Consent may be obtained by nonverbal communication.

118. Mr. Peter has obstructive sleep apnea. He has been evaluated in a sleep clinic and has been told he must use a continuous positive airway pressure (CPAP) machine at night. Mr. Peter asks the RN what this machine will do for him. Which of the following statements would be the nurse's best response?

1. "It is a machine that will stop you from snoring and waking up in the night."

2. "The machine uses air pressure to keep your airways open so that you will be able to breathe normally and get a better night's sleep."
3. "The machine increases air flow to the lungs so that your oxygen saturation does not drop and you sleep better."
4. "The machine delivers oxygen to you all night, taking the strain off your lungs and heart."

119. Audrey is sent to the school nurse by her teacher because she has pediculosis. What treatment would the nurse recommend to Audrey's parents?

1. A specifically formulated pediculicide shampoo
2. An antifungal cream
3. An over-the-counter antibiotic cream (Polysporin)
4. A salicylic acid preparation

120. Mr. Prahdeep has had radium seeds implanted in his pharyngeal area for treating cancer of the throat. While providing care for Mr. Prahdeep, which of the following actions should his nurse implement?

1. Have him cough every 2 hours
2. Maintain him in isolation
3. Use alternative communication techniques
4. Use rubber gloves when performing mouth care

121. Jaymee, age 11 years, has exercise-induced asthma. Which of the following recommendations relating to exercise would the nurse suggest to Jaymee?

1. She should participate in sports such as swimming rather than soccer.
2. She should self-administer her β_2-agonist shortly before exercise.
3. She can participate in sports, but not during cold weather.
4. If her peak flow readings are within normal ranges, she may exercise as tolerated.

122. Ms. Gianopoulos is ordered complete bedrest because she is experiencing premature labour. She begins to cry and states, "I have two small children at home. Who is going to look after them?" How should the nurse respond?

    1. "Let's talk about how you can get the help you need."
    2. "You are worried about how you will be able to manage?"
    3. "You'll be able to fix meals, and the children can go to day care."
    4. "Your husband will be able to look after the children."

123. Ms. Jaffer comes to the emergency department experiencing rapid heartbeat, shakiness, shortness of breath, and dizziness. She is diagnosed with panic disorder. Which of the following therapeutic interventions would be most effective during the initial treatment of Ms. Jaffer?

    1. Biofeedback
    2. Identification of anxiety triggers
    3. Medication with lorazepam (Ativan)
    4. Initiation of selective serotonin reuptake inhibitors

124. Mr. Loek has been diagnosed with a borderline personality disorder. What therapeutic approach by the psychiatric nurse is appropriate during counselling with Mr. Loek?

    1. Provide solutions for his behavioural problems
    2. Modify therapeutic approaches depending on his mood
    3. Discuss his ambivalent feelings toward staff members
    4. Reinforce acceptable behaviour

125. Mr. Blanche is taking isophane insulin suspension (NPH) and regular insulin daily. How should the nurse instruct him to administer these two insulin preparations?

    1. "Administer the two insulins in the same syringe only if the ratio is 1:1."

    2. "Mix the two insulins in the prescribed doses in the same syringe."
    3. "Administer the two insulins in the different syringes and at different times."
    4. "Administer each insulin in a separate syringe, using different sites for injection."

126. Clients on sodium-reduced diets need to be aware that sodium occurs naturally in foods and is added during processing. Which of the following foods would be highest in sodium?

    1. Canned tomato juice
    2. Natural cheese
    3. Fresh fish
    4. Whole-wheat pasta

127. Which of the following behaviours is an example of passive–aggressive behaviour?

    1. Pounding a wall
    2. Chronic lateness
    3. Sarcasm
    4. Piercing stares

128. Mrs. Willona is day 1 postpartum following the delivery of a healthy 4100-g infant. What instructions should the nurse provide to her about Kegel exercises?

    1. "When you are urinating or having a bowel movement, hold your breath and bear down."
    2. "Delay urinating for as long as you can to strengthen the sphincter muscles."
    3. "Tighten the muscles in your anus before you have a bowel movement."
    4. "When you are urinating, interrupt the stream by tightening your sphincter, and then continue urinating."

129. A nurse is performing a sterile wound irrigation wearing goggles, a gown, and gloves. After removing and disposing of the soiled dressings, what is the next action the nurse must perform?

    1. Discard the gloves
    2. Open the dressing tray

3. Perform hand hygiene
4. Close the room door or bed curtains

130. Ms. Vernon is hospitalized with active pulmonary tuberculosis. Which of the following diagnostic results would be the most important in determining whether the nurse can discontinue respiratory isolation and airborne precautions?

1. The two-step Mantoux tuberculin skin test is negative.
2. Ms. Vernon's chest radiograph shows improved consolidation.
3. A sputum sample is clear of acid-fast bacteria.
4. Ms. Vernon's temperature has returned to normal for 24 hours.

131. Ms. Diniz, age 85 years, is a client in a long-term care facility. The nurse suspects Ms. Diniz has developed fecal impaction. Which of the following statements by Ms. Diniz might indicate fecal impaction?

1. "I have a lot of gas pains."
2. "I don't have much of an appetite."
3. "I feel like I have to go and just can't."
4. "I haven't had a bowel movement for 2 days."

132. Toxoplasmosis in a pregnant woman can cause fetal anomalies. To prevent toxoplasmosis, which of the following measures should the nurse advise pregnant clients to avoid?

1. Contact with cat feces
2. People who have viral illnesses
3. Ingestion of freshwater fish
4. Exposure to children who have not been immunized

133. A nurse encounters a motor vehicle accident on her way home from work. She finds Mr. Cahuas under the wreckage of his car. He is conscious and breathing satisfactorily. He is lying on his back complaining of pain in his back and an inability to move his legs. What should be the first action by the nurse?

1. Leave Mr. Cahuas lying on his back with instructions not to move, and then seek help
2. Gently raise Mr. Cahuas to a sitting position to see if the pain either diminishes or increases in intensity
3. Roll Mr. Cahuas onto his abdomen, place a pad under his head, and cover him with any material available
4. Gently lift Mr. Cahuas onto a flat piece of lumber and call 9-1-1

134. Ms. Chu is diagnosed with expressive aphasia. Which of the following difficulties related to the aphasia should the nurse include in the nursing care plan?

1. Speaking or writing
2. Following specific instructions
3. Understanding speech
4. Recognizing words for familiar objects

135. A maternal–newborn community nurse speaks with a father who is concerned that there is a yellow-crusted discharge around the glans penis of his recently circumcised newborn. How should the nurse advise the father?

1. "This is a sign of an infection, and he will require antibiotics."
2. "If he is voiding normally, this is part of the healing process and just needs daily cleansing with water."
3. "This is a sign that there needs to be better cleansing of the area, so soak the penis in half-strength hydrogen peroxide."
4. "Problems such as these are one of the reasons health care providers do not recommend circumcision."

136. Mr. Edwards has a mid-thigh amputation following a severe snowboarding accident. One week after the amputation, how would the nurse best control edema in the stump?

1. Administer the prescribed diuretic
2. Restrict Mr. Edwards's oral fluid intake
3. Keep his stump elevated on a pillow
4. Rewrap the elastic bandage as necessary

137. North Beaver Creek Hospital is on alert to receive victims of an explosion in a manufacturing plant. The charge nurse reviews the triage procedure. Which of the following injuries would be the highest priority to receive care?

    1. Closed fractures of major bones
    2. Partial-thickness burns of 10% of the body
    3. Epistaxis
    4. Severe lacerations involving open fractures of major bones

138. Ms. Moss, RN, works in a cardiac step-down care unit. This is her fourth 12-hour night shift in a row. Although she has already had her break at 0400 hours, she feels ill and is so tired that she is having difficulty staying awake. All her clients are stable, are attached to monitors, and do not require any care until 0500 hours. What would be the nurse's most appropriate action?

    1. Contact her immediate nursing supervisor
    2. Put her head down on the desk in the same room as her clients
    3. Attempt to stay awake
    4. Have a co-worker who is presently on break care for her clients while she sleeps

139. On a home visit to a woman who gave birth four days prior, the visiting nurse assesses that the baby has a purulent discharge from the eyes. What is the most likely cause for the discharge?

    1. A *Chlamydia trachomatis* infection
    2. Congenital syphilis
    3. An allergic reaction to allergens in the home
    4. A reaction to the ophthalmic antibiotic ointment instilled after birth

140. A nurse works in a busy outpatient department where a team of nurses is responsible for all clients. The nurse finds that with this system, there is very little continuity of care, some interventions are missed or unnecessarily repeated, and clients are anxious because they do not have one specific nurse to speak with. What is the most appropriate action by the nurse?

    1. Advocate for a system that provides better consistency of care
    2. Ask to be assigned to a limited and specific number of clients at each shift
    3. Complain to the nursing manager that this system of care is not optimum
    4. Understand that the present system of care is necessary to efficiently manage the client numbers

141. Mrs. Scales asks the nurse what she should do to cure the upper respiratory infection (cold) she has. What would be the nurse's best advice?

    1. Go to the doctor to get a prescription for an antibiotic
    2. Ask the doctor for a prescription for an antiviral medication
    3. Drink warm fluids and try alternative therapies such as echinacea, zinc lozenges, and Cold-FX
    4. Do nothing since there's no cure for the common cold

142. An RN discusses menstruation with a group of young teenage girls. Which of the following practices would be included in the hygiene counselling regarding menstruation?

    1. "Do not bathe during menstruation."
    2. "Change tampons every 2 to 4 hours."
    3. "Use only sanitary napkins because tampons cause toxic shock syndrome."
    4. "Douche regularly with a commercial product or vinegar and water."

143. Mrs. Kyros is being treated for infertility due to endometriosis. Which of the following manifestations is characteristic of endometriosis?

    1. Amenorrhea
    2. Anovulation
    3. Dysmenorrhea
    4. Pelvic inflammation

144. A registered nurse observes another nurse fondling the breasts of a comatose female client. What should be the nurse's initial action?

1. Intervene by requesting that her colleague leave the client's room
2. Immediately report what she has observed to the unit manager
3. Report her colleague to the provincial regulatory body
4. Make a written report of what she has observed

145. Which of the following pathological conditions is a common complication of osteoporosis?

1. Spiral fractures of the radius
2. Compression fractures of the spine
3. Displaced fractures of the tibia
4. Avulsed fracture of the phalanges

146. Nurses working in a nephrology unit use automatic equipment for vital sign monitoring. At the beginning of a shift, the nurse obtains a blood pressure reading of 195/120 mm Hg for Mr. Fernandes. His readings have previously been in the range of 132/94 to 140/96 mm Hg. What should be the nurse's initial action?

1. Notify the physician
2. Administer the ordered prn antihypertensive medication
3. Change the cuff to his other arm
4. Retake the blood pressure using a manual sphygmomanometer and cuff

147. Mr. Alberto has Parkinson's disease. The nurse overhears his wife say to him, "If you take your medicines, you will be able to walk better, and you will be cured." What should the nurse say to Mr. Alberto's wife?

1. "I am glad to hear you encouraging your husband to take his medications."
2. "Has there been a problem with your husband taking his medications?"
3. "Why are you saying this to your husband when you know that, although the medications will help him, there is no cure for Parkinson's?"
4. "What is your understanding about how Parkinson's disease is affecting your husband?"

148. Which type of cancer causes the highest death rate in the Canadian population?

1. Lung
2. Breast
3. Prostate
4. Colorectal

149. Which of the following dressing materials would be most appropriate to use for a wound that has a moderate to heavy drainage and is deep, with some tunnelling?

1. An alginate dressing such as Kaltostat
2. A hydrocolloid dressing such as Tegasorb
3. A gauze dressing such as a Kling bandage
4. A foam dressing such as Allevyn

150. Linda, age 15 years, is diagnosed with idiopathic scoliosis following screening by the school nurse. What is the treatment of choice for idiopathic scoliosis?

1. An external spinal orthosis such as the Boston Brace
2. Surgical correction of the curve
3. Therapeutic exercises
4. External electrical stimulation of the spinal muscles

151. Ms. Benergan has had unprotected sex and obtains emergency contraception from a pharmacy in the form of a high-dose estrogen–progestin combination (Plan B). How does this emergency contraception prevent pregnancy?

1. If taken before ovulation, it prevents or delays ovulation.
2. If taken after ovulation, it stimulates menstruation.
3. If taken after ovulation, it causes the fertilized ovum to stop developing.
4. If taken after fertilization, it causes the ovum to abort.

152. Ms. Rogers is to have total body radiation prior to receiving a bone marrow transplant. Which of the

following topics should the nurse include in her health teaching about radiation?

1. The potential to develop blood clots
2. An increased susceptibility to infection
3. A probable loss of hair
4. The development of spontaneous fractures

153. Mr. Leslie works as an unregulated care provider in a chronic care facility. He has been trained to suction the tracheotomy of a stable long-term client and has performed this routine care for many years. Another client with a tracheotomy develops pneumonia. Mr. Leslie tells the nurse that to save her time, he can suction the client with pneumonia. Which of the following answers would be the nurse's best response?

1. Explain to Mr. Leslie that if she is very busy, he may perform the procedure but that she is ultimately responsible
2. Tell Mr. Leslie that he may not suction this client because suctioning a client with pneumonia is different from suctioning a client who has a permanent, well-established tracheotomy and is not considered routine care
3. Thank Mr. Leslie for understanding that she has a very heavy workload and let him perform the procedure
4. Tell Mr. Leslie that she will do all the suctioning in the future and that he should not be performing suctioning at all

154. A public education campaign that occurred during the 1990s following research findings about sudden infant death syndrome (SIDS) is credited with reducing the mortality from SIDS by 40%. What action did the public education campaign recommend to parents?

1. Position infants in the supine position for sleep
2. Breastfeed the infant until 6 months to confer maternal antibodies
3. Place infants in the prone position to prevent aspiration
4. Use baby monitors for high-risk infants

155. A hospitalized client, Mr. Morgan, refuses his prescribed medication because it upsets his stomach. Which of the following actions by the nurse would be most appropriate?

1. Ask Mr. Morgan's wife to convince him to take the medication
2. Put the medication in his juice as this will disguise the taste
3. Tell Mr. Morgan that if he does not take the medication, he will not get better
4. Consult with the physician or pharmacist about Mr. Morgan's refusal of the medication

156. Which of the following manifestations would be most indicative of an early sign of cervical cancer?

1. Abdominal heaviness and discomfort
2. Foul-smelling vaginal discharge
3. Pressure on the bladder
4. Bloody spotting after intercourse

157. Ms. Coton has breast cancer. She asks the nurse what the term *ERP-positive* refers to. Which of the following responses by the nurse provides correct information?

1. "It indicates whether axillary lymph nodes are involved."
2. "It states the need for supplemental estrogen."
3. "It refers to a potential response to hormone therapy."
4. "It refers to the degree of metastasis that has occurred."

158. Mr. Lemone takes nitroglycerine in the form of Nitrolingual translingual spray. How would the effectiveness of the nitroglycerine best be evaluated?

1. By the relief of anginal pain
2. By improved cardiac output
3. By a decrease in blood pressure
4. By the dilation of superficial blood vessels

159. The parents of a child who has had open-heart surgery are informed that their child is in the recovery room and is stable. They are crying and extremely worried. How can the nurse best help decrease the parents' anxiety?

1. Reassure them that their child is doing well
2. Allow them to continue to express their feelings
3. Bring them to the recovery room for several minutes
4. Encourage them to return in 1 hour when the child is transferred to the intensive care unit

160. Ms. Li has an external arteriovenous shunt for her hemodialysis. What is the most serious potential problem with an external shunt?

1. Septicemia
2. Clot formation
3. Exsanguination
4. Sclerosis of vessels

161. Which of the following behaviours produces the highest risk for the transmission of HIV?

1. Vaginal intercourse
2. Man-to-man oral sex
3. Sexual intercourse with a bisexual individual
4. Anal intercourse

162. A nurse has been nominated to participate on a task force for environmentally responsible health care. How would the task force members best promote environmental awareness in their institution?

1. Institute agency policies that incorporate "green" strategies
2. Develop brief workshops to educate the employees about environmental issues
3. Colour code green all supplies that are environmentally safe
4. Purchase recycling containers to be placed throughout the agency.

163. In the middle of an operation, a surgeon yells at a nurse, "This is the wrong instrument, you stupid nurse." What should the nurse do initially?

1. Recognize this as abuse and report the surgeon to his supervisor
2. Say to the surgeon, "This is abuse, and you will not speak to me this way."

3. File a complaint with the hospital authorities
4. After the operation is over, speak privately with the surgeon about the behaviour

164. Scott, age 16 years, participates in many athletic activities at his school. He asks the school nurse which food would be the quickest source of energy for him during his sporting events. What should the nurse recommend?

1. Glass of 2% milk
2. Slice of bread
3. Chocolate bar
4. Glass of fruit juice

165. A client with a hiatal hernia complains about having difficulty sleeping at night. What should the nurse recommend?

1. Sleeping on two or three pillows to raise his upper body
2. Reducing carbohydrates in his diet
3. Drinking a glass of milk before retiring
4. Taking an antacid such as sodium bicarbonate

166. A client is receiving intermittent feedings via a nasogastric tube. How would the nurse best evaluate whether a prior feeding has been absorbed?

1. Evaluate the intake in relation to the output
2. Aspirate for residual volume
3. Instill air into the nasogastric tube while auscultating the stomach
4. Compare the client's body weight with baseline data

167. Mr. Braccio has been admitted to hospital for alcoholic cirrhosis of the liver and portal hypertension. The nurse should be alert for which of the following potential complications?

1. Liver abscesses
2. Intestinal obstruction
3. Perforation of the duodenum
4. Hemorrhage from esophageal varices

168. A 5-month-old, pale, unresponsive infant is brought to the emergency department by his parents. Which of the following factors is the strongest indicator for a suspicion of child abuse?

   1. The story of how the child became unresponsive is not credible.
   2. The infant is thin and shows signs of failure to thrive.
   3. The parents have a previous history of neglect toward their other children.
   4. The infant has had previous fractures confirmed by X-ray.

169. Which of the following skin lesions would be of most concern to a nurse working in a dermatological clinic?

   1. A scaly erythematous patch on the elbow of Mr. LeClerc, age 24 years
   2. A sudden appearance of an oval balding patch with smooth, soft skin underneath on Venetia, age 10 years
   3. Flat, brown macules on the hands of Ms. Parsons, age 83 years
   4. A mixed pigmentation lesion with irregular borders on the back of Mr. Priestly, age 42 years

170. Following a transurethral resection of the prostate, Mr. Burn's indwelling catheter becomes obstructed. Which of the following solutions would be most appropriate for irrigating the catheter?

   1. Sterile water
   2. Hypertonic saline
   3. Sterile normal saline
   4. Genitourinary irrigating solution

171. Mr. Beauclerc is in hospital after experiencing two transient ischemic attacks. The physician discussed with him the dangers of smoking, and Mr. Beauclerc stated that he quit 2 weeks ago, after the first attack. The nurse discovers a pack of cigarettes in Mr. Beauclerc's bathrobe pocket. What would be the most appropriate action of the nurse in addressing this situation?

   1. Let Mr. Beauclerc know the cigarettes were found

   2. Admonish Mr. Beauclerc for having cigarettes
   3. Notify the physician
   4. Discard the cigarettes without making a comment

172. What is the Canadian Nurses Association?

   1. The provincial and territorial organization responsible for registering all nurses in Canada
   2. A federation of provincial and territorial associations whose mission is to advance the quality of nursing
   3. The national association whose mission is to provide collective bargaining and labour relations collaboration
   4. An association that has been delegated by federal statutes to provide self-governance within the profession of nursing

173. Ms. Serena is discharged home with her infant, who has a severe genetic disorder. When the neonatal follow-up nurse arrives to visit, Ms. Serena is crying and appears tired. Which of the following comments by the nurse would be most therapeutic?

   1. "Is everything all right? You look tired."
   2. "Tell me a little about your daily routine."
   3. "Are you having trouble looking after the baby?"
   4. "You are upset. Tell me what's wrong."

174. What is the most important factor to consider when providing environmental oxygen therapy to a premature infant?

   1. Ensure that the oxygen is administered at the appropriate flow rate
   2. Ensure that the oxygen is delivered at exactly the ordered concentration
   3. Ensure that supplemental oxygen is titrated according to oxygen saturation readings
   4. Ensure that the oxygen is sufficient to prevent hypoxia

175. A midwife and RN visit a postpartum client 3 days after her delivery. They notice that the

infant looks slightly jaundiced. What is the appropriate action by the midwife and nurse?

1. Advise the mother to discontinue breastfeeding
2. Have the mother position the infant's cot beside a sunny window
3. Advise the mother to supplement breastfeeding with glucose and water for increased fluids
4. Arrange for the infant to have a serum bilirubin test

176. Mr. and Mrs. Fenton have been married for 48 years. Recently, Mr. Fenton had a cerebrovascular accident that has left him with partial right-sided paralysis. At the rehabilitation unit, Mrs. Fenton insists on doing everything for her husband. When she leaves, he appears quite sad. Which of the following emotions is Mr. Fenton probably feeling?

1. He is losing hope for the future.
2. He is feeling the loss of his independence.
3. He is feeling guilty about being a burden to his wife.
4. He is feeling loss of his masculine role.

177. A nurse working with a rescue team following a hurricane is searching for injured people. She discovers a man lying next to a broken natural gas main. There are no signs of respirations, and he is losing a lot of blood from a wound on his left calf. What should the nurse's initial action be?

1. Treat the young man for shock
2. Start rescue breathing immediately
3. Apply surface pressure to the calf wound
4. If it can be done safely, remove the man from the immediate vicinity

178. Which of the following are manifestations or indications of atelectasis?

1. Slow, deep respirations
2. Dry, unproductive coughs
3. Rales and crackles in the lower lobes
4. Diminished breath sounds

179. Mrs. Carter sustained a Colles fracture of her wrist when she fell on an icy sidewalk. She asks the nurse why she has to have her elbow in the cast, as it is her wrist that is broken. Which of the following responses by the nurse would be the most accurate?

1. "The cast will help to keep the wrist bones aligned."
2. "The cast will stop you turning your hand up and down."
3. "It is easier to maintain this longer cast than one just on the wrist."
4. "You will soon get used to it, and it will provide support."

180. Mr. Cameron has severe frostbite on both his feet after his snowmobile broke down while he was on a hunting trip. Which of the following medications is most important to be prescribed for Mr. Cameron?

1. Tetanus antitoxin or tetanus immune globulin
2. Medicated oatmeal footbath
3. Prophylactic antibiotics
4. Narcotic analgesics

181. Ms. Atkinson is scheduled for an upper gastrointestinal series with a barium swallow. Which of the following post-test teaching points is most important for the nurse to review with Ms. Atkinson?

1. She should immediately report any nausea after the test.
2. Her stool may be colourless for up to 72 hours after the procedure.
3. There are no restrictions on diet or fluid intake after the test.
4. She will be encouraged to increase her fluid intake after the test.

182. Mr. Petrie, age 55 years, is about to be discharged home following recovery from a myocardial infarction. Mr. Petrie's partner is concerned about resuming sexual relations. Which of the following would be correct information for the nurse to give Mr. Petrie and his partner?

1. "When you feel comfortable climbing two flights of stairs, sexual activity may be resumed."
2. "This is a personal matter for both of you to discuss. You know how physical your relations are, so you can best judge when to resume sexual activity."
3. "It is usually recommended to wait about 4 to 6 months before resuming sexual relations."
4. "Sexual relations may be resumed when you can jog around a block without experiencing any significant chest pain."

183. Mr. Phillion, age 21, is on a swim team that competes internationally. He develops sinusitis, for which he receives treatment at the sports facility health clinic. He is scheduled to be in a high-profile race in 2 days. What health teaching should the clinic nurse provide to Mr. Phillion?

1. "Have warm showers twice a day, and call if you develop a fever."
2. "Take over-the-counter analgesics to relieve the pain, and stay out of the pool."
3. "Blow your nose often to keep your nasal passages open."
4. "Keep your head above the water when swimming."

184. In a group of older adults, a community nurse discusses the nutritional problems associated with aging. Which of the following statements represents correct information about older adults and nutrition?

1. Most older adults eat well and manage to get adequate nutrition for their energy needs.
2. A small but significant percentage of older adults in Canada use food banks and report being hungry due to lack of money.
3. Most older adults receive automatic supplemental governmental financial support so that they do not need to go to food banks.
4. Because of the decreased metabolic needs of older adults, most are able to achieve sufficient nutrition in their diet.

185. Ms. Cooke developed pleuritis on her right side following an automobile accident. She experiences pain when she coughs or breathes deeply. Which suggestion by the nurse would help Ms. Cooke to alleviate her pain?

1. "Turn frequently onto the unaffected side, and use a pillow as a splint when you cough."
2. "Sit up with two pillows behind you, and use the palms of your hands as a splint."
3. "Turn frequently onto the affected side, and use a pillow as a splint."
4. "Try not to breathe too deeply, and drink extra fluids to thin the secretions."

186. By what age should a newborn infant regain his or her birth weight?

1. 5 to 7 days
2. 7 to 10 days
3. 10 to 14 days
4. 14 to 21 days

187. After 4 days on an inpatient psychiatric unit, a client on suicide precautions tells the nurse, "Hey, look! I was feeling pretty depressed for a while, but I'm certainly not going to kill myself." What would be the nurse's best response?

1. "Were you really thinking of killing yourself?"
2. "You do seem to be feeling better."
3. "Why don't we sit down and talk some more about this?"
4. "That's good, but the staff will continue to observe you very carefully, just in case."

188. An international health coalition group visits an impoverished country. The group consists of a physician epidemiologist, a local community health worker, a public health nurse, and a paramedic. During their visit, an earthquake occurs a short distance away. Numerous casualties are being reported, and aid is requested to triage the victims. Of the people on the task force, who is the best health care worker to travel to the area for triage?

1. The nurse
2. The physician
3. The local community health care worker
4. The paramedic

189. A client is in the manic phase of her bipolar disorder. What would be the best approach for the nurse to assist her with her personal appearance?

    1. Encourage her to dress appropriately in her own clothing
    2. Allow her to apply makeup in whatever manner she chooses
    3. Keep cosmetics away from her because she will apply them too freely
    4. Suggest that she wear hospital clothing

190. A nurse is concerned about privatization of health care in her province, which has several private clinics where wealthy residents may pay for immediate diagnostic radiography, magnetic resonance imaging, and positron emission tomography scans. What is the most professional and effective action for the nurse to initiate?

    1. Speak with the owners of the private clinics
    2. Organize a protest march outside of a clinic
    3. Initiate a letter-writing campaign to the appropriate member of provincial or federal Parliament
    4. Discuss her concerns with her health care colleagues

191. A focus for health programming in a community is maternal–child health. It is recognized that there is a need to decrease the number of unplanned teen pregnancies. What is the best approach to decrease the number of pregnancies in this community?

    1. Education about abstinence as a birth-control choice
    2. Teaching men about the use of condoms to prevent unwanted pregnancies
    3. Providing information about abortions
    4. Increasing the availability of contraceptives.

192. Mr. Jackes tells the nurse at the urgent care clinic that he was "throwing up horribly all night long and couldn't keep anything down." What would be the nurse's best initial question?

    1. "How many times, and how much did you vomit?"
    2. "What did you have to eat last night?"

    3. "Did you take your temperature?"
    4. "Does anyone else in your family have the same symptoms?"

193. Mr. Burgess is diagnosed with gonorrhea. Which of the following statements is correct concerning this sexually transmitted infection (STI)?

    1. Gonorrhea is not a common STI.
    2. Cases of gonorrhea must be reported to health authorities.
    3. Antibiotic treatment takes several weeks to ensure a cure.
    4. Permanent damage to the testes is common.

194. Baby Liam is born at 28 weeks' gestation. What is the most common complication of prematurity?

    1. Hemorrhage
    2. Brain damage
    3. Aspiration of mucus
    4. Respiratory distress

195. Which of the following Canadians should discuss the use of a vitamin D supplement with a health care provider?

    1. Dark-skinned people
    2. People with chronic obstructive pulmonary disease
    3. People who live in southern Canada
    4. People of European descent

196. Mr. Brankston is HIV positive. He asks the nurse what antiretroviral therapy will do. Which of the following explanations by the nurse would correctly state the purpose of the therapy?

    1. "The antiretrovirals remove the virus from your body."
    2. "The antiretrovirals reduce the amount of HIV in your body and increase CD4 cells, which improve your immunity."
    3. "The antiretrovirals kill the virus just as an antibiotic does with bacteria."
    4. "The antiretrovirals prevent duplication of the virus by altering the DNA–RNA transcription phase."

197. A public health nurse participates in a task force for a charity that provides health care to an impoverished community in another country. The task force realizes that success of health care programs depends primarily on which of the following factors?

    1. Consultation with local stakeholders
    2. Fundraising capabilities
    3. Commitment of volunteers
    4. Public awareness

198. The nurse manager of a busy medical-surgical unit is concerned about meeting staffing needs over the Christmas holiday period. Many nurses have requested the same time off, and the hospital does not hire agency staff. Which of the following actions would be most successful in solving this problem?

    1. Call a meeting of the nursing staff and ask members to provide possible solutions
    2. Implement a holiday schedule that the manager feels is fair to all staff
    3. Provide senior nurses with the first opportunity to schedule their holidays
    4. Hold a lottery for nurses to win their preferred vacation days

199. Ms. Pratha, age 77 years, has been recently diagnosed with hypertension. She asks the nurse what type of exercise program she should begin. What would be the nurse's best response?

    1. "Now that you have high blood pressure, it would be unwise for you to exercise."
    2. "Begin by walking around your block, and then increase the distance as you can tolerate it."
    3. "Working out in a gym for 45 minutes three times a week under the supervision of a personal trainer would be best."
    4. "You should do all of your exercise in the evening, when your blood pressure is at its lowest."

200. A nurse is a member of an international aid group that is sending supplies to a country where a hurricane has occurred. Which of the following supplies would be most important to send to the area?

    1. Bandages and antiseptics
    2. Bottled water
    3. Oral antibiotics
    4. Prepackaged high-calorie food

END OF PRACTICE EXAM 3

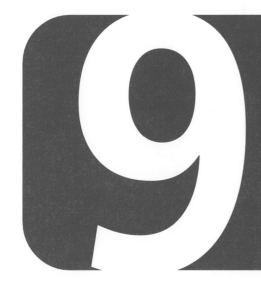

Answers and Rationales for Practice Exam 3

CASE–BASED QUESTIONS
ANSWERS AND RATIONALES

CASE 1

1. 1. Unprotected sex is a transmission route for hepatitis C but is not the most common one.
   2. Transfusions of contaminated blood were the cause of some cases of hepatitis C prior to the late 1990s, but this is not presently the most common source.
   3. There is frequently co-infection with hepatitis C and human immunodeficiency virus (HIV), but one disease does not result in the other.

   4. Hepatitis C is transmitted via blood and body fluids. More than half of hepatitis C clients are intravenous drug users.

CLASSIFICATION
Competency:
Changes in Health
Taxonomy:
Critical Thinking

2. 1. While nutritional supplements are what he needs, it is unlikely Mr. Tolea would have the financial ability to buy them.
   2. His diet does require fruit and vegetables, but it is unlikely he would be able to afford them or store them in his rooming house.

   3. Mr. Tolea requires nutritional support beyond what he can purchase himself. The strategy that has the best chance of success is to find public or private resources to provide his meals. The social worker is the health care provider with the knowledge to access appropriate resources.

   4. While it may be an option for the nurse to have the social worker try to contact his family, Mr. Tolea is estranged from them, and they may not want to support him.

CLASSIFICATION
Competency:
Health and Wellness
Taxonomy:
Critical Thinking

3. 1. Sedation is not pain management. Mr. Tolea may prefer to be awake and alert, not sedated.

   2. The purpose of palliative care is to help the client achieve a dignified, comfortable death on his own terms. The client may make decisions about sedation, analgesia, skin care, nutrition, spiritual support, and so on.

   3. Care for itchy skin that may be a result of liver failure is included in client choice.
   4. Pressure ulcers are a risk in the palliative care client, but care for these is included in provision of client choice.

CLASSIFICATION
Competency:
Changes in Health
Taxonomy:
Critical Thinking

4. 1. Terminally ill clients are the target population. Most of these clients will have received care from physicians and nurses during the course of their illness. These health care providers are best positioned to refer clients to appropriate palliative care services.

CLASSIFICATION
Competency:
Health and Wellness

2. It would be more appropriate to lobby politicians for an increase in finances for palliative services.

3. This approach may be helpful but is unlikely to be as efficient a strategy as informing health care providers.

4. Same as answer 3.

Taxonomy:
Critical Thinking

CASE 2

5. 1. This factor may cause obesity but only if it is not offset by calorie expenditure.

2. This factor may cause obesity but only if calories are not restricted.

3. When the caloric intake consistently exceeds the expenditure of calories, the excess calories will be stored in the body in the form of fat.

4. Same as answer 2.

CLASSIFICATION
Competency:
Health and Wellness
Taxonomy:
Critical Thinking

6. 1. There is no correlation between birth weight and future obesity.

2. The incidence of obese children born to obese parents (80%) is significantly higher than that of obese children born to parents of normal weight (14%).

3. This factor is predictive but is not as significant as obesity in parents.

4. Same as answer 3.

CLASSIFICATION
Competency:
Health and Wellness
Taxonomy:
Critical Thinking

7. 1. This cholesterol value is normal for an 11-year-old.

2. This value is higher than expected and may be indicative of type 2 diabetes. Childhood obesity is related to an increase in type 2 diabetes.

3. This blood pressure is normal for an 11-year-old.

4. Breathing problems do occur in overweight children, but these spirometry values are normal.

CLASSIFICATION
Competency:
Changes in Health
Taxonomy:
Application

8. 1. This calculation is incorrect.

2. Same as answer 1.

3. This calculation is correct:
$132 \times 32 = 17,424$ (this is 132 cm squared)
$58 \div 17,424 \times 10,000 = 33.3$

4. Same as answer 1.

CLASSIFICATION
Competency:
Professional Practice
Taxonomy:
Application

9.   1. Successful behaviour-modification programs assist children to identify inappropriate eating habits and to incorporate suitable physical activity, which may lead to lifelong management of the obesity.

CLASSIFICATION
Competency:
Health and Wellness
Taxonomy:
Critical Thinking

   2. Diet is one part of therapy, but it should not be severely reduced because the child will not be able to maintain the restrictions.
   3. These drugs are not recommended for children.
   4. This surgery is not recommended for children.

---

10.   1. Denying Rickhelm social interaction with his friends is a poor approach. If he is denied foods he finds enjoyable, he is not likely to stick to a diet. Many fast-food restaurants supply pamphlets with the nutritional information of their menus.

CLASSIFICATION
Competency:
Nurse–Client Partnership
Taxonomy:
Application

   2. A hamburger and fries are high in fat and calories.
   3. Same as answer 1.
   4. Same as answer 1.

---

11.   1. This question is close ended. It may also be seen by Rickhelm as intrusive.
   2. This question is close ended and will elicit a yes or no answer.
   3. This question is close ended and implies that Rickhelm should feel bad about himself.

CLASSIFICATION
Competency:
Nurse–Client Partnership
Taxonomy:
Critical Thinking

   4. This question is open ended and allows Rickhelm to discuss any problems that are occurring as a result of his weight.

CASE 3

12.   1. Various aspects of hospitalization and diagnosis could cause the client anxiety. The nurse should determine what disturbs the client most.

CLASSIFICATION
Competency:
Nurse–Client Partnership
Taxonomy:
Application

   2. Anxiety is a barrier to learning. The client would not be receptive.
   3. This approach may serve to increase his anxiety.
   4. It is likely a tracheotomy will be performed, so alternative methods of communication must be discussed; however, the nurse should initially determine what Mr. Jason's specific anxieties are.

---

13.   1. This position would neither increase nor decrease strain on the suture line.
   2. Drainage from the wound would not be affected.
   3. Providing stimulation would not be a priority; this position would not affect the degree of stimulation.

CLASSIFICATION
Competency:
Changes in Health
Taxonomy:
Application

   4. This position minimizes the discomfort associated with venous engorgement. It also promotes venous drainage by gravity, minimizing edema and improving respiratory function.

14. 1. **The client should be suctioned first to avoid secretions obstructing the outer cannula while the inner cannula is removed.**

2. This action is done following the removal of the old dressing.
3. This step is taken after the sterile field is set up.
4. The ties are cut before the inner cannula is removed.

CLASSIFICATION
Competency:
Changes in Health
Taxonomy:
Application

---

15. 1. **Administration of oxygen for a few minutes prior to suctioning reduces the risk of hypoxia, the major complication associated with suctioning.**

2. Negative pressure is applied as the catheter is withdrawn.
3. The tip of the catheter should reach the base of the tube but not far beyond.
4. When ordered, this drug is usually given by inhalation, not instillation; 3 to 5 mL of normal saline can be instilled into the tracheotomy tube to loosen secretions.

CLASSIFICATION
Competency:
Changes in Health
Taxonomy:
Application

---

16. 1. **If the dressing is too tight, impaired cerebral circulation may result.**

2. Bleeding would not cause the client to complain of tightness.
3. This statement is untrue; impaired cerebral circulation may result from a tight dressing.
4. The dressing may be removed only if indicated by the physician.

CLASSIFICATION
Competency:
Changes in Health
Taxonomy:
Critical Thinking

CASE 4

17. 1. **Holistic health care encompasses the health of the whole person— body, mind, emotions, and spirit.**

2. Primary health care is a philosophy and model for improving health that focuses on promoting health and preventing illness.
3. Spiritual health care primarily concerns the health of the spiritual aspect of the individual but does not include the physical components.
4. In socioenvironmental health care, health is closely tied to the social structure of a population.

CLASSIFICATION
Competency:
Health and Wellness
Taxonomy:
Knowledge/Comprehension

---

18. 1. **Like many infectious diseases, respiratory syncytial virus (RSV) is more readily transmitted in overcrowded conditions.**

2. Premature infants and new babies of any ethnicity are particularly at risk for the virus, but this is not the reason for the increase in incidence in Aboriginal communities.
3. Warm or changeable weather favours transmission.
4. A depressed immune system is possibly a factor but does not explain the high incidence in these communities.

CLASSIFICATION
Competency:
Health and Wellness
Taxonomy:
Critical Thinking

19.   1. This statement is not true, although the taste of high-sugar foods appeals to many.
       2. This statement is not true. High-sugar foods are sweet to taste and appealing, but there is no genetic makeup that causes a craving.

       3. Because of the high cost of transportation of food to the north, nutritional foods such as milk and fresh produce are often scarce. Sugar-filled products tend to be less expensive than those of higher nutritional value.

CLASSIFICATION
Competency:
Health and Wellness
Taxonomy:
Application

       4. While there does need to be increased and continual nutrition education, this is not the primary reason for the poor diet. The cause is socioeconomic.

20.   1. This option is not realistic, nor is it provision of optimum care. The niece may need timely information regarding birth control and may not be able to wait for several days.
       2. This statement is not necessarily true. Care should be transferred to a nonrelated caregiver if possible; however, if one is not available, care may be delivered to a relative.
       3. This option is a possibility but may not provide timely care, and a physician consultation is not necessary.

CLASSIFICATION
Competency:
Professional Practice
Taxonomy:
Critical Thinking

       4. A nurse may have to care for a family member or friend as part of her professional employment; however, this should occur only when no other caregiver is available. The nurse should reflect on whether she can maintain the boundary between professional and personal roles, clarify the boundaries to the client, and maintain confidentiality.

CASE 5

21.   1. The nurse is not yet aware if the conversation between Ms. Bennett and the counsellor is true.
       2. It is true that it is not ethical for the counsellor to accept gifts, but the nurse first needs to consult the counsellor to establish any truth to Ms. Bennett's story.
       3. It is necessary to talk to the counsellor first to establish any truth to Ms. Bennett's story.

CLASSIFICATION
Competency:
Nurse–Client Partnership
Taxonomy:
Application

       4. Given the potential for Ms. Bennett to misunderstand or misinterpret the nature of the relationship, it is the nurse's obligation to clarify the circumstances around the conversation.

22.   1. More information is required before this assumption can be made.

CLASSIFICATION
Competency:
Changes in Health
Taxonomy:
Application

       2. Grandiosity is associated with the manic phase of bipolar disorder. This often includes elaborate plans with individuals in positions of power, excessive spending of money, and misperceptions relating to the nature of relationship boundaries.

3. Same as answer 1.
4. Although the nurse will understand that Ms. Bennett's claims are likely unfounded, she will realize that they are a sign of grandiosity, characteristic of the manic phase, which is a concern.

CASE 6

23. **1. Prior to being able to assist a grieving family, the nurse must be aware of his own feelings about death.**

    2. This action may be applicable but only after the nurse reflects on his own feelings.
    3. Same as answer 2.
    4. Same as answer 2.

CLASSIFICATION
Competency:
Professional Practice
Taxonomy:
Critical Thinking

24. 1. Most agencies do require a do-not-resuscitate order (DNR), but the important first step is to determine the wishes of the client.
    2. This step may be taken if there are no directives, but the nurse should determine Mr. Braun's (or his family's) wishes so that he does not experience unwanted intervention.

    3. The nurse should determine the family and client wishes as soon as possible and communicate these to the health care team. Nurses ethically abide by the expressed wishes of the client or the client's substitute decision maker.

    4. While directives regarding end-of-life decision making are included in the Canadian Nurses Association's *Code of Ethics for Registered Nurses*, the nurse should first consult the family.

CLASSIFICATION
Competency:
Professional Practice
Taxonomy:
Critical Thinking

25. 1. This question is not therapeutic and may cause Mrs. Braun to feel defensive.

    2. This question does not accuse Mrs. Braun of denial or misunderstanding the physician's prognosis and should elicit information about what Mrs. Braun understands about her husband's situation.

    3. With this question, Mrs. Braun is able to answer yes or no, which may end the discussion and not provide the nurse with the opportunity to explore Mrs. Braun's grief.
    4. Mrs. Braun may deny her discussion with the children or may answer only yes or no; this question may make her feel defensive.

CLASSIFICATION
Competency:
Nurse–Client Partnership
Taxonomy:
Application

26. 1. This documentation is a physician responsibility and does not need to be made by the nurse.

    2. This documentation is a legal requirement.

CLASSIFICATION
Competency:
Professional Practice

3. Specific hygiene care—for example, washing the body, closing the eyes—does not need to be itemized. Documentation would need to include that care of the body was performed and by whom as well as which tubes were left in place and any personal articles left on the body.

Taxonomy:
Knowledge/Comprehension

4. Family participation should be documented, but it is not necessary to note the time of their departure.

---

27. 1. This action may happen if the nurse is not able to work through conflicts about caring for dying clients, but it should not be his first action.

2. Talking with respected colleagues may help the nurse reflect on his feelings, find support from his peers, and put his feelings of inadequacy in perspective.

CLASSIFICATION
Competency:
Professional Practice
Taxonomy:
Critical Thinking

3. Feelings of inadequacy are not part of normal grieving for a health care provider. The nurse should be able to reflect on what actions he might have performed differently, but this should not be accompanied by guilt.

4. It may help to discuss his performance with the unit manager after he has had time for self-reflection and dialogue with colleagues.

CASE 7

28. 1. Breastfeeding is contraindicated when the mother has a chemical abuse problem, most specifically involving alcohol, marijuana, or cocaine, as these substances are transmitted in breast milk.

CLASSIFICATION
Competency:
Health and Wellness
Taxonomy:
Knowledge/Comprehension

2. Women with inverted nipples are able to breastfeed.
3. Mastitis is not a contraindication unless the discomfort is intolerable to the mother.
4. Cancer is a contraindication only if the mother is receiving chemotherapy.

---

29. 1. This statement is not necessarily true. Not all bottle-fed infants are overfed.
2. Breast milk does not lack enough fat for growth.

CLASSIFICATION
Competency:
Health and Wellness
Taxonomy:
Application

3. This statement is true of breastfed infants. In fact, the head circumference of breastfed infants is larger than that of formula-fed infants, indicating superior growth parameters. There is some research that indicates the 1977 growth charts are not appropriate for breastfed infants.

4. Infant formulas are generally of equal caloric content to breast milk.

30.   1. Milk supply depends on demand. The more feedings that are required, the more milk the mother will produce. The nursing mother should be feeding her infant 8 to 12 times per day initially.

      2. Increased fluids have not been shown to increase milk production. Fifteen glasses is too much fluid.
      3. This action may stimulate the letdown reflex or help with engorgement but does not increase milk supply.
      4. This action may be of help in stimulating the letdown reflex.

CLASSIFICATION

Competency:
Health and Wellness
Taxonomy:
Application

31.   1. Jeremy should have six to eight wet diapers per day if he is receiving sufficient breast milk.

      2. This statement is correct, but this measure is not objective.
      3. This method of determining intake is outdated and has been evaluated to cause undue anxiety in mothers who are concerned about their ability to breastfeed. As well, it evaluates the intake only at one feeding.
      4. Breastfed infants at this age should have a minimum of three stools per day. However, the number of stools is not a reliable indicator of nutrition and hydration.

CLASSIFICATION

Competency:
Health and Wellness
Taxonomy:
Application

32.   1. This action may cause him to become more distressed.
      2. This action may help to wake a sleepy baby, but it will distress a fussy baby.
      3. Environmental stimuli need to be decreased, not increased.

      4. Swaddling him and allowing him to suck will help Jeremy to calm down so that he is better able to latch on to the breast.

CLASSIFICATION

Competency:
Health and Wellness
Taxonomy:
Application

33.   1. This option is not the best since there is not necessarily any need to discontinue breastfeeding.
      2. This option may have been viable if Ms. Hudson were conflicted about returning to work, but she has said that she wants to return to work. It would be better to explore her feelings about her job and the necessity of returning to work.
      3. This option is a possibility but is unnecessary since Jeremy is still just 2 weeks of age. She should continue breastfeeding exclusively for the time being.

      4. Continuing with breastfeeding after returning to work is a viable option. A lactation consultant will work with Ms. Hudson to provide individualized strategies for her and Jeremy.

CLASSIFICATION

Competency:
Nurse–Client Partnership
Taxonomy:
Application

34.   1. The La Leche League is the internationally recognized organization that provides education about breastfeeding and support to professionals and mothers.

      2. This organization provides education and support for natural childbirth.

CLASSIFICATION

Competency:
Health and Wellness
Taxonomy:
Knowledge/Comprehension

Answers Exam 3

3. This government agency mandates to protect the health and safety of Canadians; it is not specifically focused on breastfeeding.

4. This not-for-profit agency provides health care services to Canadians in the community. Breastfeeding support may be provided but is not the primary focus of the agency.

CASE 8

35. 1. Bloody drainage is expected this soon after surgery, and the physician does not need to be notified.
2. Nasogastric suction must be working and the tube must remain patent to prevent stress on the suture line.

3. Nasogastric drainage is expected to be bright red at first and gradually darkens within the first 24 hours after surgery.

4. The nasogastric tube would be irrigated with iced saline only if a physician specifically orders it.

CLASSIFICATION

Competency:
Changes in Health
Taxonomy:
Application

36. 1. Physiological normal saline is used in gastric irrigation to prevent electrolyte imbalance. Because of the fresh gastric sutures, irrigation should be slow and gentle.

2. The purpose of irrigation is to maintain the patency of the tube for gastric decompression; with a disconnection from the suction, a buildup of secretions and air can occur, or the tube can become blocked by viscous drainage.
3. Increasing the pressure may cause damage to the suture line.
4. Same as answer 2.

CLASSIFICATION

Competency:
Changes in Health
Taxonomy:
Application

37. 1. This action is not necessary unless Ms. Loates is unable to expectorate secretions.
2. Oxygen administration is generally not required unless the client has an underlying cardiac or respiratory disease.
3. Although ambulation will help to decrease the risk of pulmonary complications and a pooling of pulmonary secretions, individuals with abdominal incisions often revert to shallow breathing during physical effort. Ambulation during the first 24 hours may be limited.

4. To promote drainage of different lung regions, clients should turn every 2 hours. Deep breathing inflates the alveoli and promotes fluid drainage.

CLASSIFICATION

Competency:
Changes in Health
Taxonomy:
Application

CASE 9

38.   1. This question is close ended and would not yield the information the
nurse requires.

2. **This question is open ended and will inform the nurse of Juanita's**
understanding of what will occur when she stops treatment.

3. This question sympathizes with Juanita but does not provide the nurse
with the information she needs to confirm informed consent.
4. This action may occur but is not necessary at this point. The nurse first needs
to collect assessment data on Juanita's understanding of refusing treatment.

CLASSIFICATION

Competency:
Nurse–Client Partnership
Taxonomy:
Critical Thinking

39.   1. **According to the Canadian Nurses Association's *Code of Ethics for***
***Registered Nurses*, the nurse's first responsibility is to advocate for**
the client's wishes once an informed decision has been made.

2. It may be appropriate to refer Juanita's parents for counselling but not
for the purpose of having Juanita change her mind.
3. This action may occur if the nurse is not able to resolve her ethical
dilemma, but it is not the nurse's primary role in this situation.
4. This action may be a therapeutic approach to resolve the parents' issues
but is not the primary role of the nurse.

CLASSIFICATION

Competency:
Professional Practice
Taxonomy:
Critical Thinking

40.   1. The parents may not want to be, nor may Juanita want them to be, the
designated people to receive information. This action makes the
decision the nurse's choice, not the family's.

2. **This action achieves client and family choice and provides a clear**
communication route for the health care staff.

3. Juanita may not be able, particularly in her weakened state, to
communicate with her family.
4. This action does not solve the problem since the primary nurse still
must communicate with all family members.

CLASSIFICATION

Competency:
Nurse–Client Partnership
Taxonomy:
Critical Thinking

41.   1. The nurse does not know how the family feels.
2. It is not professional to blame poor care on staffing. The nurse does not
know what is inadequate about the care.
3. The nurse cannot change the plan of care until she has discussed with
the family exactly what is wrong with the care.

4. **This question asks the family to identify what they feel is inadequate**
about Juanita's care. By asking this question, the nurse may be able
to determine if there are facets of care that need to be improved or
if the family's lashing out is a symptom of their grief.

CLASSIFICATION

Competency:
Nurse–Client Partnership
Taxonomy:
Application

Answers Exam 3

42.   1. This action is contrary to Juanita's documented wishes.
    2. Same as answer 1.
    3. Same as answer 1.

CLASSIFICATION

Competency:

Professional Practice

Taxonomy:

Critical Thinking

    4. The nurse may not interfere with Juanita's documented wish for no resuscitation. The mother is manifesting anger in her grief and needs comforting. There is no legal basis for a lawsuit.

CASE 10

43.   1. This information is practical and honest.

    2. There is no indication that the amputation would have to be below the knee.
    3. This response avoids answering the question.
    4. This response can be construed as blaming the wife for not bringing her husband in sooner.

CLASSIFICATION

Competency:

Changes in Health

Taxonomy:

Application

44.   1. This action may be helpful but will not provide Mrs. Partilucci with the best learning experience at this time.

    2. The diabetes nurse educator is the best source of education for Mrs. Partilucci. This is a practical step to help her learning.

CLASSIFICATION

Competency:

Professional Practice

Taxonomy:

Application

    3. This action will only help her understand what is happening during this acute episode.
    4. This action dismisses Mrs. Partilucci's question and ignores her need to help her husband.

45.   1. There is a familial link.
    2. This information may not be completely correct. The timing of onset of diabetes cannot be predicted, although, in most cases, it does start to manifest after 40 years. Often the severity depends on lifestyle choices and therapeutic management.

CLASSIFICATION

Competency:

Changes in Health

Taxonomy:

Application

    3. This response is factual but not threatening and provides some information about how the son can help prevent developing type 2 diabetes.

    4. This information is not correct.

CASE 11

46.   1. It arises from melanocytes but may metastasize to any organ.

CLASSIFICATION

Competency:

Changes in Health

Taxonomy:

Knowledge/Comprehension

    2. It is not rare as it accounts for 11% of all skin cancers. It is not superficial and becomes invasive if untreated.
    3. Radiation is a risk factor, not a cause.
    4. This information is incorrect.

47.   1. It isn't known if his cancer can be cured by surgery until the extent of the tumour is known.
      2. While the surgery will remove the cancerous lesion, there is no indication that other melanomas will develop.

      3. The cure rate for cutaneous melanoma by excision is nearly 100% if the malignant cells are restricted to the epidermis and only if the entire lesion is removed prior to metastasis. At this time, it is not possible to know if there has been metastasis.

      4. This step would be unnecessary if surgery removed all the cancerous cells. This response does not answer Mr. O'Morrissey's question.

CLASSIFICATION
Competency:
Changes in Health
Taxonomy:
Application

---

48.   1. This advice is not reasonable since he works outdoors.
      2. This advice is good but does not include covering for his arms and hands.

      3. This advice is most important since, with early detection and treatment, melanoma can be cured.

      4. Sunscreen is necessary but is not as important as skin monitoring; also, the SPF should probably be 30 for increased protection.

CLASSIFICATION
Competency:
Changes in Health
Taxonomy:
Critical Thinking

CASE 12

49.   1. This description defines cystic fibrosis.
      2. This description defines emphysema.
      3. This description defines chronic bronchitis.

      4. This description defines asthma.

CLASSIFICATION
Competency:
Changes in Health
Taxonomy:
Knowledge/Comprehension

---

50.   1. Wheezing is a classic manifestation of asthma as air passes over narrowed airways. However, wheezing is an unreliable sign to gauge the severity of an attack. Minor attacks may cause audible wheezing.
      2. As the attack progresses, there may be inspiratory and expiratory wheezing, but this is not the most severe symptom.
      3. People experiencing an asthma attack will sit forward and use accessory muscles to attempt to get more air into their lungs. It is not an indicator of the severity of the attack.

      4. Severely diminished or absent breath sounds, often referred to as a "silent chest," are an ominous sign indicating severe obstruction and impending respiratory failure.

CLASSIFICATION
Competency:
Changes in Health
Taxonomy:
Critical Thinking

---

51.   1. Pulsus paradoxus is a drop in systolic pressure greater than 10 mm Hg during the inspiratory cycle.

      2. This sign is characteristic of coarctation of the aorta.

CLASSIFICATION
Competency:
Changes in Health

3. This sign is not characteristic of pulsus paradoxus. An apical heart rate is more likely to increase during an asthma attack.

4. This sign is called pulse pressure.

Taxonomy:
Knowledge/Comprehension

---

52.   1. A bronchodilator would be ordered by the physician and should be administered as quickly as possible. Oxygen may be administered prior to the order for a bronchodilator.

2. This action is necessary but probably would already have been done by the nurse. It is not the most crucial action.

3. Status asthmaticus is a life-threatening situation and could quickly lead to respiratory failure. A physician is needed immediately to direct care. Mechanical ventilation may be necessary.

4. An IV fluid bolus is not necessary for status asthmaticus.

CLASSIFICATION
Competency:
Changes in Health
Taxonomy:
Critical Thinking

---

53.   1. Normal values are PaO_2 80 to 100 mm Hg; $PaCO_2$ 35 to 45 mm Hg; and pH 7.35 to 7.45. These gases indicate a low oxygen (hypoxia), a high CO_2 (hypercapnia), and a low pH (acidosis).

2. Same as answer 1.
3. Same as answer 1.
4. Same as answer 1.

CLASSIFICATION
Competency:
Changes in Health
Taxonomy:
Critical Thinking

---

54.   1. This intervention is a component of asthma management but not the most important one.

2. The Canadian Thoracic Society and the Registered Nurses' Association of Ontario developed best practice guidelines for the management of asthma. The key component identified was appropriate education and self-management training that includes an asthma action plan.

3. This intervention is a component of the appropriate treatment of asthma but requires education for the client to manage the medication regime.

4. This intervention is an important component for monitoring the client's management of and the severity of the asthma and would be part of an action plan.

CLASSIFICATION
Competency:
Changes in Health
Taxonomy:
Critical Thinking

---

55.   1. The metered dose inhaler should be shaken five to six times, and the client should use one puff at a time.

2. Mr. Nigel should inhale as he is depressing the canister.

3. AeroChambers break up and slow down the medication particles, enhancing the amount of medication received by the client. Their use is often advantageous for children, older people, and clients who have difficulty coordinating the use of the metered dose inhaler.

4. The canister should be depressed as the client is inhaling.

CLASSIFICATION
Competency:
Changes in Health
Taxonomy:
Application

CASE 13

56.   1. This information is important but not the nurse's primary concern during admission.
2. Current substance abuse is of greater importance.

3. **The most immediate risk to Ms. Wilmox's life is what substances she may currently have in her system. All other options are valid; however, the client's medical status must be stable in order to proceed with a mental health evaluation.**

4. Ms. Wilmox has a sister and two children, so she is not without support.

CLASSIFICATION
Competency:
Changes in Health
Taxonomy:
Critical Thinking

57.   1. This action is confrontational and may prevent further cooperation.
2. This action would not be appropriate.
3. The client is always the main source of information.

4. **Presenting boundaries in a nonconfrontational, nonchallenging manner reduces the possibility that the client will feel threatened. As a result, the potential for building a therapeutic relationship with the client increases significantly.**

CLASSIFICATION
Competency:
Nurse–Client Partnership
Taxonomy:
Application

58.   1. This action is not necessary.

2. **A client always retains the right to disclosure of information; therefore, the nurse must seek permission to speak to family members or significant others. Verbal permission is adequate, and in obtaining it, the nurse builds trust and enhances the therapeutic relationship with the client. The nurse must always document a verbal consent on the client's chart.**

3. This action breaks confidentiality and could prevent further cooperation from Ms. Wilmox.
4. This action is not necessary.

CLASSIFICATION
Competency:
Professional Practice
Taxonomy:
Application

59.   1. Four-point restraints are not indicated and have not been ordered. They may prove counterproductive.

2. **The nurse's primary response should be to verbally clarify with the client that abuse of any kind is not appropriate and will not be tolerated. This gives the client the opportunity to alter her behaviour to what is more appropriate. Immediately following the nurse's verbal boundary-setting, the nurse may investigate any potential reasons for the client's change in presentation.**

3. This behaviour will escalate if ignored.
4. This intervention is not indicated in this situation.

CLASSIFICATION
Competency:
Nurse–Client Partnership
Taxonomy:
Application

CASE 14

60. 1. This method is highly recommended, particularly for heavy smokers who have not been successful with prior attempts to quit. However, one approach is not necessarily the best for all smokers.
2. This method is effective for some, but not all, smokers.
3. Same as answer 2.

4. Many factors are recognized to be important in the cessation of smoking. One method is not necessarily the best for all. By choosing an option they feel will be successful, individuals will be more motivated to continue with that method.

CLASSIFICATION
Competency:
Health and Wellness
Taxonomy:
Application

61. 1. This statement is not true.
2. This statement is not true; it is one-shot immunity.

3. There are three groups of seasonal influenza viruses, which have an ability to change over time. With each influenza season, epidemiologists predict which will be the prevalent strain and develop a vaccine particular to that strain.

4. While the vaccines are increasingly purified, this is not the reason for the need for annual immunizing.

CLASSIFICATION
Competency:
Health and Wellness
Taxonomy:
Knowledge/Comprehension

62. 1. Rituals and relaxation encourage sleep.

2. Exercising too close to bedtime releases epinephrine, which is a stimulant.
3. Over-the-counter sleep remedies are not recommended, especially for chronic insomnia.
4. Spicy meals may cause indigestion, which could interfere with sleep.

CLASSIFICATION
Competency:
Health and Wellness
Taxonomy:
Application

63. 1. This description does not define WHMIS.
2. WHMIS does not train for infection control.
3. This description does not define WHMIS.

4. Chemicals are a source of environmental risk. The Workplace Hazardous Materials Information System (WHMIS) sets the standard for control of hazardous substances in the workplace, including health care agencies.

CLASSIFICATION
Competency:
Health and Wellness
Taxonomy:
Knowledge/Comprehension

64. 1. Women are more likely than men to experience stress.

2. Each individual experiences stress differently, and there are differing stressors for each individual. Therefore, strategies must be adapted to the individual and her particular stressors.

CLASSIFICATION
Competency:
Health and Wellness
Taxonomy:
Knowledge/Comprehension

3. Stress is always present and is necessary for life. It is how an individual copes with stress that causes health problems.
4. Stress is a reality for all people.

CASE 15

65. 1. This response does nothing to relieve Ms. Magnusson's anxiety.

2. **This response addresses the client's concern about the electricity and provides a reason for the test.**

3. This response dismisses Ms. Magnusson's concerns and does not give accurate information.
4. This response is dismissive.

CLASSIFICATION
Competency:
Nurse–Client Partnership
Taxonomy:
Application

66. 1. **This response is accurate and provides information to Ms. Magnusson about how she may prevent future episodes.**

2. This response is inaccurate.
3. This response offers incorrect information.
4. Same as answer 3.

CLASSIFICATION
Competency:
Changes in Health
Taxonomy:
Application

CASE 16

67. 1. **Agency incident or risk reports are for the purpose of tracking errors and identifying system failures or deficiencies, with the purpose of decreasing medication errors.**

2. This situation may occur but would more likely be identified at a unit manager or employee level.
3. The medication error may be subpoenaed, but this is not the primary reason for their completion.
4. Although client information is included in the medication error report, specific health information related to any adverse effects should be documented in the client's health record.

CLASSIFICATION
Competency:
Professional Practice
Taxonomy:
Critical Thinking

68. 1. The physician must have ordered the medication unless it is an over-the-counter preparation, but this is not the guiding principle.
2. This consideration is important for any medication administration but is not the guiding principle for self-administration.
3. Same as answer 2.

4. **The nurse must evaluate if the individual clients have the competency to administer their own medications. If not, self-administration cannot be considered.**

CLASSIFICATION
Competency:
Professional Practice
Taxonomy:
Critical Thinking

69. 1. Many nurses work and prefer 12-hour shifts. With 8-hour shifts, they
        work more days, which for some may be just as tiring.
     2. Working too many overtime shifts can lead to nurse fatigue. But
        there may be times and situations in which overtime is an effective
        use of personnel, and if not overused, it does not contribute to nurse
        fatigue.
     3. This strategy has not been shown to prevent fatigue. Many nurses find
        that the change from days to nights contributes to fatigue.

     **4. Research has shown that individual nurses, when given an option of
        shift length and type, choose shifts that fit into their lifestyle and
        their circadian rhythm, thus decreasing fatigue.**

CLASSIFICATION
Competency:
Professional Practice
Taxonomy:
Critical Thinking

CASE 17

70. 1. Ms. LeBlanc will need constant observation and should not be isolated.
     2. This position may cause temporary supine hypotension with resultant
        bradycardia in the fetus; it could also result in aspiration should a
        seizure occur.
     3. Fluid intake depends on Ms. LeBlanc's condition and the physician's
        orders.

     **4. Absolute bed rest, a quiet room, and minimal stimulation are
        essential to reducing the risk of a seizure.**

CLASSIFICATION
Competency:
Changes in Health
Taxonomy:
Application

71. 1. Excessive muscular activity may cause a slight rise in body temperature,
        but not as high as 39°C.
     2. One elevated reading is not a conclusive sign of infection.
     3. There is no rapid fluid loss during a seizure; actually, this client has fluid
        retention.

     **4. Increased electrical charges in the brain during a seizure may
        disturb the cerebral thermoregulation centre.**

CLASSIFICATION
Competency:
Changes in Health
Taxonomy:
Application

72. **1. Severe pain accompanied by bleeding at term or close to it is
        symptomatic of complete premature detachment of the placenta
        (*abruptio placentae*). *Abruptio placentae* is a potential complication
        of eclampsia.**

     2. Bleeding caused by marginal *placenta previa* should not be painful.
     3. Clotting defects may occur after moderate and severe *abruptio
        placentae* because of the loss of fibrinogen from severe internal
        bleeding.
     4. HELLP syndrome is a laboratory diagnosis for a variant of pre-
        eclampsia that involves hepatic dysfunction characterized by *h*emolysis,
        *e*levated *l*iver enzymes, and *l*ow *p*latelets.

CLASSIFICATION
Competency:
Changes in Health
Taxonomy:
Critical Thinking

73.   1. This intervention is too time consuming; a high forceps delivery is rarely used because the forceps may further complicate the situation by tearing the cervix.

2. There is no time for insertion of a fetal monitor.

3. Immediate Caesarean delivery is the treatment of choice for complete placental separation. The risk of fetal death is too high to delay birth.

CLASSIFICATION

Competency:
Changes in Health

Taxonomy:
Application

4. This may cause further hemorrhage.

---

74.   1. Same as answer 4.
2. Same as answer 4.
3. Same as answer 4.

4. The danger of seizure in a woman with eclampsia ends when postpartum diuresis has occurred, usually 48 hours after delivery.

CLASSIFICATION

Competency:
Changes in Health

Taxonomy:
Knowledge/Comprehension

CASE 18

75.   1. *E. coli* causes diarrhea but is not as common as rotavirus.
2. Shigella causes diarrhea but is not as common as rotavirus.

3. Rotavirus is a common cause of gastroenteritis in children and infants, particularly those in day care settings.

CLASSIFICATION

Competency:
Changes in Health

Taxonomy:
Critical Thinking

4. Salmonella causes diarrhea but is not as common as rotavirus.

---

76.   1. This manifestation suggests moderate dehydration.
2. Same as answer 1.
3. Same as answer 1.

4. A rapid, thready pulse is a sign of severe dehydration and requires immediate treatment to prevent cardiovascular collapse.

CLASSIFICATION

Competency:
Changes in Health

Taxonomy:
Critical Thinking

---

77.   1. This calculation is incorrect.
2. Same as answer 1.

3. This calculation is correct:

Total fluid intake: 20 mL × 9 kg = 180 mL/hr
Oral fluids averaged over 1 hour = 120 mL ÷ 3 hours = 40 mL
IV rate = 180 mL – 40 mL = 140 mL/hr

CLASSIFICATION

Competency:
Professional Practice

Taxonomy:
Application

4. Same as answer 1.

78.   1. Oral rehydration solutions (e.g., Pedialyte, Rehydralyte, and Infalyte) are the treatment of choice for most cases of dehydration caused by diarrhea. They are safe, reduce diarrheal volume loss, provide nutrients and fluids, and shorten the duration of the disease. Infants who are breastfeeding should continue to do so, alternating feeds with the oral rehydration solution.

2. Soy formula is not necessary or recommended if he is breastfeeding. Glucose water will not treat the potential electrolyte imbalance.

3. The BRAT (*b*ananas, *r*ice, *a*pplesauce, and *t*oast) diet is no longer used for infants because it has poor nutritional value. Charlie requires more fluids than the BRAT diet and breast milk provide.

4. A lactose-free formula is not indicated since Charlie is not lactose intolerant. Breast milk will provide the necessary fluids, and its nutrients will be better digested. Apple juice may be given if tolerated, but oral rehydration solutions are more effective.

CLASSIFICATION

Competency:
Changes in Health

Taxonomy:
Application

CASE 19

79.   1. A private room with a closed door may not be safe for the nurse, and she will not want to conduct a confidential interview close to other clients.

2. Safety is the most important issue, but the assessment should provide safety and the assurance of confidentiality. This setting is not appropriate.

3. When interviewing a psychiatric client with a history of violence, the first concern for the nurse should be her own safety. If she conducts the interview in a room that provides some privacy, yet she is positioned close to a door, she will be safe, and the assessment will not be overheard by others.

4. This precaution is not necessary unless Mr. Clarkson is being violent at the time. The presence of a police officer may escalate his behaviour or intimidate him. The police officer at this point is not part of the health care team; thus, his presence would breach confidentiality.

CLASSIFICATION

Competency:
Nurse–Client Partnership

Taxonomy:
Critical Thinking

80.   1. Generally, the opposite is true.

2. Individuals with this personality disorder tend to be self-centred and impulsive and often require immediate gratification. They lack judgement and self-control and do not profit from their mistakes.

3. These people tend not to learn from their mistakes, experiences, or punishment.

4. These people are self-centred and do not have a sense of responsibility to others.

CLASSIFICATION

Competency:
Changes in Health

Taxonomy:
Application

81. 1. People with this disorder do not generally have a history of depression.
     2. They tend to be easily frustrated.
     3. They lack insight into their behaviour as well as empathy for others, which is essential in order to motivate them to change.

     4. Individuals with an antisocial personality disorder have a history of self-motivated and maladaptive behaviour.

CLASSIFICATION
Competency:
Changes in Health
Taxonomy:
Knowledge/Comprehension

82. 1. This response shifts responsibility from the issue at hand to the institution.
     2. This response does not address the statement; the client is aware of their roles.

     3. This response politely confirms the relationship as professional rather than social.

     4. Dating a client may be against her ethics, but it is the professional reason that takes precedence.

CLASSIFICATION
Competency:
Nurse–Client Partnership
Taxonomy:
Critical Thinking

CASE 20

83. 1. This type of mask is not necessary.
     2. This step is not necessary for simple access to the device.

     3. Rigorous skin preparation is necessary to prevent introducing microbes into the system. This is the most important step in preventing infection.

     4. Sterile gloves are not necessary.

CLASSIFICATION
Competency:
Changes in Health
Taxonomy:
Critical Thinking

84. **1. This entry provides the most complete information about the actions taken.**

     2. This information is incomplete.
     3. The description of dressing materials is not necessary, nor is the doctor's name.
     4. This entry provides no assessment data regarding the insertion site or condition of the skin under the dressing.

CLASSIFICATION
Competency:
Professional Practice
Taxonomy:
Critical Thinking

85. **1. The learner is responsible for recognizing her knowledge, skills, and abilities, and limits of responsibilities. The nurse preceptor must be aware of the student's abilities and knowledge base in order for the two of them to mutually develop a learning plan and provide safe care to clients.**

     2. Learners are responsible and accountable for their own practice. The nurse preceptor is not co-responsible if he has fulfilled his responsibilities as a preceptor and not put the learner in a position where she is functioning beyond her abilities.

CLASSIFICATION
Competency:
Professional Practice
Taxonomy:
Knowledge/Comprehension

3. The learner must identify the need for and act to obtain appropriate supervision.

4. The learner and the preceptor share the responsibility for errors if she is directed to provide care that the preceptor knows is beyond her level of competency.

CASE 21

86.   1. Straws should never be used because they increase the risk of aspiration.

2. This information is not necessarily accurate. Insertion of a gastrostomy tube is recommended if a full assessment by the speech therapist has shown a risk for aspiration or inadequate swallowing.

3. There is no reason for bland food if the client prefers spicy foods.

4. **This information is correct. Speech therapists perform a complete assessment of the client's eating and swallowing skills and develop a plan of care for the dysphagia.**

CLASSIFICATION

Competency:

Changes in Health

Taxonomy:

Application

87.   1. Seeing the wound is a benefit but not the main reason for this type of dressing.

2. **The moist environment promotes more rapid healing.**

3. This type of dressing does provide some protection, but it is not the main reason for choosing it.

4. Wounds may still require some debridement when this dressing is used.

CLASSIFICATION

Competency:

Changes in Health

Taxonomy:

Critical Thinking

88.   1. Trying to reorient the client to the present will only distress her.

2. This response is too complex for this type of client to understand.

3. **This response provides distraction and allows the client to express herself.**

4. This response may be appropriate if Ms. Baverstock cannot be distracted.

CLASSIFICATION

Competency:

Nurse–Client Partnership

Taxonomy:

Application

89.   1. This action is impractical and may not be possible.

2. This action is not an independent nursing action.

3. Same as answer 2.

4. **This action will ensure that she is safe and provide her with some company and interest.**

CLASSIFICATION

Competency:

Professional Practice

Taxonomy:

Application

CASE 22

90.   1. This action must be done but is not the initial action.
   2. This action will be done of there is a medical directive for the
      antipyretics. It is not the first action.

   3. **These children most likely have a communicable disease. It is**
      particularly important when working with chronically ill children that
      the symptomatic children be isolated to prevent transmission of the
      microorganisms.

   4. Same as answer 1.

CLASSIFICATION
Competency:
Professional Practice
Taxonomy:
Critical Thinking

---

91.   1. **If the child has had a previous anaphylactic response to an insect**
      bite, the nurse must be prepared to treat the expected similar
      response, which could be life threatening.

   2. This action may be done if necessary.
   3. This action will be done but is not the priority.
   4. Wasps do not generally leave stingers; however, the area should be
      inspected to see if there is one. If visible, the nurse may attempt to
      remove it. This is an important action but an assessment for anaphylaxis
      is more critical.

CLASSIFICATION
Competency:
Changes in Health
Taxonomy:
Critical Thinking

---

92.   1. This action will need to be done but is not the priority.
   2. Same as answer 1.

   3. **The nurse has an initial and primary responsibility to ensure that the**
      medication error has not caused any adverse effects in Madison.

   4. Same as answer 1.

CLASSIFICATION
Competency:
Professional Practice
Taxonomy:
Critical Thinking

---

93.   1. Nurses may be allowed to accept a gift, depending on the circumstances
      and purpose of the gift. People of some cultures would be offended by
      the nurse refusing the gift.
   2. This response implies that the nurse will take better care of Fatima
      because she has received a gift.
   3. The family may be offended by this question.

   4. **This answer does not offend the family, does not imply Fatima will**
      get special treatment, and does not create bad feelings among the
      rest of the health care team.

CLASSIFICATION
Competency:
Professional Practice
Taxonomy:
Application

---

94.   1. **This action is the most important initial action to protect the**
      children from being infected by the nurse. Chicken pox in chronically
      ill, immunosuppressed children can be very serious.

   2. This action should be done but is not the priority.

CLASSIFICATION
Competency:
Professional Practice
Taxonomy:
Critical Thinking

3. If the nurse must be in contact with anyone, he should use proper infection control practices, but it is more important that he isolate himself from the children.

4. Since the contact was 2 weeks prior, it is too late for immunization to be effective if he has contracted the disease.

CASE 23

95.   1. This response is correct but does not address Ms. Anderson's lack of information.
2. Same as answer 1.

3. **This response recognizes that Ms. Anderson still requires information before she can make an informed decision.**

4. This response may be true but avoids the issue. Ms. Anderson has not asked what the nurse would do.

CLASSIFICATION
Competency:
Nurse–Client Partnership
Taxonomy:
Critical Thinking

96.   1. **This information is correct.**

2. This information is correct but does not answer the question.
3. Production of estrogen ceases after menopause.
4. Only 5 to 10% of breast cancer cases are thought to be due to genetic causes.

CLASSIFICATION
Competency:
Changes in Health
Taxonomy:
Application

97.   1. This response offers false reassurance.
2. This response is too vague and has not answered Mr. Anderson's question.

3. **This response is practical and reliable.**

4. This response does not answer Mr. Anderson's question.

CLASSIFICATION
Competency:
Nurse–Client Partnership
Taxonomy:
Application

CASE 24

98.   1. This assessment is necessary but is not the most important.
2. Same as answer 1.

3. **Ensuring that the client has a patent airway and is able to breathe adequately is the most important assessment.**

4. Same as answer 1.

CLASSIFICATION
Competency:
Changes in Health
Taxonomy:
Critical Thinking

99. 1. This position would encourage aspiration and make it difficult for mucus to drain.

CLASSIFICATION
Competency:
Changes in Health
Taxonomy:
Application

2. **This position allows fluid to drain and permits suctioning.**

3. Same as answer 1.
4. Same as answer 1.

100. 1. **The client must be encouraged to practise good oral hygiene and have regular dental exams.**

CLASSIFICATION
Competency:
Changes in Health
Taxonomy:
Application

2. This information is not specific to this condition.
3. Same as answer 2.
4. Same as answer 2.

INDEPENDENT QUESTIONS ANSWERS AND RATIONALES

101.   1. This description describes the effect of anabolic steroids.
2. Amphetamines may actually decrease coordination.
3. Over time, use of amphetamines would cause the athlete to have a decreased ability to manage stress.

   4. This effect of amphetamines results in their abuse by athletes. Obscuring of fatigue can lead to the exceeding of physical limits and a resulting collapse.

CLASSIFICATION

Competency:

Changes in Health

Taxonomy:

Knowledge/Comprehension

---

102.   **1. Torticollis is limited neck motion, in which the neck is flexed and turned to the affected side. Treatment consists of gentle stretching exercises for the neck.**

2. This intervention does not treat torticollis.
3. This intervention does not treat torticollis and is contraindicated due to the risk of sudden infant death syndrome.
4. This intervention is a treatment for dislocation of the hips.

CLASSIFICATION

Competency:

Changes in Health

Taxonomy:

Application

---

103.   1. This question is part of the environmental assessment but is not the first question.
2. Same as answer 1.
3. Same as answer 1.

   4. This question will yield baseline information on the pattern and extent of the allergies. This information can then lead to a possible identification of triggers and a plan for management of the allergies.

CLASSIFICATION

Competency:

Professional Practice

Taxonomy:

Critical Thinking

---

104.   1. This action must be done but is not the initial step.

   2. This consideration is the priority for the nurse. People who are not ready to learn will not be able to learn, regardless of the individualization, the teaching plan, their baseline knowledge, and so on. These parents have just received a terminal diagnosis for their child and, thus, are not likely to be able to learn skills.

3. Same as answer 1.
4. Same as answer 1.

CLASSIFICATION

Competency:

Professional Practice

Taxonomy:

Critical Thinking

---

105.   1. Drug use does not necessarily lead to delirium.

   2. Delirium, temporary but acute mental confusion, is common in older adults admitted to hospital.

CLASSIFICATION

Competency:

Changes in Health

3. Depression is not an indicator for the development of delirium.

4. Ovarian cancer is not a risk for delirium

Taxonomy:
Critical Thinking

---

106. 1. Immunosuppressant action causes bone marrow depression, which decreases the number of leukocytes.

2. They do not interfere with antibody production.

3. Glucocorticoids interfere with the body's response to microorganisms but do not directly promote the spread of enteroviruses.

4. **These agents are classified as anti-inflammatory or immunosuppressive. They interfere with the release of enzymes responsible for the inflammatory response.**

CLASSIFICATION
Competency:
Changes in Health
Taxonomy:
Knowledge/Comprehension

---

107. 1. This statement is true, but because of the reference to sexually transmitted condylomas, the statement may be perceived as assigning blame and may inhibit the expression of feelings.

2. **This statement recognizes Ms. Pitre's feeling of anxiety as valid.**

3. This statement offers false reassurance. Although a condyloma is a benign wart, the papilloma virus that causes it can bring about neoplastic changes in the cervical tissue, which, if not interrupted, lead to cervical carcinoma.

4. This statement is true, but any cancer diagnosis is worrisome for people. The nurse's statement does not recognize Ms. Pitre's concerns or give her a chance to discuss her feelings.

CLASSIFICATION
Competency:
Nurse–Client Partnership
Taxonomy:
Application

---

108. 1. A wheeze is a high-pitched sound, usually louder on expiration.

2. This sound would be heard over the precordium and would be synchronized with the heartbeat.

3. **A pleural friction rub would make this sound when the parietal pleura rubs against the visceral pleura.**

4. Atelectasis has greatly reduced air entry and does not produce a rubbing sound.

CLASSIFICATION
Competency:
Changes in Health
Taxonomy:
Application

---

109. 1. **Gonorrhea is a highly contagious disease transmitted through sexual intercourse. The incubation period varies, but symptoms usually occur 2 to 10 days after contact. While all of the actions are necessary, obtaining a list of her sexual contacts is most important so that treatment may be provided to them and so that they do not infect others.**

2. Gonorrhea is a reportable sexually transmitted infection. While public health officials must be notified, it is more important to locate Ms. Chang's sexual contacts.

CLASSIFICATION
Competency:
Health and Wellness
Taxonomy:
Critical Thinking

3. Ms. Chang will need this information, but it is not the most important action.
4. The nurse may provide follow-up health teaching with Ms. Chang to help her to prevent sexual infections in the future, but this is not the most important action.

---

110. 1. There is no specific or factual information about the history of abuse.
2. This documentation does not describe the ulcer or provide any factual information about it.

3. **This documentation is specific and objective.**

4. Feelings cannot be uniformly measured.

CLASSIFICATION
Competency:
Professional Practice
Taxonomy:
Critical Thinking

---

111. 1. The client will not require turning for another 15 minutes.
2. This client should be checked hourly but can wait until 2000 hours.

3. **This client has the greatest acuity. The nurse must ensure that the hypoglycemia has been properly treated and the blood sugar is now within normal ranges.**

4. The client will not have the full effect of pain medication as yet, and this is not the most acute situation.

CLASSIFICATION
Competency:
Professional Practice
Taxonomy:
Critical Thinking

---

112. 1. **Each client should be treated as an individual regardless of any aspect of diversity.**

2. Family should be included if this is desired by the client.
3. Differences in health beliefs and practices are common but are not the most important cultural principle.
4. The nurse may not be able to have knowledge of every culture. Appropriate care may still be provided by requesting information and assistance from the client.

CLASSIFICATION
Competency:
Nurse–Client Partnership
Taxonomy:
Critical Thinking

---

113. 1. Alcohol may be consumed in moderation.
2. Alcohol does not have this effect on the pancreas.
3. Although people with type 2 diabetes may be allowed alcohol in similar amounts to people without the disease, there are other factors of which the client must be aware.

4. **The client will need to monitor the effects of alcohol on his blood sugar so that he may adjust his intake accordingly. Alcohol contains calories, which must be calculated into his daily caloric intake.**

CLASSIFICATION
Competency:
Changes in Health
Taxonomy:
Application

114.   1. Showers are preferable to tub baths since bacteria in the water may enter the urethra.

2. An increase in cranberry or blueberry juices, not apple, prevents bacteria from adhering to the wall of the bladder.
3. Voiding every hour is probably not possible or necessary. Voiding every 2 hours is recommended.
4. Intercourse is not forbidden, but it is recommended that the client void immediately afterward.

CLASSIFICATION
Competency:
Changes in Health
Taxonomy:
Application

---

115.   1. The prostate-specific antigen (PSA) is a screening test but does not necessarily confirm the presence of cancer.
2. There are several treatments recommended depending on the type and progress of the cancer: surgery, watchful waiting, external radiation, hormone therapy, insertion of radioactive pellets (brachytherapy), and others.

3. A biopsy determines if there is cancer and provides information for staging of the cancer.

4. Depending on the treatment, impotence and incontinence may be avoided.

CLASSIFICATION
Competency:
Changes in Health
Taxonomy:
Critical Thinking

---

116.   1. Often, substance use can trigger auditory and visual hallucinations, depending on the substance use pattern.

2. The client must be assessed, but there is not an immediate need.
3. There is no indication that he will become violent.
4. He is in the most likely age range for schizophrenia to appear.

CLASSIFICATION
Competency:
Changes in Health
Taxonomy:
Application

---

117.   1. Unless the care is provided in an emergency situation, consent for treatment is required; however, written consent is not necessary.
2. A signed consent is not required.
3. Same as answer 2.

4. A nurse must ask for and be granted consent before undertaking any procedure. If the procedure has been explained to the client, the client may indicate consent verbally or nonverbally by nodding the head yes or positioning the body for the procedure to be carried out.

CLASSIFICATION
Competency:
Professional Practice
Taxonomy:
Application

---

118.   1. The pressure will help with snoring, but this is not the machine's main purpose.

2. The positive pressure prevents airway collapse so that the client does not have oxygen desaturation.

CLASSIFICATION
Competency:
Changes in Health
Taxonomy:
Critical Thinking

3. The machine does help with oxygen saturation, but this is not its main purpose.

4. The machine is used to keep the airway patent, not to reduce the workload of the heart.

---

119. **1. Pediculosis is infestation by lice. Infestation by *Pediculus humanus capitis*, or head lice, is a common condition among school-aged children. The condition is treated with specifically formulated over-the-counter shampoos that kill the lice and nits.**

2. Pediculosis does not involve a fungus. It involves an arthropod (parasitic animal).

3. This treatment is used for mild abrasions and superficial infections.

4. This treatment may be used for psoriasis, not pediculosis.

CLASSIFICATION

Competency:

Changes in Health

Taxonomy:

Application

---

120. 1. This action is unnecessary.

2. During radiation therapy with radium implants, the client is placed in isolation so as to decrease the family's and staff's exposure to radiation.

3. The client will be able to speak.

4. Rubber gloves will not protect the nurse from radiation.

CLASSIFICATION

Competency:

Changes in Health

Taxonomy:

Application

---

121. 1. The goal of asthma management is that control should allow for participation in all activities.

2. This action has been shown to be effective in preventing exercise-induced asthma in 80% of clients for up to 12 hours.

3. Some children have attacks during cold weather, but if the asthma is adequately controlled, such attacks can be managed in most cases.

4. Peak flow rates may be within normal ranges in a child, but an attack can still occur during exercise.

CLASSIFICATION

Competency:

Changes in Health

Taxonomy:

Application

---

122. **1. The therapeutic regimen of bedrest includes peace of mind, which can best be achieved if the children are adequately cared for. Exploring possible options may provide practical solutions to the child care problem.**

2. This response explores the client's feelings but does not address the therapeutic regimen.

3. Complete bedrest has been prescribed, so the client should not fix meals.

4. This response offers a solution that may not be possible or acceptable rather than exploring the situation with the client.

CLASSIFICATION

Competency:

Nurse–Client Partnership

Taxonomy:

Application

123. 1. This intervention does help clients to manage panic disorders but requires counselling, which is not initially appropriate in an emergency department.
2. The client's anxiety triggers will be explored during counselling, but identifying them is not an initial intervention.

   3. Lorazepam (Ativan) is used as an initial treatment because it provides a rapid reduction in symptoms.

4. Selective serotonin reuptake inhibitors are often prescribed for clients with panic disorders; however, they would not be the initial treatment and are not as likely to be prescribed in an emergency department.

CLASSIFICATION
Competency:
Changes in Health
Taxonomy:
Critical Thinking

124. 1. Clients with a borderline personality disorder take little responsibility for themselves or their actions. They should be encouraged to solve their own problems.
2. With this disorder, it is important to maintain a consistent approach in all interactions and ensure that other staff members do so as well.
3. Clients with borderline personality disorder may idolize some staff members and devalue others. The nurse should not take sides in his disputes with other staff members.

   4. Consistent reinforcement of acceptable behaviour will enable Mr. Loek to better function in society.

CLASSIFICATION
Competency:
Changes in Health
Taxonomy:
Application

125. 1. The ratio does not affect compatibility.

   2. These types of insulin are compatible and are administered in the same syringe.

3. The two insulins may be given together at the same time.
4. This action is not required; unnecessary injections increase the risk of infection as well as cause additional discomfort.

CLASSIFICATION
Competency:
Changes in Health
Taxonomy:
Application

126. **1. Canned tomato juice is high in sodium, containing approximately 820 mg of sodium per 250 mL.**

2. Natural cheese does contain sodium but not as much as canned tomato juice.
3. Fresh fish is not high in sodium.
4. Whole-wheat pasta, if cooked in unsalted water, is low in sodium.

CLASSIFICATION
Competency:
Health and Wellness
Taxonomy:
Knowledge/Comprehension

127. 1. This example portrays aggressive behaviour.

   2. The essential feature of passive-aggressive behaviour is resistance to meeting the demands of others in terms of social and occupational functioning. Chronic lateness is an excellent example of this.

CLASSIFICATION
Competency:
Changes in Health
Taxonomy:
Knowledge/Comprehension

3. This example portrays anger or aggression but is not passive.
4. Same as answer 3.

---

128. 1. This instruction is for the Valsalva manoeuvre.
     2. It is not wise to delay voiding with a full bladder because this weakens the sphincter muscles.
     3. Kegel exercises involve the urinary sphincter, not the anal sphincter.

     4. This method is correct for performing Kegel exercises, which strengthen the urinary sphincter.

CLASSIFICATION
Competency:
Health and Wellness
Taxonomy:
Application

---

129. **1. The gloves have become contaminated by the soiled dressing and must be immediately removed to prevent transmission of microorganisms.**

     2. The dressing tray should not be opened while the nurse is wearing soiled gloves.
     3. Hand hygiene should be performed before putting on the gloves. It is not necessary to perform hand hygiene at this point unless the nurse contaminates her hands while removing the soiled gloves.
     4. The door or curtain should have been closed prior to applying the gown, gloves, and goggles.

CLASSIFICATION
Competency:
Professional Practice
Taxonomy:
Application

---

130. 1. This test determines exposure to the tubercle bacillus. Once an individual has been infected, the test will always be positive.
     2. This test does not provide information about communicability.

     3. The absence of bacteria in the sputum indicates that the disease can no longer be spread by the airborne route.

     4. Absence of fever is not evidence that the disease cannot be transmitted.

CLASSIFICATION
Competency:
Changes in Health
Taxonomy:
Knowledge/Comprehension

---

131. 1. Flatulence may occur as a result of immobility, not just obstruction.
     2. Anorexia may occur with an impaction, but it may also be caused by other conditions.

     3. Because of the presence of feces in the colon, a client with a fecal impaction has the urge to defecate but is unable to.

     4. The frequency of bowel movements varies for individuals; it may be normal for this individual not to have one for several days.

CLASSIFICATION
Competency:
Changes in Health
Taxonomy:
Application

---

132. **1. _Toxoplasma gondii_, a protozoan, can be transmitted by exposure to infected cat feces or by ingestion of undercooked, contaminated meat.**

     2. Toxoplasmosis is not related to viral illnesses.

CLASSIFICATION
Competency:
Changes in Health

3. *Toxoplasma gondii* is a parasite of warm-blooded animals; fish are not considered the source of contamination.

4. Toxoplasmosis is not related to diseases included in childhood immunizations.

Taxonomy:
Knowledge/Comprehension

---

133. **1. To avoid additional spinal cord damage, the victim must be moved with great care. Moving a person whose spinal cord has been injured could cause irreversible paralysis. The nurse requires assistance from emergency health care workers who have the appropriate equipment.**

2. A back injury is suspected; therefore, the person should not be moved.

3. A back injury precludes changing the person's position.

4. A flat board would be indicated; however, one rescuer alone could not safely move the victim.

CLASSIFICATION

Competency:
Changes in Health

Taxonomy:
Critical Thinking

---

134. **1. Damage to Broca's area, located in the posterior frontal region of the dominant hemisphere, causes problems in the motor aspect of speech.**

2. This difficulty is associated with receptive aphasia, not expressive aphasia; receptive aphasia is associated with disease of Wernicke's area of the brain.

3. Understanding speech is associated with receptive aphasia.

4. Same as answer 2.

CLASSIFICATION

Competency:
Changes in Health

Taxonomy:
Knowledge/Comprehension

---

135. 1. This manifestation is not a sign of infection.

2. This manifestation is part of the normal healing process. The penis does not require any further care, other than gentle cleansing with water.

3. This manifestation is not a sign of a need for better cleansing. Hydrogen peroxide is not necessary and would irritate the skin.

4. This statement is implied criticism of the father for having the child circumcised and is not a therapeutic response.

CLASSIFICATION

Competency:
Changes in Health

Taxonomy:
Application

---

136. 1. This action would have a systemic effect on fluid balance; edema of the stump is a localized response to inflammation.

2. Same as answer 1.

3. Prolonged immobilization of the residual extremity in one position can lead to a flexion contracture of the hip.

4. Elastic bandages compress the stump, preventing edema and promoting stump shrinkage and moulding; the bandage must be rewrapped when it loosens.

CLASSIFICATION

Competency:
Changes in Health

Taxonomy:
Application

137.   1. Individuals with these injuries could wait for treatment per the triage routine.
2. Same as answer 1.
3. Same as answer 1.

4. Individuals with these injuries require urgent care as they may experience severe blood loss and risk of infection.

CLASSIFICATION
Competency:
Changes in Health
Taxonomy:
Critical Thinking

---

138.   **1. This action is the professional choice. If she is ill or too tired to function, she must consult with the supervisor, who will decide what solution is appropriate.**

2. This action would be considered professional misconduct.
3. The nurse may not be able to stay awake. She is jeopardizing the safety of her clients, particularly if she is ill.
4. This action is not reasonable. The co-worker is in need of a break and should not be asked or told to look after the nurse's clients. If the co-worker offers to cover for the nurse and the co-worker is feeling refreshed, it may be allowable.

CLASSIFICATION
Competency:
Professional Practice
Taxonomy:
Critical Thinking

---

139.   **1. This type of conjunctivitis occurs about 3 to 4 days after birth. If it is not treated, chronic follicular conjunctivitis with conjunctival scarring will likely result.**

2. Congenital syphilis does not manifest as eye discharge.
3. Allergies are uncommon in newborns due to the transmission of maternal antibodies.
4. This chemical conjunctivitis occurs within the first 48 hours, and the discharge is not purulent.

CLASSIFICATION
Competency:
Changes in Health
Taxonomy:
Knowledge/Comprehension

---

140.   **1. The role of the professional nurse includes advocating for quality environments to promote safe, holistic client care.**

2. This problem is with the system and will not be solved by the nurse's having a limited client assignment.
3. It is more professional and effective to advocate than to complain. The manager may not be receptive to complaints.
4. The status quo does not allow for the provision of quality care. There may be alternatives that would address quality care and client numbers.

CLASSIFICATION
Competency:
Professional Practice
Taxonomy:
Critical Thinking

---

141.   1. Colds are caused by viruses; therefore, antibiotics have no effect.
2. Antiviral medications are neither recommended nor effective for colds.

CLASSIFICATION
Competency:
Health and Wellness
Taxonomy:
Knowledge/Comprehension

3. Warm or hot fluids help keep mucus fluid and clear the nose. Anecdotal and some research evidence suggest that echinacea, zinc lozenges, and Cold-FX work for some people.

4. Although there is no cure, Mrs. Scales can be encouraged to rest, increase her fluids, and treat specific symptoms.

---

142. 1. This statement repeats a myth. Regular bathing is even more important during menstruation.

2. Changing tampons every 2 to 4 hours helps prevent toxic shock syndrome.

3. Tampons may be worn, provided they are changed frequently.
4. Douches are not recommended because they alter the natural flora of the vagina and may introduce microorganisms.

CLASSIFICATION
Competency:
Changes in Health
Taxonomy:
Application

---

143. 1. Endometriosis does not cause amenorrhea.
2. Endometriosis does not cause anovulation.

3. Endometriosis is the presence of aberrant endometrial tissue outside the uterus. The tissue responds to ovarian stimulation, bleeds during menstruation, and causes severe pain.

4. Pelvic inflammation usually results from infection.

CLASSIFICATION
Competency:
Changes in Health
Taxonomy:
Knowledge/Comprehension

---

144. 1. The nurse's initial action is to stop the abuse.

2. This action will have to be done but is not the priority.
3. Reporting the abuse to the regulatory body is a nurse's legal responsibility, but it is not the initial action.
4. A written report will have to be made, but stopping the abuse is the most important action initially.

CLASSIFICATION
Competency:
Professional Practice
Taxonomy:
Critical Thinking

---

145. 1. This type of fracture is caused by twisting of the limb. It is seen in cases of child abuse.

2. Bone fragility causes the spinal vertebrae to weaken, leading to multiple compression fractures that cause pain and reduce height.

3. This type of fracture is caused by direct force to the bone.
4. This type of fracture pulls bone and other tissues from the usual attachments and does not commonly occur with osteoporosis.

CLASSIFICATION
Competency:
Changes in Health
Taxonomy:
Application

146. 1. This action is not the initial action. The physician would likely request that the nurse retake the client's blood pressure using a manual system.
2. The client's blood pressure should be retaken manually to confirm the findings prior to medication administration.
3. This action is an option but is unlikely to change the reading.

4. **Automatic monitoring systems malfunction on occasion. Aberrant recordings should be checked manually.**

CLASSIFICATION
Competency:
Professional Practice
Taxonomy:
Critical Thinking

147. 1. This statement would indicate to the wife that she was correct in what she was telling her husband.
2. This question voices an assumption and may make Mrs. Alberto feel defensive.
3. This question is aggressive and sounds punitive.

4. **There may be many reasons for Mrs. Alberto's telling her husband incorrect information. By using an open-ended question asking for information, the nurse should be able to identify and correct misinformation.**

CLASSIFICATION
Competency:
Nurse–Client Partnership
Taxonomy:
Application

148. 1. **According to the Canadian Cancer Society, lung cancer is the leading cause of cancer deaths in Canada.**

2. Breast cancer accounts for a high incidence of cancer in women, but in the overall population, it does not cause as many deaths as lung and colon cancers.
3. Prostate cancer accounts for a high incidence of cancer in men, but in the overall population, it does not cause as many deaths as lung and colon cancers.
4. Colorectal cancer, which may be effectively treated if caught in the early stages, is the second-largest cause of cancer death.

CLASSIFICATION
Competency:
Health and Wellness
Taxonomy:
Knowledge/Comprehension

149. 1. **An alginate would be the preferred choice for this type of wound.**

2. A hydrocolloid dressing is for minimal to moderately draining wounds and is good for preventing friction.
3. A gauze dressing is a good choice for protection or when autolytic debridement is required.
4. Foams provide protection and can be used for absorption in exuding wounds, but they are not used when tunnelling is present.

CLASSIFICATION
Competency:
Changes in Health
Taxonomy:
Knowledge/Comprehension

150. 1. **Use of an individually fitted spinal orthosis (a brace) is generally successful in halting or slowing the progression of most curvatures while the child reaches skeletal maturity.**

2. Surgery is required only for severe scoliosis.

CLASSIFICATION
Competency:
Changes in Health
Taxonomy:
Knowledge/Comprehension

3. Exercises have been proven to be of limited use with scoliosis, although they do help to prevent atrophy of spinal and abdominal muscles.
4. This treatment has not proven to be effective.

---

151. **1. Emergency contraception pills stop or delay the release of an egg from the ovary. They should be taken within 72 hours of unprotected sex in order to be effective.**

2. It does not stimulate menstruation.
3. It will not prevent a fertilized ovum from developing but may stop it implanting in the uterus.
4. It does not terminate a pregnancy and will not work if the woman is already pregnant.

CLASSIFICATION
Competency:
Changes in Health
Taxonomy:
Knowledge/Comprehension

---

152. 1. Blood clots are not usually a side effect of body irradiation.

2. Total body radiation causes depression of the bone marrow, resulting in a decreased white blood cell count and a susceptibility to infection.

3. Chemotherapy is more likely to cause loss of hair.
4. Bone density is not affected, and susceptibility to fractures is not increased.

CLASSIFICATION
Competency:
Changes in Health
Taxonomy:
Application

---

153. 1. The nurse should not be delegating this task.

2. This response offers correct information and explains why she cannot delegate the task.

3. Allowing an unregulated care provider to perform this task is irresponsible and constitutes professional malpractice.
4. Taking this action is unnecessary since Mr. Leslie has been performing suctioning safely for some time.

CLASSIFICATION
Competency:
Professional Practice
Taxonomy:
Critical Thinking

---

154. **1. Research has shown that positioning infants in the supine position for sleep has reduced the mortality from SIDS by 40%.**

2. This action will help the infant's general health but has not been proven to have a significant effect on SIDS.
3. It was previously believed that placing children in the prone position would prevent asphyxia. This belief has been discredited.
4. This action may be recommended for high-risk premature infants who have a history of apnea, but it was not part of the public awareness campaign.

CLASSIFICATION
Competency:
Health and Wellness
Taxonomy:
Knowledge/Comprehension

---

155. 1. This action places the nursing responsibility on the wife and does not solve the problem.
2. Mr. Morgan has refused the medication because of the adverse effects, not the taste.

CLASSIFICATION
Competency:
Professional Practice

3. This action could be considered a threat.

4. The pharmacist may be able to recommend or the physician prescribe a different medication that will not cause digestive distress.

Taxonomy:
Application

---

156. 1. Discomfort is a late sign.
    2. Discharge becomes foul smelling only after there is necrosis and infection; it is not an early sign.
    3. Pressure is not an early symptom because the cancer must be extensive to cause pressure.

    4. Any abnormal vaginal bleeding may indicate cervical cancer.

CLASSIFICATION
Competency:
Changes in Health
Taxonomy:
Knowledge/Comprehension

---

157. 1. This term does not refer to involvement of lymph nodes.
    2. Estrogen contributes to tumour growth; supplements are not indicated.

    3. Estrogen receptor protein–positive (ERP-positive) tumours have a more dramatic response to hormonal therapies that reduce estrogen.

    4. This term is unrelated to metastasis.

CLASSIFICATION
Competency:
Changes in Health
Taxonomy:
Knowledge/Comprehension

---

158. **1. Cardiac nitrates relax the smooth muscles of the coronary arteries so that they dilate and deliver more blood to relieve ischemic pain.**

    2. Although cardiac output may improve because of improved oxygenation of the myocardium, this is not a basis for evaluating the drug's effectiveness.
    3. Although the dilation of blood vessels and a subsequent drop in blood pressure may occur, this is not the basis for evaluating the drug's effectiveness.
    4. Although superficial vessels dilate, lowering the blood pressure and creating a flushed appearance, this is not a basis for evaluating the drug's effectiveness.

CLASSIFICATION
Competency:
Changes in Health
Taxonomy:
Application

---

159. 1. This action will not necessarily provide reassurance. The parents have a need to actually see for themselves that their child is stable.
    2. This action is therapeutic but unlikely to reduce the parents' anxiety; seeing their child would be more therapeutic.

    3. This action provides the best reassurance, as long as the parents know what to expect in the recovery room.

    4. There is an immediate need to reduce the parents' anxiety; time away will not meet this need.

CLASSIFICATION
Competency:
Nurse–Client Partnership
Taxonomy:
Application

160. 1. Although a potential complication, this problem does not pose the same immediate threat to life as does exsanguination.
    2. Same as answer 1.

    3. **Because an external shunt provides circulatory access to a major artery and vein, special safety precautions must be taken to prevent exsanguination.**

    4. Same as answer 1.

CLASSIFICATION
Competency:
Changes in Health
Taxonomy:
Critical Thinking

---

161. 1. HIV can be transmitted in vaginal fluids during unprotected vaginal intercourse, but this is not the most high-risk behaviour.
    2. HIV may be transmitted via oral sex with either gender, but this is not the most high-risk behaviour.
    3. HIV transmission depends on sexual behaviour, not sexual orientation.

    4. **Anal intercourse is an extremely high-risk behaviour because HIV may enter the bloodstream via small tears in the fragile lining of the anus.**

CLASSIFICATION
Competency:
Health and Wellness
Taxonomy:
Critical Thinking

---

162. 1. People respond more positively to policies when they understand them. Just instituting policies without providing education about them is less effective.

    2. **Education would increase employees' awareness of environmental issues and help them to understand the importance of the "green" initiatives.**

    3. This strategy is not practical.
    4. This action is valuable, but employees may not use the containers if they are not educated about and "buy into" the program.

CLASSIFICATION
Competency:
Health and Wellness
Taxonomy:
Critical Thinking

---

163. 1. The surgeon's action constitutes abuse and should be reported, but reporting it is not the nurse's first action.

    2. **The nurse's first action when encountering abuse is to intervene and speak up.**

    3. This action may be taken but is not the nurse's first action.
    4. Intervention is best when it is immediate. Due to the abusive behaviour, the nurse should not confront the surgeon in private.

CLASSIFICATION
Competency:
Professional Practice
Taxonomy:
Critical Thinking

---

164. 1. Milk contains fat and protein—both of which require a longer digestion time—and lactose, which is a disaccharide.
    2. Bread contains carbohydrates, which require a longer time to digest because they must be converted to simple sugars.

CLASSIFICATION
Competency:
Health and Wellness
Taxonomy:
Critical Thinking

3. Chocolate bars do not contain the high proportion of simple sugars found in orange juice; they also contain fat, which takes longer to digest.

4. **Fruit juice has a higher proportion of simple sugars, which are quickly absorbed and are then readily available for conversion to energy.**

---

165. 1. **Sleeping on pillows raises the upper torso and prevents reflux of the gastric contents through the hernia.**

2. This action would have no effect on the mechanical problem of the stomach entering the thoracic cavity.
3. Increasing the contents of the stomach before lying down would aggravate the symptoms associated with a hiatal hernia.
4. The effect of antacids is not long-lasting enough to promote a full night's sleep; also, sodium bicarbonate is not the antacid of choice.

CLASSIFICATION
Competency:
Changes in Health
Taxonomy:
Application

---

166. 1. This action evaluates fluid balance and is best performed over a 24-hour period.

2. **The presence of 50 mL or more of undigested formula may indicate impaired absorption; the volume of the next feeding may need to be reduced or the feeding postponed to reduce the risk of aspiration.**

3. This action is a method for evaluating the correct placement of the nasogastric tube.
4. Although weighing the client regularly is important in evaluating overall nutritional progress, it cannot provide information about absorption of a particular feeding.

CLASSIFICATION
Competency:
Changes in Health
Taxonomy:
Critical Thinking

---

167. 1. Liver abscesses may occur as a complication of intestinal infections. They are not related to portal hypertension or cirrhosis.
2. An intestinal obstruction is not related to portal hypertension or cirrhosis. It may be caused by manipulation of the bowel during surgery, peritonitis, neurological disorders, or organic obstruction.
3. Perforation of the duodenum is usually caused by peptic ulcers. It is not a direct result of portal hypertension or cirrhosis.

4. **The elevated pressure within the portal circulatory system causes elevated pressure in areas of portal systemic collateral circulation (most important, in the distal esophagus and proximal stomach). Hemorrhage is a possible life-threatening complication.**

CLASSIFICATION
Competency:
Changes in Health
Taxonomy:
Knowledge/Comprehension

---

168. 1. This factor is a "red flag" but is not the most indicative finding.
2. This factor is a possible sign of neglect but is not a confirmation of abuse.

CLASSIFICATION
Competency:
Health and Wellness

3. This factor is a definite risk factor for this infant for neglect, but it is not the most indicative finding.

Taxonomy:
Critical Thinking

4. Previous fractures without adequate explanation in a child under 1 year of age is highly suggestive of abuse.

---

169. 1. This manifestation describes psoriasis.
2. This manifestation is alopecia areata. It is a benign condition with an unknown cause, but the client usually has a complete regrowth of the hair.
3. These manifestations are normal in an aging person and are commonly known as liver spots.

CLASSIFICATION
Competency:
Changes in Health
Taxonomy:
Critical Thinking

4. This manifestation describes malignant melanoma.

---

170. 1. Sterile water is a hypotonic solution, which may be absorbed by body tissues.
2. Isotonic, not hypertonic, solutions are used because they are similar to body fluids.

3. Although other solutions may be ordered, irrigations of the bladder usually employ sterile normal saline (0.9% NaCl), which is a solution of approximately the tonicity of normal body fluids.

CLASSIFICATION
Competency:
Changes in Health
Taxonomy:
Application

4. Genitourinary irrigators usually contain an antimicrobial agent such as neomycin sulphate plus polymyxin B sulphate (Neosporin). Indiscriminate use of such agents leads to the emergence of resistant strains of microorganisms.

---

171. **1. An honest nurse–client relationship should be maintained so that trust can develop.**

2. This action is punitive and will not assist the nurse in working with Mr. Beauclerc to stop smoking.
3. Through this action, the nurse is deferring professional responsibility to another health care provider.
4. This action does nothing to establish communication about feelings or motivation behind the client's behaviour.

CLASSIFICATION
Competency:
Nurse–Client Partnership
Taxonomy:
Critical Thinking

---

172. 1. Each province and territory is responsible for registering its nurses.

2. This description accurately describes the role of the Canadian Nurses Association.

3. This description describes a nursing union.
4. Each provincial, not federal, government delegates regulation to a provincial college of nurses.

CLASSIFICATION
Competency:
Professional Practice
Taxonomy:
Knowledge/Comprehension

173.   1. It is obvious that things are not right, and Ms. Serena would be tired.
       2. This comment does not deal with the mother's concerns.
       3. This question may be interpreted as criticism and could make Ms. Serena feel defensive.

       4. This comment acknowledges Ms. Serena's feelings. An open-ended, unbiased question provides an opportunity for the nurse to collect as much data as possible.

CLASSIFICATION
Competency:
Nurse–Client Partnership
Taxonomy:
Critical Thinking

174.   1. For premature infants, oxygen is generally administered according to concentration, rather than flow rate.
       2. This factor is important, but the delivery must be flexible, depending on the oxygen saturations.

       3. Oxygen must be constantly titrated and adjusted according to the levels in the blood in order to prevent hypoxia, which can lead to brain damage, or hyperoxia, which can result in retrolental fibroplasia.

       4. This factor is important, but hypoxia is only a hazard of too little oxygen.

CLASSIFICATION
Competency:
Changes in Health
Taxonomy:
Critical Thinking

175.   1. Frequent breastfeeding is recommended.
       2. This action may be recommended for mild hyperbilirubinemia since the sun will help to decrease the bilirubin in the blood. However, because the extent of the hyperbilirubinemia is not known, this treatment may be inadequate.
       3. A glucose and water mixture is to be avoided in jaundiced breastfed infants because it will decrease the amount of breast milk they drink.

       4. The degree of jaundice is determined by serum bilirubin measurements. Although most newborn jaundice is benign, this cannot be determined without an actual level.

CLASSIFICATION
Competency:
Changes in Health
Taxonomy:
Critical Thinking

176.   1. This emotion cannot be assumed from the situation described.

       2. Changes in self-image and family role can initiate a grieving process with a variety of emotional responses.

       3. Same as answer 1.
       4. This emotion may be present, but it is only part of his general loss of independence.

CLASSIFICATION
Competency:
Nurse–Client Partnership
Taxonomy:
Critical Thinking

177.   1. This action will be necessary once the victim is moved and his breathing is re-established in a safe environment.
       2. Breathing is the priority once further injury is avoided.

CLASSIFICATION
Competency:
Professional Practice

3. This wound would be treated after the victim is removed from danger and patency of the airway is verified.

4. **The first action should be to remove the victim from a source of potential further injury from the broken gas main.**

---

178. 1. A client suffering atelectasis would have rapid, shallow respirations to compensate for poor gas exchange.
2. Atelectasis results in a loose, productive cough.
3. The distal lobes will have diminished sounds due to collapsed alveoli.

CLASSIFICATION
Competency:
Changes in Health
Taxonomy:
Application

4. **Because atelectasis involves the collapsing of the alveoli distal to the bronchioles, breath sounds would be diminished in the lower lobes.**

---

179. 1. Immobilization of the wrist would achieve this outcome. In addition to the wrist bones' being aligned, the hand must not move at the wrist. Only an elbow cast can accomplish this.

CLASSIFICATION
Competency:
Changes in Health
Taxonomy:
Application

2. **The elbow is immobilized to prevent pronation and supination of the wrist.**

3. A longer cast is not easier to manage.
4. This response does not answer the question, and "provide support" is vague.

---

180. 1. **Frostbite can allow the *Clostridium tetani* bacillus to enter the body. Depending on Mr. Cameron's immunization status, prophylactic tetanus antitoxin or tetanus immune globulin would be administered.**

CLASSIFICATION
Competency:
Changes in Health
Taxonomy:
Application

2. This treatment would be contraindicated at this stage since there may be open sores.
3. Antibiotic treatment may be initiated, but it would not be the most important concern.
4. Pain medications will likely be necessary, but the most important concern is tetanus prophylaxis.

---

181. 1. Nausea sometimes occurs with the swallowing of barium. It does not need to be reported.
2. This information is correct but does not pose any risk to the client. It is not as important as the need for increased fluids.
3. This information is correct but is not most important.

CLASSIFICATION
Competency:
Changes in Health
Taxonomy:
Application

4. **Increased fluid intake is required after the procedure to flush the barium out of the system and prevent impaction.**

182.   **1. This information is correct. Sexual intercourse is not more taxing than climbing two flights of stairs.**

2. This response avoids answering the client's partner's question.
3. A wait of 4 to 6 months is unnecessary.
4. Jogging may not be possible for the client and is not an accurate reflection of when relations may be resumed.

CLASSIFICATION

Competency:
Changes in Health

Taxonomy:
Application

---

183.   **1. The showers will help thin the secretions. A fever would indicate infection, which would require antibiotic therapy.**

2. It is unrealistic to ask Mr. Phillion not to swim if he is part of a competitive team. Taking over-the-counter medications may disqualify him from the competition.
3. Frequent nose blowing may irritate the lining of the nasal passage and will not help the sinusitis.
4. It is unlikely that Mr. Phillion would be able to keep his head out of the water during competitive swimming.

CLASSIFICATION

Competency:
Changes in Health

Taxonomy:
Application

---

184.   1. Fewer than 40% of older adults eat the recommended servings of fruit and vegetables on a daily basis.

2. This statement reflects the reality of older adults living in a community.

3. Although Canada offers Old Age Security to older adults, this payment is sometimes not sufficient to cover housing and food expenses.
4. Metabolic demands are decreased, but this does not equate to older adults' getting adequate nutrition.

CLASSIFICATION

Competency:
Health and Wellness

Taxonomy:
Application

---

185.   1. Turning onto the unaffected side will not splint the chest wall.
2. The hands may be used, but the semi-Fowler position provides no support to the chest wall.

3. This method is best. Turning onto the affected side splints the chest wall and reduces the stretching of the pleura.

4. Deep breathing needs to be encouraged; fluid intake will help, but secretions are not indicated in the question.

CLASSIFICATION

Competency:
Changes in Health

Taxonomy:
Application

---

186.   1. A newborn will likely not regain his or her birth weight by this age.
2. Same as answer 1.

CLASSIFICATION

Competency:
Health and Wellness

Taxonomy:
Knowledge/Comprehension

3. **A newborn is most likely to regain birth weight by 10 to 14 days. This guideline is important for parents who are anxious concerning infant feeding and growth.**

4. A newborn should have regained his or her birth weight before the age of 14 to 21 days.

---

187. 1. This response would make the client wonder if the nurse had any knowledge or understanding of his diagnosis.
      2. This response cuts off any further communication of feelings; it ignores what the client has expressed to the nurse.

CLASSIFICATION
Competency:
Nurse–Client Partnership
Taxonomy:
Application

3. **Sitting down with the client indicates a willingness to talk and to give attention in a relaxed manner.**

4. This response does not provide the client an opportunity to discuss his suicidal feelings.

---

188. 1. As a public health nurse, the nurse may not have the necessary triage skills.
      2. As an epidemiologist, the physician may not have the necessary triage skills.
      3. The local health care worker is trained to provide simple health care aid and likely does not have the necessary advanced triage skills.

CLASSIFICATION
Competency:
Professional Practice
Taxonomy:
Critical Thinking

4. **The paramedic is trained in triage and emergency first aid. It is within the scope of practice for the paramedic to provide appropriate care to casualty victims.**

---

189. 1. **Having the client dress appropriately helps keep her more in touch with reality.**

CLASSIFICATION
Competency:
Changes in Health
Taxonomy:
Application

2. This approach may cause the client to be a target of ridicule by the other clients.
3. This approach could be perceived as punitive.
4. This approach may not be acceptable to the client and does not help her to make appropriate clothing decisions.

---

190. 1. This action is an option, but it is unlikely to have any effect.
      2. This action is an option, but it is not the most professional one.

CLASSIFICATION
Competency:
Professional Practice
Taxonomy:
Critical Thinking

3. **Advocating healthy public policy is the foundation of health promotion. Nurses should persuade decision makers to adopt options that preserve the *Canada Health Act*.**

Answers Exam 3

4. This action is an option and may assist to develop a network of like-minded individuals. However, they still need to bring their concerns to the local government.

191.
1. This approach is an option, but research has shown abstinence education does not reduce the number of unwanted pregnancies.
2. This approach is an option; however, in most societies, it is women who take the responsibility for effective birth control.
3. This approach serves to reduce unwanted pregnancies after the fact and may not be an ethical option for some clients.

4. **Research has shown there are fewer unplanned pregnancies when contraceptives are readily and easily available.**

CLASSIFICATION
Competency:
Health and Wellness
Taxonomy:
Critical Thinking

192.
1. **The first step in the nursing process is to validate data. Asking this question will provide the nurse with specific information on the severity of the vomiting.**

2. This question will be asked but is not the first question.
3. Same as answer 2.
4. Same as answer 2.

CLASSIFICATION
Competency:
Changes in Health
Taxonomy:
Critical Thinking

193.
1. Gonorrhea is common. In 2002, 7185 cases were reported in Canada.

2. **Gonorrhea is a reportable sexually transmitted infection.**

3. Usually, a single dose of medication is sufficient to cure the client.
4. Gonorrhea does not cause permanent damage to the testes.

CLASSIFICATION
Competency:
Changes in Health
Taxonomy:
Application

194.
1. This complication may occur as a consequence of severe respiratory distress syndrome.
2. This complication is not a primary concern unless severe hypoxia occurred during labour; it would be difficult to diagnose at this time.
3. This complication may be a problem, but generally the air passageway is well suctioned at birth.

4. **Immaturity of the respiratory tract in preterm infants can be evidenced by a lack of functional alveoli; smaller lumens, increasing the possibility of the collapse of the respiratory passages; weakness of respiratory musculature; and insufficient calcification of the bony thorax, leading to respiratory distress.**

CLASSIFICATION
Competency:
Changes in Health
Taxonomy:
Critical Thinking

195.
1. **Vitamin D is produced by the skin when it is exposed to solar UVB rays. People with dark skin tend to produce less and should have their health care provider monitor their vitamin D levels.**

CLASSIFICATION
Competency:
Health and Wellness

2. There is no reason people with chronic obstructive pulmonary disease require vitamin D supplements.

3. It is people who live in more northern climates, where there is less sunshine, who may require supplements.

4. People of European descent are most likely to have light skin and be able to produce greater amounts of vitamin D than darker-skinned people.

Taxonomy:
Knowledge/Comprehension

---

196. 1. This therapy does not remove the virus.

2. **Raising the CD4 count and reducing the viral load are the purposes of the therapy. This answer is in language easily understood by Mr. Brankston.**

3. Antiretrovirals do not kill the virus.

4. This statement is not accurate and is too complex an answer for Mr. Brankston.

CLASSIFICATION
Competency:
Changes in Health
Taxonomy:
Knowledge/Comprehension

---

197. 1. **Local stakeholders know their community and what strategies the community will accept.**

2. Fundraising is important to finance programs, but the programs will not be successful if the local community does not accept them.

3. Volunteers are important members of the programs but will be noneffective if the local community does not support their efforts.

4. Public awareness will highlight the necessity of the task force's programs, but the local community must support the programs.

CLASSIFICATION
Competency:
Health and Wellness
Taxonomy:
Critical Thinking

---

198. 1. **This strategy would provide the staff with the opportunity to be involved in coming to a democratic solution, which may be perceived as a fair approach.**

2. This action may not be perceived by staff as a fair solution.

3. This strategy is often implemented by managers but may not be viewed as a fair approach by less senior members of the nursing staff.

4. A lottery may be an effective solution but only if agreed upon by the entire nursing staff.

CLASSIFICATION
Competency:
Professional Practice
Taxonomy:
Critical Thinking

---

199. 1. It is important for clients with hypertension to exercise.

2. **This regimen starts with mild exercise and increases as Ms. Pratha increases her fitness level.**

3. This recommendation is unnecessary and may be harmful.

4. Blood pressure is not lower in the evening.

CLASSIFICATION
Competency:
Changes in Health
Taxonomy:
Application

Answers Exam 3

200.   1. These supplies are important for treating wounds from the hurricane but not as important as bottled water.

2. **Contaminated water occurs quickly in disaster areas due to lack of sanitation and hygiene practices. Diseases such as dysentery and cholera occur from drinking contaminated water. Clean water is also necessary for cleansing of wounds. Water purification tablets will also be required.**

CLASSIFICATION
Competency:
Health and Wellness
Taxonomy:
Critical Thinking

3. Antibiotics will be needed but are not as important as water.
4. Food will be needed but is not as important as clean water.

END OF ANSWERS AND RATIONALES TO PRACTICE EXAM 3

Scoring Sheets

COMMON ERRORS WHEN FILLING IN SCORING SHEETS

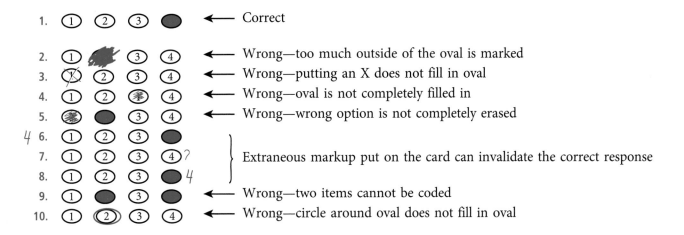

1. ① ② ③ ●   ←— Correct

2. ① ▓ ③ ④   ←— Wrong—too much outside of the oval is marked
3. ⊗ ② ③ ④   ←— Wrong—putting an X does not fill in oval
4. ① ② ▒ ④   ←— Wrong—oval is not completely filled in
5. ▒ ● ③ ④   ←— Wrong—wrong option is not completely erased
4 6. ① ② ③ ●   ⎫
7. ① ② ③ ④?   ⎬ Extraneous markup put on the card can invalidate the correct response
8. ① ② ③ ● 4   ⎭
9. ① ● ③ ●   ←— Wrong—two items cannot be coded
10. ① ⊘ ③ ④   ←— Wrong—circle around oval does not fill in oval

EXAM 1 SCORING SHEETS

CASE-BASED QUESTIONS

1. ① ② ③ ④	26. ① ② ③ ④	51. ① ② ③ ④	76. ① ② ③ ④
2. ① ② ③ ④	27. ① ② ③ ④	52. ① ② ③ ④	77. ① ② ③ ④
3. ① ② ③ ④	28. ① ② ③ ④	53. ① ② ③ ④	78. ① ② ③ ④
4. ① ② ③ ④	29. ① ② ③ ④	54. ① ② ③ ④	79. ① ② ③ ④
5. ① ② ③ ④	30. ① ② ③ ④	55. ① ② ③ ④	80. ① ② ③ ④
6. ① ② ③ ④	31. ① ② ③ ④	56. ① ② ③ ④	81. ① ② ③ ④
7. ① ② ③ ④	32. ① ② ③ ④	57. ① ② ③ ④	82. ① ② ③ ④
8. ① ② ③ ④	33. ① ② ③ ④	58. ① ② ③ ④	83. ① ② ③ ④
9. ① ② ③ ④	34. ① ② ③ ④	59. ① ② ③ ④	84. ① ② ③ ④
10. ① ② ③ ④	35. ① ② ③ ④	60. ① ② ③ ④	85. ① ② ③ ④
11. ① ② ③ ④	36. ① ② ③ ④	61. ① ② ③ ④	86. ① ② ③ ④
12. ① ② ③ ④	37. ① ② ③ ④	62. ① ② ③ ④	87. ① ② ③ ④
13. ① ② ③ ④	38. ① ② ③ ④	63. ① ② ③ ④	88. ① ② ③ ④
14. ① ② ③ ④	39. ① ② ③ ④	64. ① ② ③ ④	89. ① ② ③ ④
15. ① ② ③ ④	40. ① ② ③ ④	65. ① ② ③ ④	90. ① ② ③ ④
16. ① ② ③ ④	41. ① ② ③ ④	66. ① ② ③ ④	91. ① ② ③ ④
17. ① ② ③ ④	42. ① ② ③ ④	67. ① ② ③ ④	92. ① ② ③ ④
18. ① ② ③ ④	43. ① ② ③ ④	68. ① ② ③ ④	93. ① ② ③ ④
19. ① ② ③ ④	44. ① ② ③ ④	69. ① ② ③ ④	94. ① ② ③ ④
20. ① ② ③ ④	45. ① ② ③ ④	70. ① ② ③ ④	95. ① ② ③ ④
21. ① ② ③ ④	46. ① ② ③ ④	71. ① ② ③ ④	96. ① ② ③ ④
22. ① ② ③ ④	47. ① ② ③ ④	72. ① ② ③ ④	97. ① ② ③ ④
23. ① ② ③ ④	48. ① ② ③ ④	73. ① ② ③ ④	98. ① ② ③ ④
24. ① ② ③ ④	49. ① ② ③ ④	74. ① ② ③ ④	99. ① ② ③ ④
25. ① ② ③ ④	50. ① ② ③ ④	75. ① ② ③ ④	100. ① ② ③ ④

EXAM 1 SCORING SHEETS

INDEPENDENT QUESTIONS

101. ① ② ③ ④	126. ① ② ③ ④	151. ① ② ③ ④	176. ① ② ③ ④
102. ① ② ③ ④	127. ① ② ③ ④	152. ① ② ③ ④	177. ① ② ③ ④
103. ① ② ③ ④	128. ① ② ③ ④	153. ① ② ③ ④	178. ① ② ③ ④
104. ① ② ③ ④	129. ① ② ③ ④	154. ① ② ③ ④	179. ① ② ③ ④
105. ① ② ③ ④	130. ① ② ③ ④	155. ① ② ③ ④	180. ① ② ③ ④
106. ① ② ③ ④	131. ① ② ③ ④	156. ① ② ③ ④	181. ① ② ③ ④
107. ① ② ③ ④	132. ① ② ③ ④	157. ① ② ③ ④	182. ① ② ③ ④
108. ① ② ③ ④	133. ① ② ③ ④	158. ① ② ③ ④	183. ① ② ③ ④
109. ① ② ③ ④	134. ① ② ③ ④	159. ① ② ③ ④	184. ① ② ③ ④
110. ① ② ③ ④	135. ① ② ③ ④	160. ① ② ③ ④	185. ① ② ③ ④
111. ① ② ③ ④	136. ① ② ③ ④	161. ① ② ③ ④	186. ① ② ③ ④
112. ① ② ③ ④	137. ① ② ③ ④	162. ① ② ③ ④	187. ① ② ③ ④
113. ① ② ③ ④	138. ① ② ③ ④	163. ① ② ③ ④	188. ① ② ③ ④
114. ① ② ③ ④	139. ① ② ③ ④	164. ① ② ③ ④	189. ① ② ③ ④
115. ① ② ③ ④	140. ① ② ③ ④	165. ① ② ③ ④	190. ① ② ③ ④
116. ① ② ③ ④	141. ① ② ③ ④	166. ① ② ③ ④	191. ① ② ③ ④
117. ① ② ③ ④	142. ① ② ③ ④	167. ① ② ③ ④	192. ① ② ③ ④
118. ① ② ③ ④	143. ① ② ③ ④	168. ① ② ③ ④	193. ① ② ③ ④
119. ① ② ③ ④	144. ① ② ③ ④	169. ① ② ③ ④	194. ① ② ③ ④
120. ① ② ③ ④	145. ① ② ③ ④	170. ① ② ③ ④	195. ① ② ③ ④
121. ① ② ③ ④	146. ① ② ③ ④	171. ① ② ③ ④	196. ① ② ③ ④
122. ① ② ③ ④	147. ① ② ③ ④	172. ① ② ③ ④	197. ① ② ③ ④
123. ① ② ③ ④	148. ① ② ③ ④	173. ① ② ③ ④	198. ① ② ③ ④
124. ① ② ③ ④	149. ① ② ③ ④	174. ① ② ③ ④	199. ① ② ③ ④
125. ① ② ③ ④	150. ① ② ③ ④	175. ① ② ③ ④	200. ① ② ③ ④

EXAM 2 SCORING SHEETS

CASE-BASED QUESTIONS

1. ① ② ③ ④   26. ① ② ③ ④   51. ① ② ③ ④   76. ① ② ③ ④
2. ① ② ③ ④   27. ① ② ③ ④   52. ① ② ③ ④   77. ① ② ③ ④
3. ① ② ③ ④   28. ① ② ③ ④   53. ① ② ③ ④   78. ① ② ③ ④
4. ① ② ③ ④   29. ① ② ③ ④   54. ① ② ③ ④   79. ① ② ③ ④
5. ① ② ③ ④   30. ① ② ③ ④   55. ① ② ③ ④   80. ① ② ③ ④
6. ① ② ③ ④   31. ① ② ③ ④   56. ① ② ③ ④   81. ① ② ③ ④
7. ① ② ③ ④   32. ① ② ③ ④   57. ① ② ③ ④   82. ① ② ③ ④
8. ① ② ③ ④   33. ① ② ③ ④   58. ① ② ③ ④   83. ① ② ③ ④
9. ① ② ③ ④   34. ① ② ③ ④   59. ① ② ③ ④   84. ① ② ③ ④
10. ① ② ③ ④   35. ① ② ③ ④   60. ① ② ③ ④   85. ① ② ③ ④
11. ① ② ③ ④   36. ① ② ③ ④   61. ① ② ③ ④   86. ① ② ③ ④
12. ① ② ③ ④   37. ① ② ③ ④   62. ① ② ③ ④   87. ① ② ③ ④
13. ① ② ③ ④   38. ① ② ③ ④   63. ① ② ③ ④   88. ① ② ③ ④
14. ① ② ③ ④   39. ① ② ③ ④   64. ① ② ③ ④   89. ① ② ③ ④
15. ① ② ③ ④   40. ① ② ③ ④   65. ① ② ③ ④   90. ① ② ③ ④
16. ① ② ③ ④   41. ① ② ③ ④   66. ① ② ③ ④   91. ① ② ③ ④
17. ① ② ③ ④   42. ① ② ③ ④   67. ① ② ③ ④   92. ① ② ③ ④
18. ① ② ③ ④   43. ① ② ③ ④   68. ① ② ③ ④   93. ① ② ③ ④
19. ① ② ③ ④   44. ① ② ③ ④   69. ① ② ③ ④   94. ① ② ③ ④
20. ① ② ③ ④   45. ① ② ③ ④   70. ① ② ③ ④   95. ① ② ③ ④
21. ① ② ③ ④   46. ① ② ③ ④   71. ① ② ③ ④   96. ① ② ③ ④
22. ① ② ③ ④   47. ① ② ③ ④   72. ① ② ③ ④   97. ① ② ③ ④
23. ① ② ③ ④   48. ① ② ③ ④   73. ① ② ③ ④   98. ① ② ③ ④
24. ① ② ③ ④   49. ① ② ③ ④   74. ① ② ③ ④   99. ① ② ③ ④
25. ① ② ③ ④   50. ① ② ③ ④   75. ① ② ③ ④   100. ① ② ③ ④

EXAM 2 SCORING SHEETS

INDEPENDENT QUESTIONS

101. ① ② ③ ④	126. ① ② ③ ④	151. ① ② ③ ④	176. ① ② ③ ④
102. ① ② ③ ④	127. ① ② ③ ④	152. ① ② ③ ④	177. ① ② ③ ④
103. ① ② ③ ④	128. ① ② ③ ④	153. ① ② ③ ④	178. ① ② ③ ④
104. ① ② ③ ④	129. ① ② ③ ④	154. ① ② ③ ④	179. ① ② ③ ④
105. ① ② ③ ④	130. ① ② ③ ④	155. ① ② ③ ④	180. ① ② ③ ④
106. ① ② ③ ④	131. ① ② ③ ④	156. ① ② ③ ④	181. ① ② ③ ④
107. ① ② ③ ④	132. ① ② ③ ④	157. ① ② ③ ④	182. ① ② ③ ④
108. ① ② ③ ④	133. ① ② ③ ④	158. ① ② ③ ④	183. ① ② ③ ④
109. ① ② ③ ④	134. ① ② ③ ④	159. ① ② ③ ④	184. ① ② ③ ④
110. ① ② ③ ④	135. ① ② ③ ④	160. ① ② ③ ④	185. ① ② ③ ④
111. ① ② ③ ④	136. ① ② ③ ④	161. ① ② ③ ④	186. ① ② ③ ④
112. ① ② ③ ④	137. ① ② ③ ④	162. ① ② ③ ④	187. ① ② ③ ④
113. ① ② ③ ④	138. ① ② ③ ④	163. ① ② ③ ④	188. ① ② ③ ④
114. ① ② ③ ④	139. ① ② ③ ④	164. ① ② ③ ④	189. ① ② ③ ④
115. ① ② ③ ④	140. ① ② ③ ④	165. ① ② ③ ④	190. ① ② ③ ④
116. ① ② ③ ④	141. ① ② ③ ④	166. ① ② ③ ④	191. ① ② ③ ④
117. ① ② ③ ④	142. ① ② ③ ④	167. ① ② ③ ④	192. ① ② ③ ④
118. ① ② ③ ④	143. ① ② ③ ④	168. ① ② ③ ④	193. ① ② ③ ④
119. ① ② ③ ④	144. ① ② ③ ④	169. ① ② ③ ④	194. ① ② ③ ④
120. ① ② ③ ④	145. ① ② ③ ④	170. ① ② ③ ④	195. ① ② ③ ④
121. ① ② ③ ④	146. ① ② ③ ④	171. ① ② ③ ④	196. ① ② ③ ④
122. ① ② ③ ④	147. ① ② ③ ④	172. ① ② ③ ④	197. ① ② ③ ④
123. ① ② ③ ④	148. ① ② ③ ④	173. ① ② ③ ④	198. ① ② ③ ④
124. ① ② ③ ④	149. ① ② ③ ④	174. ① ② ③ ④	199. ① ② ③ ④
125. ① ② ③ ④	150. ① ② ③ ④	175. ① ② ③ ④	200. ① ② ③ ④

EXAM 3 SCORING SHEETS

CASE-BASED QUESTIONS

1. ① ② ③ ④	26. ① ② ③ ④	51. ① ② ③ ④	76. ① ② ③ ④
2. ① ② ③ ④	27. ① ② ③ ④	52. ① ② ③ ④	77. ① ② ③ ④
3. ① ② ③ ④	28. ① ② ③ ④	53. ① ② ③ ④	78. ① ② ③ ④
4. ① ② ③ ④	29. ① ② ③ ④	54. ① ② ③ ④	79. ① ② ③ ④
5. ① ② ③ ④	30. ① ② ③ ④	55. ① ② ③ ④	80. ① ② ③ ④
6. ① ② ③ ④	31. ① ② ③ ④	56. ① ② ③ ④	81. ① ② ③ ④
7. ① ② ③ ④	32. ① ② ③ ④	57. ① ② ③ ④	82. ① ② ③ ④
8. ① ② ③ ④	33. ① ② ③ ④	58. ① ② ③ ④	83. ① ② ③ ④
9. ① ② ③ ④	34. ① ② ③ ④	59. ① ② ③ ④	84. ① ② ③ ④
10. ① ② ③ ④	35. ① ② ③ ④	60. ① ② ③ ④	85. ① ② ③ ④
11. ① ② ③ ④	36. ① ② ③ ④	61. ① ② ③ ④	86. ① ② ③ ④
12. ① ② ③ ④	37. ① ② ③ ④	62. ① ② ③ ④	87. ① ② ③ ④
13. ① ② ③ ④	38. ① ② ③ ④	63. ① ② ③ ④	88. ① ② ③ ④
14. ① ② ③ ④	39. ① ② ③ ④	64. ① ② ③ ④	89. ① ② ③ ④
15. ① ② ③ ④	40. ① ② ③ ④	65. ① ② ③ ④	90. ① ② ③ ④
16. ① ② ③ ④	41. ① ② ③ ④	66. ① ② ③ ④	91. ① ② ③ ④
17. ① ② ③ ④	42. ① ② ③ ④	67. ① ② ③ ④	92. ① ② ③ ④
18. ① ② ③ ④	43. ① ② ③ ④	68. ① ② ③ ④	93. ① ② ③ ④
19. ① ② ③ ④	44. ① ② ③ ④	69. ① ② ③ ④	94. ① ② ③ ④
20. ① ② ③ ④	45. ① ② ③ ④	70. ① ② ③ ④	95. ① ② ③ ④
21. ① ② ③ ④	46. ① ② ③ ④	71. ① ② ③ ④	96. ① ② ③ ④
22. ① ② ③ ④	47. ① ② ③ ④	72. ① ② ③ ④	97. ① ② ③ ④
23. ① ② ③ ④	48. ① ② ③ ④	73. ① ② ③ ④	98. ① ② ③ ④
24. ① ② ③ ④	49. ① ② ③ ④	74. ① ② ③ ④	99. ① ② ③ ④
25. ① ② ③ ④	50. ① ② ③ ④	75. ① ② ③ ④	100. ① ② ③ ④

EXAM 3 SCORING SHEETS

INDEPENDENT QUESTIONS

101.	①	②	③	④	126.	①	②	③	④	151.	①	②	③	④	176.	①	②	③	④
102.	①	②	③	④	127.	①	②	③	④	152.	①	②	③	④	177.	①	②	③	④
103.	①	②	③	④	128.	①	②	③	④	153.	①	②	③	④	178.	①	②	③	④
104.	①	②	③	④	129.	①	②	③	④	154.	①	②	③	④	179.	①	②	③	④
105.	①	②	③	④	130.	①	②	③	④	155.	①	②	③	④	180.	①	②	③	④
106.	①	②	③	④	131.	①	②	③	④	156.	①	②	③	④	181.	①	②	③	④
107.	①	②	③	④	132.	①	②	③	④	157.	①	②	③	④	182.	①	②	③	④
108.	①	②	③	④	133.	①	②	③	④	158.	①	②	③	④	183.	①	②	③	④
109.	①	②	③	④	134.	①	②	③	④	159.	①	②	③	④	184.	①	②	③	④
110.	①	②	③	④	135.	①	②	③	④	160.	①	②	③	④	185.	①	②	③	④
111.	①	②	③	④	136.	①	②	③	④	161.	①	②	③	④	186.	①	②	③	④
112.	①	②	③	④	137.	①	②	③	④	162.	①	②	③	④	187.	①	②	③	④
113.	①	②	③	④	138.	①	②	③	④	163.	①	②	③	④	188.	①	②	③	④
114.	①	②	③	④	139.	①	②	③	④	164.	①	②	③	④	189.	①	②	③	④
115.	①	②	③	④	140.	①	②	③	④	165.	①	②	③	④	190.	①	②	③	④
116.	①	②	③	④	141.	①	②	③	④	166.	①	②	③	④	191.	①	②	③	④
117.	①	②	③	④	142.	①	②	③	④	167.	①	②	③	④	192.	①	②	③	④
118.	①	②	③	④	143.	①	②	③	④	168.	①	②	③	④	193.	①	②	③	④
119.	①	②	③	④	144.	①	②	③	④	169.	①	②	③	④	194.	①	②	③	④
120.	①	②	③	④	145.	①	②	③	④	170.	①	②	③	④	195.	①	②	③	④
121.	①	②	③	④	146.	①	②	③	④	171.	①	②	③	④	196.	①	②	③	④
122.	①	②	③	④	147.	①	②	③	④	172.	①	②	③	④	197.	①	②	③	④
123.	①	②	③	④	148.	①	②	③	④	173.	①	②	③	④	198.	①	②	③	④
124.	①	②	③	④	149.	①	②	③	④	174.	①	②	③	④	199.	①	②	③	④
125.	①	②	③	④	150.	①	②	③	④	175.	①	②	③	④	200.	①	②	③	④

Bibliography

Arnold, E., & Boggs, K. (2007). *Interpersonal relationships: Professional communication skills for nurses* (5th ed.). St. Louis, MO: Saunders/Elsevier.

Bowen, A., & Muhajarine, N. (2006). Antenatal depression. *The Canadian Nurse, 102*(9), 26–30.

Burgess, A. (1997). *Psychiatric nursing: Promoting mental health.* Stamford, CT: Appleton & Lange.

Canadian Cancer Society. (2009). *Early detection and screening. Facts for men* [Monograph]. Author.

Canadian Mental Health Association. (2005). *Understanding mental illness: Resource manual.* Toronto, ON: Author.

Canadian Nurses Association. (2008). *Code of ethics for registered nurses.* Ottawa, ON: Author.

Canadian Nurses Association. (2010). *Blueprint for the Canadian registered nurse examination, June 2010–May 2015.* Ottawa, ON: Author.

Canadian Nurses Association. (2010). *The Canadian registered nurse examination prep guide* (5th ed.). Ottawa, ON: Author.

Charting defensively. (2000, May). *Nursing, 30*(5), 28–29.

College of Nurses of Ontario. (1999). You asked us. *Communiqué.*

College of Nurses of Ontario. (2002). *Practice standard: Decisions about procedures and authority, revised 2009* (Publication No. 41071). Toronto, ON: Author.

College of Nurses of Ontario. (2002). *Practice standard: Therapeutic nurse–client relationship, revised 2009* (Publication No. 41033). Toronto, ON: Author.

College of Nurses of Ontario. (2005). *Practice standard: Resuscitation, revised 1999* (Publication No. 42001). Toronto, ON: Author.

College of Nurses of Ontario. (2005). *Reference document: Legislation and regulation: Professional misconduct* (Publication No. 42007). Toronto, ON: Author.

College of Nurses of Ontario. (2006). Summarized discipline decisions. *The Standard, 31*(3), 34–39.

College of Nurses of Ontario. (2009). *Practice guideline: Culturally sensitive care* (Publication No. 41017). Toronto, ON: Author.

College of Nurses of Ontario. (2009). *Practice guideline: Refusing assignments and discontinuing nursing services* (Publication No. 41070). Toronto, ON: Author.

College of Nurses of Ontario. (2009). *Practice guideline: Restraints* (Publication No. 41043). Toronto, ON: Author.

College of Nurses of Ontario. (2009). *Practice guideline: Supporting learners* (Publication No. 44034). Toronto, ON: Author.

College of Nurses of Ontario. (2009). *Practice guideline: Working with unregulated care providers* (Publication No. 41014). Toronto, ON: Author.

College of Nurses of Ontario. (2009). *Practice standard: Documentation* (Publication No. 41001). Toronto, ON: Author.

College of Nurses of Ontario. (2009). *Practice standard: Infection prevention and control* (Publication No. 41002). Toronto, ON: Author.

College of Nurses of Ontario. (2009). *Practice standard: Medication* (Publication No. 41007). Toronto, ON: Author.

College of Nurses of Ontario. (2010, spring). Here we go again! Pandemics and the ethical challenges they bring. *The Standard, 35*(1), 13–15.

College of Nurses of Ontario. (2010, spring). The practice assessment. *The Standard, 35*(1), 18–19.

College of Nurses of Ontario. (2010, spring). Recognizing family needs. *The Standard, 35*(1), 36–37.

College of Registered Nurses of Nova Scotia. (2004). *Entry-level competencies for registered nurses in Nova Scotia.* Halifax, NS: Author.

Day, R., Paul, P., Williams, B., Smeltzer, S., & Bare, B. (2007). *Brunner & Suddarth's textbook of medical-surgical nursing* (1st Canadian ed.). Philadelphia, PA: Lippincott Williams & Wilkins.

Dipchand, A., Friedman, J., Bismilla, Z., Gupta, S., & Lam, C. (Eds.). (2010). *The Hospital for Sick Children handbook of pediatrics* (11th ed.). Toronto, ON: Saunders.

Dobbelsteyn, J. (2006, April). Nursing in First Nations and Inuit communities in Atlantic Canada. *Can Nurse, 102*(4), 32–35.

Dovgan, V. (2008). *Nursing and back injury.* Unpublished student presentation, Toronto, ON: Ryerson University.

Dudek, S. G. (2006). *Nutrition essentials for nursing practice* (5th ed.). Philadelphia, PA: Lippincott Williams & Wilkins.

Fortinash, K., & Holoday Worret, P. (2008). *Psychiatric mental health nursing* (4th ed.). St. Louis, MO: Mosby/ Elsevier.

Government of Canada. (2006). *Pandemic influenza.* Retrieved from www.pandemicinfluenza.gc.ca.

Hales, D., & Lauzon, L. (2007). *An invitation to health* (1st Canadian ed.). Toronto, ON: Thomson Nelson.

Handbook of signs and symptoms (3rd ed.). (2006). Philadelphia, PA: Lippincott Williams & Wilkins.

Hebert, M. (2000). A national education strategy to develop nursing informatics competencies. *Nursing Leadership (CJNL), 13*(2), 11–14.

Hockenberry, M. (2006). *Wong's nursing care of infants and children* (7th ed.). St. Louis, MO: Mosby/Elsevier.

Jurisdictional Collaborative Process. (2006). *A report of the 2004–2006 jurisdictional competency project: Competencies in the context of entry-level registered nurse practice.* Vancouver, BC: College of Registered Nurses of British Columbia.

Keatings, M., & Smith, O. (2010). *Ethical and legal issues in Canadian nursing* (3rd ed.). Toronto, ON: Elsevier.

Langford, R., & Thompson, J. (2005). *Mosby's handbook of diseases* (3rd ed.). St. Louis, MO: Mosby/Elsevier.

Lewis, S., Heitkemper, M., Dirksen, S., Barry, M., Goldsworthy, S., & Goodridge, D. (2010). *Medical-surgical nursing in Canada* (2nd Canadian ed.). Toronto, ON: Elsevier.

Lowdermilk, E., & Perry, S. (2006). *Maternity and women's health care* (8th ed.). St. Louis, MO: Mosby/Elsevier.

Marshall-Henty, J., Sams, C., & Bradshaw, J. (2009). *Mosby's comprehensive review for the Canadian RN exam* (1st Canadian ed.). Toronto, ON: Mosby/Elsevier.

McCarthy, K. (2006). Understanding the challenges, witnessing primary health care in action. *The Canadian Nurse, 102*(4), 9–11.

McConnell, E. A. (2003). Clinical do's and don'ts: Using proper body mechanics. *Nursing, 32,* 20.

Mosby's medical, nursing, and allied health dictionary (6th ed.). (2002). St. Louis, MO: Mosby.

Nelson, A., & Baptiste, A. S. (2006, November/December). Evidence-based practices for safe patient handling and movement. *Orthopaedic Nursing, 25*(6), 366–379.

Nelson, A., Fragala, G., & Menzel, N. (2003). Myths and facts about back injuries in nursing. *The American Journal of Nursing, 103,* 32–41.

Obermeyer, M. (2006). Are you a culturally competent preceptor? *Nursing, 36*(6), 54–55.

O'Neill, P. (2002). *Caring for the older adult: A health promotion perspective.* Philadelphia, PA: W.B. Saunders/ Elsevier.

Pagana, K., & Pagana, T. (2009). *Mosby's manual of diagnostic and laboratory tests* (4th ed.). St. Louis, MO: Mosby/Elsevier.

Pennington, S., Gafner, G., Schilit, R., & Bechtel, B. (1993). Addressing ethical boundaries among nurses. *Nursing Management, 24*(6), 36–39.

Perry, S., Hockenberry, M., Lowdermilk, D., & Wilson, D. (2010). *Maternal child nursing care* (4th ed.). Maryland Heights, MO: Mosby/Elsevier.

Perry, A., & Potter, P. (2010). *Canadian fundamentals of nursing* (revised 4th ed.). Toronto, ON: Elsevier.

Perry, A., & Potter, P. (2010). *Clinical nursing skills and techniques* (7th ed.). St. Louis, MO: Mosby/Elsevier.

Potter, P. A., Griffin Perry, A., Ross-Kerr, J. C., & Wood, M. J. (2006). *Canadian fundamentals of nursing* (3rd ed.). St. Louis, MO: Mosby.

Professional guide to diseases (7th ed). (2001). Pennsylvania, PA: Springhouse.

Registered Nurses' Association of Ontario. (2002). *Nursing best practice guidelines project.* Toronto, ON: Author.

Roberts, G. (1986, December). Tips for taking and passing examinations. *Laboratory Medicine, 17*(12), 756–758.

Santulli, E. (2004). No strain? No pain! *Hospital Nursing, 34,* 7–8.

Saunders, N., & Friedman, J. (Eds.). (2006). *Caring for kids.* Toronto, ON: Key Porter Books.

Saxton, D., Nugent, P., Pelikan, P., Marshall-Henty, J., & Vernon, P. (2003). *Mosby's Canadian comprehensive review of nursing* (2nd ed.). Toronto, ON: Mosby/Elsevier.

Siegel, B. (1996). *The world of the autistic child.* New York, NY: Oxford University Press.

Skidmore-Roth, L. (2007). *Mosby's nursing drug reference* (20th ed.). St. Louis, MO: Mosby/Elsevier.

Skidmore-Roth, L. (2010). *Mosby's drug guide for nurses with 2010 update* (8th ed.). St. Louis, MO: Mosby/Elsevier.

Skidmore-Roth, L. (2010). *Mosby's handbook of herbs and natural supplements* (4th ed.). St. Louis, MO: Mosby/Elsevier.

University Health Network. (2001). *What is VRE? Information for patients and families* [Monograph]. Toronto: Author.

Appendix
The Canadian Registered Nurse Examination Competencies

ASSUMPTIONS

Throughout the development of the CRNE competencies, the following assumptions were established:

1. The CRNE competencies are directed toward the professional practice of the entry-level registered nurse in Canada.
2. Entry-level registered nurses practise in a manner consistent with:
   (a) professional nursing standards of the regulatory body;
   (b) nursing codes of ethics;
   (c) scope of nursing practice applicable in the jurisdiction; and
   (d) common law and provincial/territorial and federal legislation that direct practice. (Jurisdictional Collaborative Process, 2006)
3. The CRNE competencies are each of equal importance for safe, ethical and effective practice of entry-level registered nurses.
4. The entry-level registered nurse is a generalist whose practice, autonomy and proficiency will be enhanced by reflective practice, evidence-informed knowledge, and collaboration and support from registered nurse colleagues, other health-care team members and employers.
5. The entry-level registered nurse is prepared to practise safely and competently along the continuum of care in situations of health and illness across a client's lifespan.
6. The entry-level registered nurse and the client are partners in the decision-making process related to the client's health.
7. The CRNE competencies are grounded within the context of the client's health, the principles of primary health care, current and emerging health trends, determinants of health, the Canadian health-care system and professional nursing practice.
8. The practice environment of entry-level registered nurses can be any setting, program or circumstance in which nursing is practised (e.g., hospitals, communities, homes, clinics, schools, industries, residential facilities, telehealth, correctional facilities). (Jurisdictional Collaborative Process, 2006).
9. The nursing process is used by registered nurses to think critically and to make sound and reasonable decisions (Potter, Griffin Perry, Ross-Kerr, and Wood, 2006) and is reflected throughout the competencies.
10. The entry-level registered nurse has a leadership role in the health-care system. Leadership is not limited to formalized roles. (College of Registered Nurses of Nova Scotia, 2004; Jurisdictional Collaborative Process, 2006).
11. The entry-level registered nurse uses information and communication technologies to interpret, organize and utilize data to influence nursing practice, improve client outcomes and contribute to knowledge development in nursing. (Hebert, 2000).

1. PROFESSIONAL PRACTICE

Registered nursing competencies in this category focus on personal professional growth, as well as intraprofessional, interprofessional and intersectoral practice responsibilities. Each registered nurse is accountable for safe, compassionate, competent and ethical nursing practice. Professional practice occurs within the context of the *Code of Ethics for Registered Nurses* (CNA, 2008), provincial/territorial standards of practice and scope of practice, legislation and common law. Registered nurses are expected to demonstrate professional conduct as reflected by the attitudes, beliefs and values espoused in the *Code of Ethics for Registered Nurses*.

Professional registered nurse practice is self-regulating. Nursing practice requires professional judgment, interprofessional collaboration, leadership, management skills, cultural safety, advocacy, political awareness and social responsibility. Professional practice includes awareness of the need for, and the ability to ensure, continued professional development. This ability involves the capacity to perform self-assessments, seek feedback and plan self-directed learning activities that ensure professional growth. Registered nurses are expected to use knowledge and research to build an evidence-informed practice.

The registered nurse:

PP-1   Practises in a manner consistent with the values in the *Code of Ethics for Registered Nurses* (2008) (e.g., providing safe, compassionate, competent and ethical care; promoting health and well-being; promoting and respecting informed decision-making; preserving dignity; maintaining privacy and confidentiality; promoting justice; being accountable). (CNA, 2008)

PP-2   Practises in a manner that recognizes and respects the intrinsic worth of clients (e.g., providing privacy, respecting diversity and vulnerabilities, relieving suffering, respecting and fostering cultural expression, appropriately using chemical and physical restraints, accepting a client's report of pain). (CNA, 2008)

PP-3   Applies ethical and legal principles related to maintaining client confidentiality in all forms of communication: written, oral and electronic (e.g., blogs, social networking sites, camera phones, text messaging, e-documentation, electronic health records). (Jurisdictional Collaborative Process, 2006)

PP-4   Uses professional judgment when accessing, organizing and using electronic resources (e.g., for own professional development, nursing practice, text messaging, personal digital assistant).

PP-5   Maintains clear, concise, accurate, objective and timely documentation.

PP-6   Uses established communication protocols within and across health-care agencies and with other service sectors (e.g., preserving privacy, maintaining confidentiality, following appropriate channels of communication). (Jurisdictional Collaborative Process, 2006)

PP-7   Advocates for equitable treatment and allocation of resources for the client (e.g., assisting vulnerable and marginalized clients to gain access to quality health care, facilitating and monitoring the quality of care, facilitating appropriate and timely responses by health-care team members, challenging questionable decisions).

PP-8   Demonstrates accountability for own actions and decisions.

PP-9   Practises within the scope of practice of the registered nurse.

PP-10   Articulates the registered nurse's scope of practice to others (e.g., the client, health-care team members, the public, community leaders, politicians).

PP-11   Provides rationale for nursing actions and decisions based on professional judgment and theoretical and evidence-informed knowledge from nursing and related disciplines.

PP-12   Uses professional judgment when following agency policies, procedures and protocols (e.g., when to use chemical and physical restraints, when to consult another member of the health-care team).

PP-13   Uses professional judgment in the absence of agency policies, procedures and protocols.

PP-14   Integrates continuous quality improvement into nursing practice (e.g., identifying and reporting when a policy, procedure or protocol is unsafe, obsolete or unnecessary; participating in audits; participating in quality improvement committees). (Jurisdictional Collaborative Process, 2006)

PP-15   Uses evidence and critical inquiry to challenge, change, enhance or support nursing practice (e.g., questioning accepted practice, participating in research).

PP-16   Takes action when aware of potential or actual abuse of the client by health-care professionals, family or others.

PP-17   Takes action when aware of potential or actual abusive situations to protect self and colleagues from injury (e.g., aggressive behaviours, bullying, workplace incivility, non-abuse policies). (Jurisdictional Collaborative Process, 2006)

PP-18   Recognizes and reports errors, near misses and sentinel events and takes action to minimize harm (e.g., client incorrectly identified, error in drug administration).

PP-19   Intervenes when unsafe practice of nursing colleagues and other members of the health-care team is identified (e.g., talking to colleague, stopping the unsafe practice, reporting to appropriate authority).

PP-20   Uses conflict resolution strategies.

PP-21   Implements strategies for continuing competence based on reflective practice, identified strengths, limitations and learning needs.

PP-22   Is accountable when assigning nursing activities to other health-care providers consistent with competence, expertise, education, role description/agency policy, legislation and the client's needs (e.g., assessment, planning, implementation and evaluation of workload assignment).

PP-23   Manages workloads effectively (e.g., time management, prioritizing, assignment).

PP-24   Seeks appropriate assistance when unsafe workload is identified.

PP-25   Collaborates and builds partnerships with nursing colleagues and other members of the health-care team to provide health services.

PP-26   Understands the roles and contributions of other health-care team members (e.g., scope of practice, role description, consultation).

PP-27   Shares knowledge and provides constructive feedback to colleagues (e.g., peer assessment, continuing competence, nursing students, mentorship, interprofessional rounds).

PP-28   Manages resources in an effective and efficient manner (e.g., human, material, technological, financial).

2. NURSE–CLIENT PARTNERSHIP

Registered nursing competencies in this category focus on therapeutic use of self, communication skills, nursing knowledge and collaboration to achieve the client's identified health goals. The nurse–client partnership is a purposeful, goal-directed relationship between nurse and client that is directed at advancing the best interest and health outcome of clients. The therapeutic partnership is central to all nursing practice and is grounded in an interpersonal process that occurs between the nurse and client (Registered Nurses' Association of Ontario, 2002). The nurse approaches this partnership with self-awareness, trust, respect, openness, empathy and sensitivity to diversity, reflecting the uniqueness of the client.

The registered nurse:

NCP-1   Applies the principles of a therapeutic nurse–client relationship and responds appropriately (e.g., openness, non-judgmental attitude, active listening, self-awareness).

NCP-2   Uses therapeutic verbal and non-verbal communication techniques with the client.

NCP-3   Establishes a therapeutic relationship with the client (e.g., maintaining professionalism, maintaining boundaries).

NCP-4   Fosters an environment that encourages questioning and exchange of information.

NCP-5   Analyzes the impact of personal values and assumptions on interactions with clients (e.g., cultural safety, ethical issues).

NCP-6   Applies principles of effective group processes (e.g., group roles, group phases, group dynamics, establishing group norms).

NCP-7 Demonstrates sensitivity to and respect for diversity in health practices and beliefs (e.g., sexual orientation, gender identity, child birth practices, dietary differences, gender, beliefs, values, spirituality, culture, language).

NCP-8 Ensures that the client's informed consent has been obtained prior to providing nursing care, including involving others in the care (e.g., implied consent for nursing care).

NCP-9 Supports the informed choice of the client in making decisions about care (e.g., right to refuse, right to request care, right to choose, right to participate in research).

NCP-10 Facilitates and respects the client's informed choice to use alternative or complementary therapies (e.g., aromatherapy, acupressure, therapeutic touch, nutritional supplements, diets).

NCP-11 Collaborates with clients in developing strategies to accommodate or modify health practices (e.g., integrating traditional food into a diabetic diet, modifying built environments, promoting healthy choices in schools).

NCP-12 Provides care that is supportive to the client experiencing loss (e.g., loss of health, amputation, natural disaster, chronic illness, death).

NCP-13 Promotes the client's positive self-concept (e.g., supporting cultural and spiritual preferences, validating the client's strengths, promoting the use of effective coping techniques, building community capacity).

NCP-14 Uses principles/strategies related to teaching and learning to meet the client's learning needs (e.g., assessing readiness to learn, identifying strategies for change, establishing an environment conducive to learning, evaluating learning process, using theoretical approaches, using social marketing).

3. HEALTH AND WELLNESS

Registered nursing competencies in this category focus on recognizing and valuing health and wellness. The category encompasses the concept of population health and the principles of primary health care. Registered nurses partner with clients to develop personal skills, create supportive environments for health, strengthen community action, reorient health services and build healthy public policy. Nursing practice is influenced by continuing competency, determinants of health, life phases, demographics, health trends, economic and political factors, evidence-informed knowledge and research.

The registered nurse:

HW-1 Collaborates with clients to identify priority areas for health promotion (e.g., healthy public policy, environmental health, stress management, social justice).

HW-2 Assists clients in understanding links between health promotion strategies and health (e.g., education programs regarding cancer risks, health fairs, anti-smoking campaigns, handwashing campaigns, ergonomics).

HW-3 Collaborates with key partners in health promotion activities (e.g., community leaders, public- and private-sector organizations, special interest groups).

HW-4 Collaborates with clients to prioritize needs and develop prevention strategies (e.g., safe needle exchange, condoms in public places, reading nutritional labels).

HW-5 Collaborates with clients and other health-care providers to respond to rapidly changing complex health risks (e.g., SARS outbreak, Norwalk virus, antibiotic-resistant organisms, pandemic).

HW-6 Collaborates with clients to identify appropriate groups and resources for mutual aid, support and community action (e.g., poverty, homelessness, marginalized and vulnerable populations).

HW-7   Collaborates with other health-care team members to implement strategies that prevent violence, abuse and neglect (e.g., using screening tools, providing information).

HW-8   Collaborates with other health-care team members in implementing strategies related to the prevention and early detection of prevalent diseases (e.g., cardiovascular disease, cancer, diabetes, communicable disease).

HW-9   Collaborates with other health-care team members in implementing strategies related to the prevention of addictive behaviours (e.g., smoking, substance use, gambling).

HW-10   Collaborates with other health-care team members in implementing strategies to promote mental health (e.g., stress management, support groups, coping strategies, public policy, crisis intervention).

HW-11   Coordinates activities with the client and others to facilitate continuity of care (e.g., cardiac rehabilitation, breastfeeding support, nutrition program).

HW-12   Promotes and utilizes safety measures to prevent injury to clients (e.g., accessibility of a call bell, supervision, diffusion of potentially violent situations, suicide prevention, least restraint, falls prevention, seat belts, bicycle helmets, smoke alarms, infant car seats).

HW-13   Promotes healthy lifestyle practices (e.g., physical activity and exercise, nutrition, rest/sleep, stress management, sexual health, family planning, contraception, hygiene, waste disposal, food preparation, infection prevention and control, smoking cessation, mental health).

HW-14   Implements strategies related to the safe and appropriate use of medication (e.g., overuse or underuse of antibiotics, polypharmacy, complementary medicine, over-the-counter medication, medication reconciliation).

HW-15   Takes action to address actual or potential risk factors related to health (e.g., food access, unsafe sexual practices, inactivity, smoking).

HW-16   Takes action to address actual or potential environmental risk factors (e.g., incidents and accidents, environmental contaminants, mechanical equipment, infectious diseases).

HW-17   Takes action to address actual or potential risks of abuse (e.g., intimate partner violence, older adult abuse, child abuse, sexual abuse, bullying, substance abuse, workplace incivility).

HW-18   Participates in preventive strategies related to workplace safety (e.g., occupational health and safety practice, latex sensitivity protocols, needleless systems, musculoskeletal injury prevention, protective equipment, WHMIS, managing aggressive and violent behaviour, pandemic planning, healthy workplace environment initiative).

HW-19   Incorporates determinants of health into the plan of care (e.g., adequate income, food and water safety, adequate housing and shelter).

HW-20   Incorporates research about health risks and risk/harm reduction to support evidence-informed practice (e.g., second-hand smoke, Pap smears).

HW-21   Uses the appropriate protocol when there is risk of communicable disease transmission (e.g., education on hand hygiene, isolation protocol, adhering to reporting protocols, encouraging needle exchange program, participating in immunization programs).

HW-22   Supports the client in role change and/or developmental transitions (e.g., parenting groups, retirement, job loss, puberty, menopause).

HW-23   Documents relevant data related to health promotion, risk reduction and injury and illness prevention (e.g., needs assessment, program planning, implementation, evaluation).

HW-24   Uses safety measures to protect self, colleagues and clients from injury (e.g., non-scented products, harassment, psychological abuse, physical aggression, safe walking buddy system, falls prevention, workplace incivility).

HW-25   Provides education about immunization programs.

HW-26   Provides evidence-informed health-related information to clients (e.g., credible electronic sources, relevant and current information).

HW-27   Uses data collection techniques that are appropriate to the client and the situation (e.g., community assessment, assessment tools).

4. CHANGES IN HEALTH

Registered nurse competencies in this category focus on care across the lifespan of the client who is experiencing changes in health. The competencies in this category thus focus on health promotion and illness prevention activities, as well as on acute, chronic, rehabilitative, palliative and end-of-life care. Such nursing actions may be delivered across a range of settings. Essential aspects of nursing care include critical inquiry, safety, solution-focused approaches, reflective practice and evidence-informed decision-making. Registered nurses collaborate with clients and other health-care professionals to identify health priorities and empower clients to improve their own health. In responding to and managing health situations, nurses promote optimal quality of life and development of self-care capacity and dignity during illness and during the dying and death process.

The registered nurse:

CH-1   Collaborates with clients in a holistic assessment (e.g., physical, emotional, mental, spiritual, cognitive, developmental, environmental, meaning of health). (Jurisdictional Collaborative Process, 2006)

CH-2   Involves clients in identifying their health needs, strengths, capacities and goals (e.g., the use of community development and empowerment principles, networking strategies, understanding of relational power, community capacity assessment).

CH-3   Collects assessment data from a range of appropriate sources (e.g., the client, previous and current health records, nursing care plans, collaborative plans of care, family members, significant others, substitute decision-makers, census data, epidemiological data, evidence-informed data, referrals, other health-care providers).

CH-4   Uses appropriate assessment techniques for data collection, (e.g., observation, inspection, auscultation, palpation, percussion, selected screening tests, pain scales, interview, consultation, focus group, measuring and monitoring).

CH-5   Validates data collected with the client and appropriate sources (e.g., medication reconciliation, health history, consultations, referrals).

CH-6   Analyzes data to establish relationships and draw conclusions from the various data collected (e.g., determining relationship between health assessment and laboratory values).

CH-7   Applies knowledge from nursing and other disciplines concerning current health situations (e.g., the health-care needs of older adults, vulnerable and/or marginalized populations, health promotion and injury prevention, pain prevention and management, end-of-life care, addiction, blood-borne pathogens, traumatic stress syndrome). (Jurisdictional Collaborative Process, 2006)

CH-8   Applies knowledge from the health sciences (e.g., physiology, pathophysiology, psychopathology, pharmacology, microbiology, epidemiology, genetics, immunology, nutrition, sociology). (Jurisdictional Collaborative Process, 2006)

CH-9   Identifies actual and potential changes in health (e.g., pain management, disability, immobility).

CH-10   Collaborates with the client in developing and implementing the plan of care (e.g., setting priorities, establishing target dates, selecting relevant interventions, developing teaching plans, administration of insulin, home IV and TPN programs, referring to self-care groups).

CH-11   Incorporates the client's personal strengths and resources in meeting self-care needs (e.g., healthy habits, personal beliefs, complementary and alternative therapies, social supports, coping strategies).

CH-12   Uses evidence-informed knowledge to assist the client to understand interventions and their relationship to expected outcomes (e.g., possible risks and benefits, discomforts, inconveniences, costs).

CH-13   Individualizes the plan of care to apply interventions consistent with the client's capacities, identified priorities and health situation (e.g., geriatric care, palliative care).

CH-14   Collaborates with the client during the care process to prepare for transfer and discharge (e.g., discharge teaching and planning, transfer of care).

CH-15   Documents nursing practice (e.g., assessment data, written plan, actual care, evaluation).

CH-16   Applies technology in accordance with available resources and the client's needs (e.g., relevant web-based material, e-documentation, telehealth, patient lifts, home IV pumps).

CH-17   Supports the client through transitions related to health situations (e.g., new diagnoses, chronic illness, dying process).

CH-18   Facilitates physical, psychological and psychosocial adjustment (e.g., therapeutic communication, counselling, appropriate referral, chronic disease management).

CH-19   Facilitates the involvement of family and significant others in collaboration with the client.

CH-20   Prevents and minimizes complications (e.g., turning and positioning, early detection and intervention).

CH-21   Evaluates changes in the client's health status (e.g., decreased oxygen saturation, decreased urine output).

CH-22   Manages multiple nursing interventions simultaneously (e.g., prioritizing and organizing interventions).

CH-23   Communicates accurate and relevant information about the client's health situation to appropriate health-care team members.

CH-24   Intervenes in a timely manner to changes observed in the client's health situation.

CH-25   Evaluates the effectiveness of nursing interventions in collaboration with the client (e.g., learning needs, comparing actual outcomes to anticipated outcomes).

CH-26   Modifies plan of care based on an ongoing holistic assessment of the client's changing health situation.

CH-27   Initiates urgent inclusion of the health-care team members in response to the client's changing health status (e.g., hemorrhage, imminent birth, low blood pressure, drug reactions).

CH-28   Coordinates activities with the client and other members of the health-care team to promote continuity and consistency of care within and across settings (e.g., referrals, unit reports, community health centres, air and ground transport).

CH-29   Consults with other health-care team members to analyze and plan care in complex health situations (e.g., obesity, comorbidities, chemical exposure, burns, cancer, complex family situations). (Jurisdictional Collaborative Process, 2006)

CH-30   Prepares the client for diagnostic procedures and treatments (e.g., explanation, evidence-informed information, tests, obtaining specimens).

CH-31   Provides preoperative and postoperative care.

CH-32   Promotes oxygenation (e.g., positioning, deep breathing and coughing exercises, oxygen therapy, oral and nasal suctioning).

CH-33   Promotes circulation (e.g., active or passive exercises, positioning, mobilization, cast care).

CH-34   Promotes and monitors fluid balance (e.g., intake and output, weight, non-invasive hemodynamic measurement, measuring abdominal girth).

CH-35   Promotes and manages adequate nutrition (e.g., burns, inflammatory bowel disease, diabetes, HIV/AIDS, infant gastric reflux, obesity, malnutrition).

CH-36   Administers and manages parenteral and enteral nutrition (e.g., TPN, nasogastric tube).

CH-37   Promotes and manages adequate urinary elimination (e.g., stoma care, bladder retraining, self-catheterization, bladder irrigation, bladder catheterization, pharmacological measures).

CH-38   Promotes and manages adequate bowel elimination (e.g., bowel retraining, ostomy care, enema, rectal tubes, pharmacological measures, dietary measures).

CH-39   Promotes and ensures a client's proper body alignment (e.g., proper positioning, external immobilizing devices).

CH-40   Promotes mobility (e.g., active and passive exercises, early ambulation, activities of daily living, prosthetic and mobilizing devices, use of ergonomics).

CH-41   Promotes and maintains tissue integrity (e.g., providing skin and wound care).

CH-42   Promotes and maintains comfort (e.g., the nurse's presence, warm and cold application, touch, positioning).

CH-43   Determines and implements appropriate sensory stimulation for the client's health situation (e.g., touch with unconscious client, minimizing environmental stimuli, sensory stimulation for premature infant in isolette, adolescent in isolation).

CH-44   Evaluates safe use of prescribed and non-prescribed medication (e.g., safe dosage and route, food–drug interactions, drug–drug interactions, age, weight).

CH-45   Takes action with unsafe medication packaging and/or orders.

CH-46   Calculates medication dosage.

CH-47   Administers medication (e.g., right client, drug, dose, route and time; documentation; client's rights; right reason; allergies).

CH-48   Evaluates client's response to medication (e.g., desired effects, adverse effects, interactions).

CH-49   Assesses when a p.r.n. medication is indicated (e.g., analgesics, inhalers, antihypertensives, antianginals, laxatives, antianxiety agents).

CH-50   Takes action when desired responses to medication are not attained.

CH-51   Assists the client to manage pain with non-pharmacological measures (e.g., applying heat and cold, touch, massage, visual imagery, turning and positioning).

CH-52   Assists the client to manage pain with pharmacological agents or devices (e.g., non-opiates, opiates, epidural analgesia, patient-controlled analgesia [PCA]).

CH-53   Collects and communicates accurate medication information (e.g., medication reconciliation upon admission, at transfer of care, at discharge).

CH-54   Administers blood and blood products safely.

CH-55   Manages central venous access devices (e.g., implanted devices, PICC lines, infusion pumps).

CH-56   Manages drainage tubes and collection devices (e.g., chest tubes and vacuum drainages).

CH-57   Inserts, maintains and removes nasogastric tubes.

CH-58   Inserts, maintains and removes peripheral intravenous therapy.

CH-59   Applies routine/standard precautions.

CH-60   Intervenes in a rapidly changing health situation: acute cardiovascular event (e.g., myocardial infarction, unstable angina).

CH-61   Intervenes in a rapidly changing health situation: acute neurological event (e.g., brain attack [stroke], trans-ischemic attack [TIA], seizure, head injury).

CH-62   Intervenes in a rapidly changing health situation: shock (e.g., hypovolemic, anaphylactic, neurogenic, cardiogenic, septic and hemodynamic deterioration).

CH-63   Intervenes in a rapidly changing health situation: acute respiratory event (e.g., acute asthma, pulmonary embolus, pulmonary edema).

CH-64   Intervenes in a rapidly changing health situation: cardiopulmonary arrest.

CH-65   Intervenes in a rapidly changing health situation: perinatal (antepartum, intrapartum, postpartum, newborn).

CH-66   Intervenes in a rapidly changing health situation: diabetes crisis (e.g., diabetic coma, hyperglycemia, hypoglycemia, ketoacidosis).

CH-67   Intervenes in a rapidly changing health situation: mental health crisis (e.g., psychotic episode, neuroleptic malignant syndrome, suicide ideation, delirium, acute onset of extrapyramidal side-effects).

CH-68   Intervenes in a rapidly changing health situation: trauma (e.g., burns, fractures).

CH-69   Intervenes in a rapidly changing health situation: postoperatively (e.g., malignant hyperthermia, hemorrhage, wound dehiscence).

CH-70   Intervenes in a rapidly changing health situation: acute renal failure (e.g., nephrotoxins).

CH-71   Provides supportive care to meet hospice, palliative or end-of-life care needs of dying clients (e.g., symptom control, spiritual care, advocacy, family counselling, support for clients and significant others, advance care planning, grief and bereavement counselling). (Jurisdictional Collaborative Process, 2006)

CH-72   Intervenes to meet spiritual needs (e.g., assessing for spiritual distress, providing time for prayer or meditation, appropriate referral, cultural safety).

CH-73   Facilitates with the client to explore and access community resources (e.g., self-help groups, geriatric day programs, respite care, finances, transportation, social networks).

CH-74   Facilitates the client's development of independence and safety in activities of daily living (e.g., removal of scatter rugs, keeping essential furniture on one level of the house, raised toilet seat, ordering specialized equipment such as a walker and special utensils, consulting with other health-care team members).

CH-75   Facilitates social well-being of the client (e.g., encouraging and creating opportunities for social participation, encouraging development of new interests and support systems, facilitating of peer-to-peer helping model).

CH-76   Facilitates the client's reintegration into family and community (e.g., adaptation to role transitions, physical mobility, self-help groups).

CH-77   Provides supportive care to clients with chronic health situations (e.g., outpatient clinics, adult day care, respite care, pain management, symptom management, polypharmacy, group therapy, addictions counselling).

CH-78   Demonstrates understanding of organizational responses and appropriate nursing roles in emergency community disasters and emerging global health issues (e.g., mass casualty response, bioterrorism, pandemic, emergency preparedness/disaster planning, food and water safety).

CH-79   Takes appropriate nursing actions in disaster situations (e.g., mass casualty response, bioterrorism).

STUDY NOTES

STUDY NOTES

STUDY NOTES

STUDY NOTES